"Judy Koenigsberg contributes significantly to the discourse on rupture repair, something dear to my heart. She does so in a unique and unified way, proposing a transtheoretical, psycholinguistic model that should prove useful to therapists across levels and traditions. Her book is rich with clinical detail and wisdom."

J. Christopher Muran, PhD, Dean and Full Professor,
The Gordon F. Derner School of Psychology, Adelphi University
Principal Investigator, Mount Sinai Beth Israel
Psychotherapy Research Program

"As in her previous books on anxiety and depression, Dr. Koenigsberg returns to explore and emphasize the primacy of the therapeutic relationship and the potential vulnerabilities.

In her very well referenced book she discusses ruptures and termination with a transtheoretical eye to the commonalities of these issues in all dyadic psychotherapies. New therapists, in particular, will find the review of therapeutic strategies very helpful."

Judith Tanner, MD, *Clinical Assistant Professor of*
Psychiatry and Behavioral Sciences, Northwestern University

"Judy Koenigsberg has written an outstanding volume that cannot help but advance the therapeutic enterprise. While reading it, I found myself constantly thinking about my own patients and how relevant and helpful the material in this book is to the therapy I conduct. At its core, it sensitizes therapists to the occurrence of both obvious and subtle ruptures and, most significantly, gives them excellent strategies to repair them. This book deserves to be disseminated widely among therapists of all professional backgrounds and theoretical persuasions and to patients and potential patients as well."

Stanley B. Messer, PhD, *Distinguished Professor Emeritus and*
Former Dean of the Graduate School of Applied and
Professional Psychology, Rutgers University

Navigating Ruptures, Repairs, and Termination Within the Therapeutic Process

This book explores the importance of the therapeutic relationship, the tensions or disagreements that may emerge during a therapy session, and how they can be repaired.

Dr. Koenigsberg introduces a two-part transtheoretical, psycholinguistic model that focuses on the connection between ruptures and the termination phase of therapy, emphasizing the verbal and nonverbal nuances of language, to understand what is happening in the therapeutic alliance. With a reliance on psycholinguistic elements, this model can guide therapists who wish to reduce the premature termination of patients from therapy. Written in an accessible format, it provides case examples, including the patient's and therapist's inner experiences, and defines and describes the phases of therapy so that difficult transitions in the therapeutic process can be navigated with skill and compassion.

This text is essential for providing early career as well as more seasoned therapists with excellent strategies to repair their therapeutic relationships with clients.

Judy Z. Koenigsberg, PhD, is a clinical psychologist, licensed in Illinois, who has practiced integrated psychology for 30 years. Dr. Koenigsberg holds graduate degrees in psychology and linguistics. After earning her PhD from Northwestern University, Dr. Koenigsberg was employed as a clinical psychologist at the University of Chicago. Later, she taught research methodology to graduate students in the social sciences at Loyola University, Chicago. Her recent books, *Anxiety Disorders: Integrated Psychotherapy Approaches* and *Depressive Disorders: Integrated and Unified Psychotherapy Approaches*, are published by Routledge/Taylor & Francis. Judy's articles in psychology and sociology have been published in peer reviewed journals, and her course, "Listening to the language of Your Patients: Integrating Psycholinguistic Concepts into Clinical Practice," is designed for mental health practitioners.

Navigating Ruptures, Repairs, and Termination Within the Therapeutic Process

JUDY Z. KOENIGSBERG

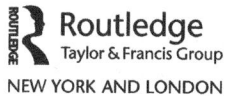
Routledge
Taylor & Francis Group

NEW YORK AND LONDON

Designed cover image: Artjafara © Getty Images

First published 2024
by Routledge
605 Third Avenue, New York, NY 10158

and by Routledge
4 Park Square, Milton Park, Abingdon, Oxon, OX14 4RN

Routledge is an imprint of the Taylor & Francis Group, an informa business

Library of Congress Cataloging-in-Publication Data
Names: Koenigsberg, Judy Z., author.
Title: Navigating ruptures, repairs, and termination within the
therapeutic process / Judy Z. Koenigsberg.
Description: New York, NY : Routledge, 2024. |
Identifiers: LCCN 2023044429 (print) | LCCN 2023044430 (ebook) |
ISBN 9780367652333 (pbk) | ISBN 9780367652340 (hbk) |
ISBN 9781003128489 (ebk)
Subjects: LCSH: Psychotherapy–Termination. | Therapeutic alliance. |
Nonverbal communication. | Psychotherapist and patient.
Classification: LCC RC489.T45 K64 2024 (print) |
LCC RC489.T45 (ebook) | DDC 616.89/14–dc23/eng/20231227
LC record available at https://lccn.loc.gov/2023044429
LC ebook record available at https://lccn.loc.gov/2023044430

ISBN: 978-0-367-65234-0 (hbk)
ISBN: 978-0-367-65233-3 (pbk)
ISBN: 978-1-003-12848-9 (ebk)

DOI: 10.4324/9781003128489

Typeset in Dante and Avenir
by Newgen Publishing UK

I dedicate this book to my loving grandchildren, with special thanks to my dear grandson, Meir Koenigsberg, for his many acts of kindness: his caring, his responsiveness, his support, his uplifting spirit, and for keeping in touch on a weekly basis; to my husband, David Koenigsberg, MD, for his help; to my best friend, Susan Solny, Decorative Arts Historian, for valuing my work; and to Thetis Cromie, PhD, for her responsiveness, understanding, caring, support, superior talent, and the depth of her insight.

Contents

Foreword

The necessity of many creatures to be attached to their fellow creatures, be they animal or human, in order to thrive and survive has emerged as a predominant theme in psychology in recent decades. Within clinical and counseling psychology and related therapeutic disciplines, this has led to a focus on the nature and importance of the relationship that is established early on between therapist and patient (or client). From the point of view of theory, there is now an enhanced appreciation of psychodynamic/relational, person-centered, interpersonal, and experiential approaches and, even within the more technique-oriented models such as cognitive-behavioral therapies, a recognition of the importance of building a solid relationship or attachment for therapy to succeed. From a research perspective, there are many individual studies and meta-analyses that demonstrate a moderate-sized but very consistent correlation between the strength of the therapeutic alliance and therapy outcome.

In such a context, the present volume by Judy Koenigsberg on Navigating Ruptures, Repairs, and Termination Within the Therapeutic Process is most timely and welcome. Its outlook grows out of the general psychological literature on the nature and personal styles of attachment, as well as the more specific work by authors such as Jeremy Safran, Christopher Muran, and Catherine Eubanks on ruptures. These can occur fairly frequently in the therapeutic relationship and the author points out the necessity of repairing them if therapy is to proceed to a successful conclusion. One very useful conception the author draws upon in discussing the nature and purpose of the relationship is the bonds, goals, and tasks established by the therapist and patient (cf. Edward Bordin). The bond is the fundamental building block of therapy which, once formed, allows the participants to fashion therapeutic goals and ways to achieve them.

Ruptures in relationships often result from two fundamental but opposing human needs: Communion and agency. Communion refers to the human need for relatedness and togetherness, while agency encompasses the need for individuality and self-expression. In everyday life ruptures stem from disagreements leading to arguments, which can disrupt friendships and marriages temporarily or permanently. This happens in therapy as well and it is critical that therapists pick up the signals when it does occur so that they can repair the breach and, when applicable, use it as an example of the difficulties patients are experiencing in their lives. Two frequent signals that a rupture is in process is the patient withdrawing from or confronting the therapist. The attachment style of the patient can affect which of these or other indicators of ruptures occur. Koenigsberg gives copious examples of the causes of such ruptures, how they manifest themselves, and how to repair them. The way in which she achieves this is very creative and of great value to the practicing clinician. Based on cases with which she is familiar, she imagines the inner thoughts of both therapist and patient as the rupture occurs and what the therapist should do to repair it. The therapist, says Koenigsberg (following Eubanks), has to possess a certain degree of humility to recognize their own contribution to the rupture and acknowledge it. Therapy patients will also profit from reading these internal dialogues, with which they can readily identify.

Of special interest in this volume is a focus on the termination process of therapy, which is of particular relevance to the book's major theme of rupture and repair. The author points to different types of termination, e.g., premature or mutual, patient or therapist initiated, planned or unplanned, and so forth, and explores how the patient's ambivalence or resistance can lead to ruptures which, in turn, can result in premature termination. The research she reports concludes that the stronger the therapeutic alliance, the less likely premature dropout will occur. Furthermore, she illustrates via case vignettes how different patient diagnoses and therapist theories lead to different termination experiences.

There are other features of this book that make it stand out in the literature on therapy process. Koenigsberg demonstrates how microaggressions, a concept referring to the subtle interpersonal biases and prejudices experienced all-too-frequently by members of minority groups in America such as Blacks, Asians, Muslims and Jews, can also occur within the therapy dyad via the therapist's insensitive words or body language. This is another source of potential rupture in the therapy that requires prompt attention lest it lead to a failed therapy. Regarding major theoretical models in the field, the author is eclectic and integrative in the way she addresses similarities and differences among these approaches. For example, she shows how the therapeutic relationship is a common factor across all forms of therapy, the latter being one of the major forms of psychotherapy integration alongside theoretical integration, technical eclecticism, and assimilative integration. In this connection, Daniel Fishman and I have mapped out different models of the therapeutic relationship and their implications for integrative practice. In essence, we argue that the relationship is more a common theme than it is a common factor in so far as it is handled differently in varying models of therapy.

Other worthy features of this book are its frequent references to the current research bearing on the topic at hand. This provides a scientific basis for the clinical concepts employed as well as for the recommended interventions. Reference is made to teletherapy, a current mode of practice necessitated by the pandemic, in which patient and therapist meet in a virtual space via the computer. Fortunately, this mode has been found to lead to results that are as robust as in-person psychotherapy.

In a final section, Koenigsberg presents a sophisticated transtheoretical, psycholinguistic model of ruptures and repairs that is truly integrative in the best sense of that word. No stranger to integrative and unified models of therapy, she has previously published well-received books on integrative approaches to depression and anxiety. She encourages therapists to attend to linguistic and paralinguistic concepts, verbal and nonverbal modes of communication, to better understand the ruptures that occur and how to address them. In the last chapter in this section, she applies her model to the crucial termination process when, optimally, consolidation takes place. How she connects the concrete processes of therapy, illustrated in the case examples, with the theory of the rupture-repair cycle is a valuable contribution of her book.

In brief, Koenigsberg has written an outstanding volume that cannot help but advance the therapeutic enterprise. As I was reading it, I found myself constantly thinking about my own patients and how relevant and helpful the material in this book is to the therapy I conduct. At its core, it sensitizes therapists to the occurrence of both obvious and subtle ruptures and, most significantly, gives them strategies to repair them. This book deserves to be disseminated widely among therapists of all professional backgrounds and theoretical persuasions and to patients and potential patients as well.

Stanley B. Messer, PhD
Distinguished Professor Emeritus, Rutgers University

Preface

Are you a therapist who has experienced tension or a disagreement with a patient who has dropped out of therapy? Are you a patient who wishes to quit therapy, or have you already dropped out of therapy because you have experienced a fall-out in the therapeutic relationship? If you are thinking about beginning therapy, do you have ambiguous feelings about calling a therapist or meeting your therapist for the first time? If so, join the club. Many individuals have experienced these challenging moments. These delicate, or not so delicate, moments of tension can be perplexing for clients and therapists.

The book, *Navigating Ruptures, Repairs, and Termination Within the Therapeutic Process*, explores the difficult moments or impasses that may emerge during a therapy session, the importance of the therapeutic relationship, the bond between the therapist and the client, the inner experiences of patients and therapists, how breaks in the relationship may be repaired, the termination process, and the connection between breaks in the relationship and the termination phase of therapy. A focus on the inner thoughts and experiences of patients and therapists is underscored throughout the book. The last two chapters of the book suggest the use of a transtheoretical, psycholinguistic model that can inform therapists about how their moment-to-moment interactions and choices, particularly during a rupture or at a time of tension in the therapeutic relationship, can make a difference for patients.

Consider the following example of a rupture or a potential impasse and a near premature termination by a client in a therapeutic setting. Mateo, a 26-year-old patient, is meeting with his therapist for his third therapy session. A few weeks ago, his girlfriend broke off their engagement. Mateo is disappointed and has not felt connected to his therapist. He is thinking about discontinuing therapy. Mateo's thoughts: *"I don't think I'm gaining much from this therapy."* Mateo says (angrily), "I'm not getting much here." Therapist's thoughts: *"Mateo has complained from the start. I wonder if his pushing me away is connected to his recent breakup."* The therapist says, "Can you tell me what's going on?" Mateo's thoughts: *"I'm out of here. I'm getting nothing."* Mateo walks out the door and goes into the waiting room. The therapist is thinking: *"I can let him go, or wait for a bit, or perhaps he needs to see that someone cares."* The therapist exits his office, enters the waiting room, and says to Mateo who is sitting with his head down in the waiting room: *"I care."* Mateo is thinking: *"Wow. Someone cares enough to get up from his chair."* Mateo walks back into the therapist's office. Over the course of the next year, Mateo and the therapist gradually develop a strong working and therapeutic alliance. Ruptures or disagreements during therapy are often make or break events for patients and therapists and may steer the future course of therapy.

The therapeutic alliance is the bond between the therapist and the patient that facilitates the patient's investment in the therapeutic process and the patient's experiences of deep emotions (Fisher et al., 2016; Goldfried, 2012). It is the "quintessential integrative" factor, and it is recognized by therapists with different theoretical approaches as an important variable in psychotherapy (Wolfe & Goldfried, 1988, p. 449). Acknowledged by therapists with different perspectives as the essence of psychotherapy, the therapeutic alliance is underscored throughout the book, *Navigating Ruptures, Repairs, and Termination Within the Therapeutic Process*. Muran and colleagues (2009, p. 234) point out that the alliance is strongly correlated with outcome in therapy irrespective of the type of treatment employed (e.g., Horvath & Symonds, 1991; Martin et al., 2000). Some of the extensive literature on the therapeutic alliance and its relationship to outcome in therapy is included in the book. The relationship between a therapist and a patient is a critical part of the treatment process in that it facilitates the acceptance of interventions and interpretations so that the patient can grow (Auchincloss, 2016; Horvath & Symonds, 1991). The therapeutic alliance and patients' experiences of working their emotional concerns during therapy have been demonstrated to decrease their anguish outside of or beyond therapy (Fisher et al., 2016).

The book, *Navigating Ruptures, Repairs, and Termination Within the Therapeutic Process*, can help readers to discover how the creation of the alliance begins to set the stage for potential ruptures or tensions to emerge, and ultimately for the termination process to evolve. For example, research has shown that in psychotherapy with patients with borderline personality disorder, a psychotherapist's contribution to the treatment contract and to the therapeutic alliance is associated with treatment length (Yeomans et al., 1994). Sensitivity to potential ruptures in the therapeutic alliance, the process of short circuiting them, and working toward their resolution can contribute to retention and outcome in treatment (Muran et al., 2009). For example, Muran and colleagues (2009) found that a rupture repair or resolution that is elevated and a rupture intensity that is lower are correlated with elevated alliance ratings and the quality of sessions. Furthermore, they suggested that a rupture resolution or repair that is elevated is associated with greater retention in therapy, and a rupture intensity that is lower is associated with good interpersonal functioning. The book, *Navigating Ruptures, Repairs, and Termination Within the Therapeutic Process*, speaks to the need for a strong bond between therapists and clients without which therapists will find it challenging, if not impossible, to process a rupture, potentially leading to clients' premature termination or dropout from therapy, a negative event that therapists wish to avoid. Much evidence has demonstrated that an alliance that is not strong is associated with a patient's unilateral or premature termination (Muran et al., 2009; Samstag et al., 1998; Tryon & Kane, 1990, 1993, 1995).

Ruptures can manifest as disagreements and as other rifts in the therapeutic relationship between a therapist and a client (Safran & Muran, 2000). Why study ruptures or tensions in the alliance? What do these breaches or impasses offer to therapists and patients? Ruptures or strains in the therapeutic alliance facilitate learning on the part of therapists and patients, and each member of the dyad, client and therapist, can learn to recognize how to navigate the needs of the self and the other in the face of a confrontation in the therapeutic relationship (Coutinho et al., 2011; Safran & Segal, 1990). In order to navigate ruptures or misattunements in a way that is not defensive, therapists need to cultivate humility, and it is the humility of therapists that can inspire patients (Eubanks et al., 2023). For example, the therapist described at the beginning of this section could have been aggressive in confronting his client, Mateo, who expressed anger and dissatisfaction with the therapist, or, in a more passive way, could have let Mateo linger in the waiting room and/or walk out altogether. Instead, he chose to repair the confrontation rupture by refraining to react with hostility, by showing Mateo that he cared, thereby facilitating the exploration of Mateo's emotions in subsequent sessions. Some therapists will find it easier than others to fully engage their patients, to empathize with their patients' suffering, to take responsibility for recognizing their contribution to a rupture. Therapists with a healthy degree of humility may be in a better position to navigate ruptures when patients like Mateo confront them angrily. Sometimes therapists' personal issues will interfere with their ability to cope with their clients' expression of anger. For these therapists, contributing factors may be their own family-of-origin issues (Coutinho et al., 2011).

The book, *Navigating Ruptures, Repairs, and Termination Within the Therapeutic Process,* is written for therapists and patients who wish to understand more about tensions, breaks, or ruptures in therapy and beyond and their association with the termination phase of therapy, a phase of therapy that, to this date, has not been extensively explored. Many parts of the book are written in an accessible style and are buttressed by past and contemporary research. Throughout the book, the inner experiences of therapists and patients are provided, and these inner thoughts and feelings, at times, offered as vignettes, are supported by the literature on ruptures and termination. Any case, vignette, illustration, example, and/or conversation in the book includes practice experiences that do not represent any specific case but are based on a sum total of many similar cases. Fictional cases, conversations, or examples are included as well. Sometimes the term, client, and at other times, the term, patient, is used interchangeably. Readers who are therapists may be able to relate the discussions in the book to their own work and experiences, and to the way they address their clients whom they meet in their practices. Readers who are or who have been patients may find some of the material relevant to their own experiences in therapy.

Part I, "Ruptures and Repairs," consists of Chapters 1 and 2. Chapter 1, "What Are Therapeutic Relationship Ruptures?" defines ruptures as empathic failures (Kohut, 1984) or as tensions (Safran & Muran, 2006) that relate to outcome in therapy (Safran et al., 2011). This chapter introduces the concept of a therapeutic relationship rupture and expands the definition to include disagreements, fall outs, breakups, and estrangements that may occur both within and beyond the therapeutic alliance (e.g., Muran et al., 2023). Examples that offer the inner experiences of the therapist and patient are illustrated throughout this chapter.

Chapter 2, "Ruptures and Repairs in the Therapeutic Relationship: Diagnostic and Theoretical Considerations," addresses three types of ruptures. They are: 1) Disagreements that entail psychotherapy tasks; 2) Disagreements about the goals of psychotherapy treatment; and 3) Tensions in the therapist-patient relationship (Bordin, 1979; Safran et al., 2011). The focus is on the navigation of these ruptures within a specific therapy session and/or throughout the treatment. Emphasis is given to ruptures in the therapeutic relationship for patients with different emotional and personality disorders and how therapists of different theoretical orientations navigate these ruptures. Whereas Chapter 1 focuses on the ruptures themselves, Chapter 2 addresses the process of repair or resolution of the ruptures. Examples of the inner experiences of the therapist and patient are included throughout Chapter 2.

There has not been extensive research on the termination process of therapy. It is more difficult to explore the ending phase of therapy than the beginning and mid-phases because of the lack of material addressing the termination phase. Part II, "Termination," consists of Chapters 3 and 4. Chapter 3, "Definition, Types, and Duration of the Termination Process," defines the termination process, outlines the different types of terminations, e.g., mutual, premature, the result of illness or death, a move, or the end of time-limited therapy, and illustrates the effects of the termination phase on clients. An exploration of the connection between ruptures or breaks in the therapeutic alliance and unilateral or premature terminations is included in the chapter along with examples of the inner cognitions of therapists and patients during the termination phase of therapy.

In Chapter 4, "Termination Across Different Diagnoses and Theories," the focus is on the different types of termination that evolve for patients with different emotional and personality disorders and how therapists with different theoretical orientations navigate the termination process with their patients. Examples of the inner experiences of therapists with different theoretical orientations and of the inner thoughts of patients with different emotional difficulties during the termination process are included in the chapter.

Part III, "A Transtheoretical Model," consists of Chapters 5 and 6. Chapter 5, "The I_{rt} – CARE Transtheoretical, Psycholinguistic Model of Ruptures and Repairs," proposes a transtheoretical, psycholinguistic model that encourages therapists to consolidate the work of the therapeutic process across various theories. In the I_{rt} – CARE Transtheoretical, Psycholinguistic Model of Ruptures and Repairs, the letter "I" stands for inner or immediacy, and corresponds on a microcosmic level, for example, to the caring that Mateo's therapist conveyed to him, and on a macrocosmic level to the I or responsibility that therapists, in general, need to take for their own contributions to ruptures and for client dropout from therapy. The letter I for inner (or C for covert) represents the backbone of the model. According to this transtheoretical framework, the subscript "r" of I_{rt} stands for rupture; the subscript "t" of I_{rt} stands for termination; the letter "C" in the word CARE stands for covert, curiosity, or compassion; the letter "A" in the word CARE stands for awareness, alliance, attunement, or authenticity; the letter "R" in the word CARE stands for repair or resolution; and the letter "E" of the word CARE stands for empathy or ending.

The overarching psycholinguistic model, with its emphasis on the covert (C) or inner (I) experiences of patients and therapists, provides a framework that therapists can use to understand the dynamic interplay between patients and therapists and considers the critical phases in the therapy process so that the difficult moment-to-moment transitions during a rupture can be navigated with skill and compassion. Conscious and unconscious communications by therapists and patients are considered in this chapter.

Chapter 5, "The I_{rt} – CARE Transtheoretical, Psycholinguistic Model of Ruptures and Repairs" (the first part of The I_{rt} – CARE Transtheoretical, Psycholinguistic Model of Ruptures, Repairs, and Termination), underscores how therapists think and speak about their work, provides a blueprint that emphasizes the verbal, paralinguistic, and nonverbal dynamics of the therapeutic process, and explores the notion of verbal and nonverbal synchrony between therapists and patients. For example, acoustic data can signal markers for ruptures, and these acoustic markers include speech and vocal parameters that measure the physical characteristics of speech production, e.g., fundamental frequency (F0) (pitch of the sound), articulation rate, shimmer, and pause proportion (e.g., De Cheveigné & Kawahara, 2002; Dolev-Amit et al., 2022; Rochman & Amir, 2013). The I_{rt} – CARE Transtheoretical, Psycholinguistic Model of Ruptures and Repairs in Chapter 5 encourages psychotherapists to avail themselves of linguistic and paralinguistic concepts to study the communication of their patients in order to understand the rupture and repair process. It aims to help therapists establish clarity about their intention for a particular phase of the therapy, and for each intervention that therapists introduce, it encourages their reflections, for example: Why am I doing what I am doing? What is my goal or hope for what I propose? What possible interventions are available, and does the intervention that I am proposing fit clients' individual needs? The I_{rt} – CARE Transtheoretical, Psycholinguistic Model of Ruptures and Repairs emphasizes the delicate and, at times, not so delicate moment to moment interactions between clients and therapists and suggests a psycholinguistic framework that can provide therapists with an opportunity to study the details of these challenging and sensitive moments within the framework of the dyadic dialogue.

Chapter 6, "The I_{rt} – CARE Transtheoretical Psycholinguistic Model of Termination: The Termination or the Ending Process of Therapy" (the second part of The I_{rt} – CARE Transtheoretical, Psycholinguistic Model of Ruptures, Repairs, and Termination), focuses on the relationship between verbal and nonverbal synchrony between therapist and patient and the termination phase of therapy. For example, it has been suggested that nonverbal synchrony may help to spot patients who are likely to drop out of therapy

(Paulick et al., 2018; Rubel et al., 2015). Previous chapters discuss the relationship between ruptures or impasses and client unilateral termination, early ending of therapy, or dropout from therapy. It has been shown that ruptures or disagreements that have not been repaired or resolved can lead to a poor therapeutic relationship, to poor outcome, and to a patient's premature termination from therapy (Henry et al., 1986; Safran et al., 2005; Safran & Kraus, 2014). Chapter 6, "The I_{rt} – CARE Transtheoretical, Psycholinguistic Model of Termination: The Termination or the Ending Process of Therapy," discusses the process used to navigate termination in the context of differing theoretical orientations and proposes a transtheoretical, psycholinguistic model that can be useful across theories. The chapter focuses on the relationship between linguistic and paralinguistic signals and premature termination from therapy.

Chapter 6 addresses how therapists can help patients during the termination process regardless of whether the ending is an agreed ending by the therapist and the patient or a unilateral ending by the therapist or the patient, which may be a therapy ending that may not be a positive event. The I_{rt} – CARE Transtheoretical, Psycholinguistic Model of Termination: The Termination or the Ending Process of Therapy, the portion of the model offered in Chapter 6, embraces a psycholinguistic framework that underscores the verbal and nonverbal nuances of language along with paralinguistic features, discusses the synchrony or alignment between patients and therapists, and describes the relationship between the aforementioned explicit and covert language components and the termination process. The transtheoretical model, with its emphasis on the internal experiences of patients and therapists, provides a blueprint for the termination process, and entails a compass that can guide therapists and patients as they navigate difficult transitions, particularly during the termination phase. Goals of the model include encouragement for psychotherapists to take responsibility for their contribution to client dropout, for therapists to learn how to navigate therapy endings with finesse, and for therapists to develop the ability to think about their thoughts and their work as they move through the termination process.

References

Auchincloss, E. L. (2016). New developments of the therapeutic alliance (TA): Good news for psychodynamic psychiatry. *Psychodynamic Psychiatry, 44*(1), 105–116. https://doi.org/10.1521/pdps.2016.44.1.105

Bordin, E. S. (1979). The generalizability of the psychoanalytic concept of the working alliance. *Psychotherapy: Theory, Research and Practice, 16*(3), 252–260. https://doi.org/10.1037/h0085885

Coutinho, J., Ribeiro, E., Hill, C., & Safran, J. (2011). Therapists' and clients' experiences of alliance ruptures: A qualitative study. *Psychotherapy Research, 21*(5), 525–540. https://doi.org/10.1080/10503307.2011.587469

De Cheveigné, A., & Kawahara, H. (2002). YIN, a fundamental frequency estimator for speech and music. *The Journal of the Acoustical Society of America, 111*(4), 1917–1930. https://doi.org/10.1121/1.1458024

Dolev-Amit, T., Nof, A., Asaad, A., Tchizick, A., & Zilcha-Mano, S. (2022). The melody of ruptures: Identifying ruptures through acoustic markers. *Counselling Psychology Quarterly, 35*(4), 724–743. https://doi.org/10.1080/09515070.2020.1860906

Eubanks, C. F., Samstag, L. W., & Muran, J. C. (2023). Conclusion: Don't be afraid to get messy – Points of convergence in rupture and repair. In C. F. Eubanks, L. W. Samstag, & J. C. Muran (Eds.), *Rupture and repair in psychotherapy: A critical process for change* (pp. 305–317). American Psychological Association. https://doi.org/10.1037/0000306-013

Fisher, H., Atzil-Slonim, D., Bar-Kalifa, E., Rafaeli, E., & Peri, T. (2016). Emotional experience and alliance contribute to therapeutic change in psychodynamic therapy. *Psychotherapy, 53*(1), 105–116. https://doi.org/10.1037/pst0000041

Goldfried, M. R. (2012). The corrective experience: A core principle for therapeutic change. In L. G. Castonguay & C. E. Hill (Eds.), *Transformation in psychotherapy: Corrective experience across cognitive behavioral, humanistic, and psychodynamic approaches* (pp. 13–29). American Psychological Association. https://doi.org/10.1037/13747-002

Henry, W. P., Schacht, T. E., & Strupp, H. H. (1986). Structural analysis of social behavior: Application to a study of interpersonal process in differential psychotherapeutic outcome. *Journal of Consulting and Clinical Psychology, 54*(1), 27–31. https://doi.org/10.1037/0022-006X.54.1.27

Horvath, A. O., & Symonds, B. D. (1991). Relation between working alliance and outcome in psychotherapy: A meta-analysis. *Journal of Counseling Psychology, 38*(2), 139–149. https://doi.org/10.1037/0022-0167.38.2.139

Kohut, H. (1984). *How does analysis cure?* University of Chicago Press.

Martin, D. J., Garske, J. P., & Davis, M. K. (2000). Relation of the therapeutic alliance with outcome and other variables: A meta-analytic review. *Journal of Consulting and Clinical Psychology, 68*(3), 438–450. https://doi.org/10.1037/0022-006X.68.3.438

Muran, J. C., Eubanks, C. F., & Samstag, L. W. (2023). Introduction: Rupture in a wicked and wonderful world. In C. F. Eubanks, L. W. Samstag, & J. C. Muran (Eds.), *Rupture and repair in psychotherapy: A critical process for change* (pp. 3–20). American Psychological Association. https://doi.org/10.1037/0000306-001

Muran, J. C., Safran, J. D., Gorman, B. S., Samstag, L. W., Eubanks-Carter, C., & Winston, A. (2009). The relationship of early alliance ruptures and their resolution to process and outcome in three time-limited psychotherapies for personality disorders. *Psychotherapy: Theory, Research, Practice, Training, 46*(2), 233–248. https://doi.org/10.1037/a0016085

Paulick, J., Deisenhofer, A.-K., Ramseyer, F., Tschacher, W., Boyle, K., Rubel, J., & Lutz, W. (2018). Nonverbal synchrony: A new approach to better understand psychotherapeutic processes and drop-out. *Journal of Psychotherapy Integration, 28*(3), 367–384 https://doi.org/10.1037/int0000099

Rochman, D., & Amir, O. (2013). Examining in-session expressions of emotions with speech/vocal acoustic measures: An introductory guide. *Psychotherapy Research, 23*(4), 381–393. https://doi.org/10.1080/10503307.2013.784421

Rubel, J., Lutz, W., Kopta, S. M., Köck, K., Minami, T., Zimmermann, D., & Saunders, S. M. (2015). Defining early positive response to psychotherapy: An empirical comparison between clinically significant change criteria and growth mixture modeling. *Psychological Assessment, 27*(2), 478–488. https://doi.org/10.1037/pas0000060

Safran, J. D., & Kraus, J. (2014). Alliance ruptures, impasses, and enactments: A relational perspective. Psychotherapy, *51*(3), 381–387. https://doi.org/10.1037/a0036815

Safran, J. D., & Muran, J. C. (2000). *Negotiating the therapeutic alliance: A relational treatment guide.* Guilford.

Safran, J. D., & Muran, J. C. (2006). Has the concept of the alliance outlived its usefulness? *Psychotherapy, Theory, Research, Practice, Training, 43*(3), 286–291. https://doi.org/10.1037/0033-3204.43.3.286

Safran, J. D., Muran, J. C., & Eubanks-Carter, C. (2011). Repairing alliance ruptures. *Psychotherapy, 48*(1), 80–87. https://doi.org/10.1037/a0022140

Safran, J. D., Muran, J. C., Samstag, L. W., & Winston, A. (2005). Evaluating an alliance-focused treatment for potential treatment failures. Psychotherapy: Theory, Research, Practice, Training, 42(4), 512–531. https://doi.org/10.1037/0033-3204.42.4.512

Safran, J. D., & Segal, Z. V. (1990). *Interpersonal process in cognitive therapy.* Jason Aronson.

Samstag, L. W., Batchelder, S. T., Muran, J. C., Safran, J. D., & Winston, A. (1998). Early identification of treatment failures in short-term psychotherapy: An assessment of therapeutic alliance and interpersonal behavior. *Journal of Psychotherapy Practice & Research, 7*(2), 126–143.

Tryon, G. S., & Kane, A. S. (1990). The helping alliance and premature termination. *Counselling Psychology Quarterly, 3*(3), 233–238. https://doi.org/10.1080/09515079008254254

Tryon, G. S., & Kane, A. S. (1993). Relationship of working alliance to mutual and unilateral termination. *Journal of Counseling Psychology, 40*(1), 33–36. https://doi.org/10.1037/0022-0167.40.1.33

Tryon, G. S., & Kane, A. S. (1995). Client involvement, working alliance, and type of therapy termination. *Psychotherapy Research, 5*(3), 189–198. https://doi.org/10.1080/10503309512331331306

Wolfe, B. E., & Goldfried, M. R. (1988). Research on psychotherapy integration: Recommendations and conclusions from an NIMH workshop. *Journal of Consulting and Clinical Psychology, 56*(3), 448–451. https://doi.org//0022-006x.56.3.448

Yeomans, F. E., Gutfreund, J., Selzer, M. A., Clarkin, J. F., Hull, J. W., & Smith, T. E. (1994). Factors related to drop-outs by borderline patients: Treatment contract and therapeutic alliance. *The Journal of Psychotherapy Practice and Research, 3*(1), 16–24.

Acknowledgments

I thank Stanley Messer, PhD, Distinguished Professor Emeritus, Rutgers University, and Former Dean of the Graduate School of Applied and Professional Psychology, Rutgers University, for writing a gracious foreword for this book. His generous, personable, grounded, supportive, and highly integrative style inspires.

I am grateful to Marilyn Susman, PhD, Professor Emerita, Loyola University, Chicago, for her valuable contribution to this book. It was Professor Susman's influence that led to the use of the inner experiences of therapists and patients, an important element in the presentation of the concepts, a focus of her teaching and research at Loyola University, Chicago.

Thank you to the following individuals who have endorsed the book, *Navigating Ruptures, Repairs, and Termination Within the Therapeutic Process*:

Judith Tanner, MD, Clinical Assistant Professor of Psychiatry and Behavioral Sciences, Northwestern University;

J. Christopher Muran, PhD, Dean and Full Professor, The Gordon F. Derner School of Psychology, Adelphi University, and Principal Investigator, Mount Sinai Beth Israel Psychotherapy Research Program;

Stanley Messer, PhD, Distinguished Professor Emeritus, Rutgers University and Former Dean of the Graduate School of Applied and Professional Psychology, Rutgers University.

Thank you, mentors, colleagues, and friends: Mark Paris, PhD, ABPP; Vladimir Nacev, PhD, ABPP; Andre Marquis, PhD; JoAnn Hoeppner, PhD; John Crites, PhD (deceased); Terrence Koller, PhD, ABPP; Gloria Berkwits,

MD; Daniel Barnes, PhD; Jack Dunietz, MD; Michelle Rodoletz, PhD; Jill Jefferson-Miller, geologist; and Kathryn Choate, MPT, CFMT, FAAOMPT, for your kindness and support and for having taken an interest in me and my career. A special thank you to Nell Logan, PhD, ABPP, for her support, deep insight, and caring.

With lots of love to my grandchildren for easing my mind and heart. I thank my daughter, Rachel Tzipporah Klein, MS, CGC, and my son-in-law, Ari Klein, MBA, for their visits. Thank you, Mom (deceased) and Dad (deceased), for providing me with the wherewithal and courage to pursue a path that women in my time and milieu were not encouraged to pursue.

There are many individuals to thank. I am grateful to Sarah Rae, Editor, Mental Health, at Routledge/Taylor & Francis, and her team for promoting this book and for providing valuable assistance and support throughout the project. Thank you, Pragati Sharma, Editorial Assistant, Mental Health, at Routledge/Taylor & Francis, for your dedicated work on this book project. I appreciate the work of Kris Šiošytė, Senior Production Editor at Taylor & Francis Books, Jill Harper, Project Manager at Newgen Publishing UK, and Lesley Cooper, Copy Editor and Proofreader at Wee Bear Editing for their efforts that helped to bring this work to fruition.

Part I

Ruptures and Repairs

Glen sits down in the therapist's office during his third session and begins to text. The therapist waits. After several minutes Glen says, "I am furious at my friend. I repeatedly call him to get together. He rarely returns my calls. I tried to take your advice several times, but my efforts are fruitless." The therapist, too, feels frustrated by the course of the therapy.

During the first two sessions, the therapist explored with Glen the history of his former friendships and relationships with his colleagues at work, and his present situation with his friend seems similar to what has occurred in the past. The therapist seeks to help Glen to become aware of his feelings and of his tendency to withdraw. Glen wishes to know only how he can fix the friendship with his friend. The therapist wishes to help Glen resolve the conflict and understands that this moment is critical in the therapeutic process. In the meantime, Glen looks down and begins to text again.

An alliance rupture occurs when the connection between Glen and the therapist deteriorates leading to a breakdown in their cooperation on the goals and tasks of the therapy. A withdrawal rupture takes place as Glen sits down, moves away from the therapist, and begins to text.

Ruptures are bound to occur because of the behavior of either the therapist or the patient or a misattunement between the two members of the dyad. In this case, the therapist and the patient are frustrated with the therapy process to date. The therapist is aware of the tension between them and knows that he needs to be attuned and empathetic if he is to repair the rupture. The therapist's focus is on the therapeutic alliance, and he is aware that it is a crucial aspect for continuing the work with Glen.

DOI: 10.4324/9781003128489-1

There is a robust, positive relationship between the therapeutic or working alliance and treatment outcome in psychotherapy (Flückiger et al., 2018). It is important for a therapist to create a strong therapeutic alliance with a patient. Psychotherapy has been viewed as a process that is cooperative, a milieu where the therapist and patient explore the patient's experiences within a joint space that promotes a reflective view (Knox, 2019). It is in this creative or transcendent space that a patient and a therapist can work on changes in the patient's current and earlier experiences (Knox, 2019). It is the quality of the interaction between a therapist and a patient that comprises the therapeutic alliance rather than the theoretical orientation that the therapist uses that creates change, and it is the relational communication and the intersubjective minute-minute kernels of interchanges that have the power to repair ruptures (Fuchs & De Jaegher, 2009; Knox & Lepper, 2014; Knox, 2019).

When the therapeutic alliance holds tension, a potential rupture may occur (Norcross & Hill, 2004). Bordin (1979, 1994) proposes that the rupture and repair process of the alliance strengthens the therapeutic relationship and is critical for the alliance. A therapist's ability to recognize alliance ruptures early in the therapy process (or early in the moment-to-moment interaction) is crucial, and the healing of these ruptures can facilitate change (Safran et al., 1990). A risk factor for potentially negative outcomes in therapy has been found to be a therapist's inability to perceive and repair ruptures in the therapeutic alliance (Knox, 2019; Parry et al., 2016). The difficulty in seeing the process of ruptures and their resolutions during a therapeutic interaction may involve the subtlety of the interaction that creates the tension.

Part I, "Ruptures and Repairs," includes Chapters 1 and 2. Chapter 1, "What Are Therapeutic Relationship Ruptures?" explains the importance of the therapeutic alliance and describes how ruptures relate to the psychotherapy process over the longer term. The chapter introduces the fall outs, breakups, and estrangements that may occur within and beyond the therapeutic alliance. Chapter 1 offers examples that describe the inner experiences of the therapist and patient before, during, and after a therapeutic relationship rupture.

Chapter 2, "Ruptures and Repairs in the Therapeutic Relationship: Diagnostic and Theoretical Considerations," addresses different types of ruptures and their repairs. The chapter describes how to navigate these ruptures within a specific therapy session and throughout the treatment, including ruptures in the therapeutic relationship for patients with different emotional disorders, and discusses how therapists with different theoretical orientations seek to resolve these ruptures. Chapter 2 provides examples of the inner experiences of the therapist and the patient during therapist-initiated repairs.

References

Bordin, E. S. (1979). The generalizability of the psychoanalytic concept of the working alliance. *Psychotherapy: Theory, Research and Practice, 16*(3), 252–260. https://doi.org/10.1037/h0085885

Bordin, E. S. (1994). Theory and research on the therapeutic working alliance: New directions. In A. O. Horvath & L. S. Greenberg (Eds). *The working alliance: Theory, research, and practice* (pp. 13–37). Wiley.

Flückiger, C., Del Re, A. C., Wampold, B. E., & Horvath, A. O. (2018). The alliance in adult psychotherapy: A meta-analytic synthesis. *Psychotherapy, 55*(4), 316–340. https://doi.org/10.1037/pst0000172

Fuchs, T., & De Jaegher, H. (2009). Enactive intersubjectivity: Participatory sense-making and mutual incorporation. *Phenomenology and the Cognitive Sciences, 8*(4), 465–486. https://doi.org/10.1007/s11097-009-9136-4

Knox, J. (2019). The harmful effects of psychotherapy: When the therapeutic alliance fails. *British Journal of Psychotherapy, 35*(2), 245–262. https://doi.org/10.1111/bjp.12445

Knox, J., & Lepper, G. (2014). Intersubjectivity in therapeutic interaction: A pragmatic analysis. *Psychoanalytic Psychotherapy, 28*(1), 33–51. https://doi.org/10.1080/02668734.2013.840331

Norcross, J. C., & Hill, C. E. (2004). Empirically supported therapy relationships. *The Clinical Psychologist, 57*(3), 19–24. https://psycnet.apa.org/record/533282009-008

Parry, G. D., Crawford, M. J., & Duggan, C. (2016). Iatrogenic harm from psychological therapies – Time to move on [Editorial]. *The British Journal of Psychiatry, 208*(3), 210–212. https://doi.org/10.1192/bjp.bp.115.163618

Safran, J. D., Crocker, P., McMain, S., & Murray, P. (1990). Therapeutic alliance rupture as a therapy event for empirical investigation. *Psychotherapy: Theory, Research, Practice, Training, 27*(2), 154–165. https://doi.org/10.1037/0033-3204.27.2.154

What Are Therapeutic Relationship Ruptures? **1**

Introduction

During the seventh therapy session, a therapist discloses a personal piece of information about himself to the client, Tabatha. Hoping to allay her anxiety, he says, "When I was a young student, I became nervous, and asked the driver of the car to pull over; however, it was too late. I literally lost my breakfast in the car on my way to the test. Years later, the professor called on me to read my paper in front of colleagues, and I had difficulty getting the words out in front of a group of my peers. I exited the room in shame." The therapist's intention for self-disclosure was to empathize with the client and to encourage her to open up further about her thoughts and anxieties. The therapist notices that the opposite effect has taken place. Tabatha looks down for several minutes and no longer seems engaged in the conversation. The therapist is hoping to re-engage the client, and says, "Can you tell me what you're thinking?" The client is thinking: *I thought he said this therapy is about me. Why then would I want to know about his personal problems? I'm feeling uncomfortable knowing his stuff. It distracts from my own problems. Why couldn't he, at least, have realized how burdened I feel about my problems without my having to attend to his stuff?* Looking down uncomfortably, Tabatha says, "Okay." And then looks away. A withdrawal rupture has occurred in the therapeutic alliance.

The therapeutic alliance refers to the agreement between a therapist and a patient about the goals and tasks of therapy and to the bond between the patient and the therapist (Bordin, 1979). The aforementioned vignette depicts a rupture or a disturbance in the relationship between the therapist and

DOI: 10.4324/9781003128489-2

the client, Tabatha, and tension ensues. A rupture in the alliance refers to an impasse in the therapeutic relationship between a client and a therapist in the space of the goals, or the tasks, or the bond (Safran & Muran, 2000; Zlotnick et al., 2020). In the aforementioned scenario, the client, Tabatha, has inner thoughts about the situation, but does not express them to the therapist. Instead, Tabatha becomes silent and moves away from the therapist. The scenario includes a withdrawal rupture or break in the therapeutic alliance, a type of misunderstanding described later in the chapter. Chapter 2 includes ideas for rupture resolution or repair where the client and the therapist, comprising a therapeutic dyad, continue their work in therapy to the same extent as prior to the rupture, sometimes, at a more advanced or deeper level, thereby strengthening the therapeutic alliance.

There are different types of alliance ruptures or strains in the quality of the alliance. Alliance ruptures are composed of confrontation ruptures, moves that oppose the therapy work or the therapist, and withdrawal ruptures, moves that are away from the therapy work or the therapist (Eubanks, Muran, et al., 2018; Eubanks, Muran, et al., 2019; Eubanks et al., 2021). Whereas the patient complains about the therapist or the therapy during a confrontation rupture or disengages from the therapist or the therapy during a withdrawal rupture, the patient enacts withdrawal and confrontation behaviors during mixed ruptures (Mylona & Avdi, 2021). The patient, Tabatha, in the previous section, looked down and away from the therapist and did not express herself during a withdrawal rupture. Here is another brief example of a withdrawal rupture, breach, or impasse that can occur in the therapeutic alliance. A later section of this chapter more fully describes this type of tension. A therapist and a patient, Eric, have a solid relationship. The patient has been in psychodynamic therapy for approximately three months. Today, the psychodynamic therapist is riding along on her bicycle and encounters Eric taking a walk. She says, "Hi," and rides on. Eric is thinking: *I thought she was out there for me. She seemed so cold. I'm a bit concerned about my next session.* During the next therapy session, the therapist notices that the patient enters the room and is pouting and looking away from her. She cannot figure out why Eric is withdrawing from her. She asks him about his week. He mutters, "Fine." She then asks if she has done something to upset him. The therapist notices his unwillingness to speak, which is different than his usual, friendly interaction with her. Again, a withdrawal rupture has occurred, this time, in an otherwise solid therapeutic relationship. Then, the patient looks away and meekly whispers, "You barely noticed me this morning."

The aforementioned examples that include the clients, Tabatha and Eric, described withdrawal ruptures. The following example depicts a different type of rupture or break: A confrontation rupture also known as an impasse, a misunderstanding, or a break in the therapeutic alliance. A later section of this chapter describes more fully the confrontation rupture. During the first seven sessions with the client, Heather, the therapeutic relationship has been characterized by a good deal of contention. Heather, who looks a bit pale, tells a cognitive-behavioral therapist that she is not feeling well today. The cognitive-behavioral therapist says, "Last week, we talked about paying your bill on time. You are now two months overdue." Heather is thinking: *I feel physically ill with a headache today. How can I focus on this stuff at this time? I wish she knew better. She's really a pain now. I'll put her in her place.* Heather responds angrily, "You care only about being paid. Didn't you hear that I said that I have a headache today? How much money do you need!" A confrontation rupture has taken place between a client and a cognitive-behavioral therapist. In this scenario, rather than moving away from the therapist, as in the aforementioned situations of Tabatha and Eric where withdrawal ruptures occur, Heather opposes the therapist and a confrontation rupture ensues.

Ruptures, breaches, impasses, tensions, or misunderstandings may be familiar experiences in our relationships generally. They can be personal as well as professional. Many have experienced a time in conversation with a friend or colleague where the dialogue flowed, but then something was said, and there was tension or disagreement. Thoughts may be: *How can that person speak like that to me?* There is a shift in the interaction, a recognition that the tension has the potential to cause a rupture in the relationship, and we do not know what to do. In an attempt to repair a rupture, we may find that one rupture may follow another, and we find ourselves stuck sometimes, in a morass that we, ourselves, have created. Both the client, Heather, in the therapy session of the previous section and her therapist may feel vulnerable and at a loss after the rupture has occurred. The book, *Navigating Ruptures, Repairs, and Termination Within the Therapeutic Process,* presents some ways to think about ruptures, misunderstandings, or misalliances in therapy and beyond and how to cope with the challenges of these disagreements when they occur. Chapter 5 includes a transtheoretical or overarching psycholinguistic model of the rupture and repair process in the therapeutic alliance that can help therapists to become aware of deeper processes that may be evolving during therapy sessions.

First, this chapter, "What are Therapeutic Relationship Ruptures," attends to an introduction to the ruptures themselves, what they are, and how they impact the therapeutic alliance. Luo and colleagues (2022, p. 642) point out that the transtheoretical term "ruptures" refers to impasses, negative interactions, or disruptions between clients and patients, and the term, ruptures, is transtheoretical in that they have the potential to occur in different types of therapy, regardless of the theoretical orientation of the therapist, e.g., cognitive-behavioral, humanistic, psychodynamic, systems (e.g., Safran & Muran, 2006; Safran et al., 2011a). When ruptures occur in the therapeutic relationship, they are of concern to patients and therapists alike. The patient can feel misunderstood, and the therapist feels discomfort not knowing what exactly caused the shift in atmosphere and then worrying about how to repair the breach. Safran & Kraus (2014, p. 381) note that terms such as "misunderstanding events," "empathic failures," and "transference-countertransference enactments" have been used to describe alliance ruptures (e.g., Safran et al., 2011a). (Countertransference has been conceptualized as the unconscious, conflictual reactions of the therapist to the transference of the patient (Gelso & Hayes, 2007; Reich, 1951, 1960)). Some psychodynamic therapists see ruptures as defense mechanisms (Abbass & Town, 2023). The bottom line is that ruptures can be a source of hurt, for therapists and patients alike. Therapeutic alliance ruptures can be a threat to the therapeutic alliance and can threaten the outcome of therapy (Luo et al., 2022). Ruptures in the therapeutic alliance are a common ground for therapists, regardless of their theoretical orientation, and it is an important task for therapists to address them when they occur (Eubanks et al., 2023).

The literature that reflects the importance of the therapeutic alliance is extensive. Chapter 1, "What are Therapeutic Relationship Ruptures," addresses the association between the alliance and ruptures and between the therapeutic alliance and outcome in therapy. Wampold and colleagues (2017, p. 42) point out that the therapeutic alliance, a pantheoretical term, includes the bond between the therapist and the client and an understanding between the therapist and the client about the goals and tasks of therapy (e.g., Bordin, 1979; Hatcher & Barends, 2006; Horvath, 2006; Horvath & Luborsky, 1993). The strong bond or the working alliance between the therapist and the patient is a key factor in the success of therapy (Hill & Knox, 2009). Rubel and colleagues (2018, p. 354) note that when patients report a strong therapeutic alliance the outcomes are significantly more successful (e.g., Flückiger et al., 2012; Horvath et al., 2011). Eubanks, Burckell, and colleagues (2018, p. 61) point out that the alliance is an integrative or fundamental common factor because it is not restricted to one therapeutic perspective (e.g., Wolfe & Goldfried, 1988). For example, Borelli and colleagues (2019, p. 9) assert that the therapeutic alliance derives from psychoanalysis and accounts for approximately a quarter to almost 60% of the modification of symptoms of depression in cognitive behavior therapy (CBT) (e.g., Gaston et al., 1991; Gaston et al., 1998).

There is a connection between ruptures or feelings of being misunderstood and the therapeutic relationship. Kline and colleagues (2019, p. 1087) point out that there is a relationship between ruptures which have not been addressed and alliances that deteriorate, leading to poor outcomes in therapy (e.g., Safran et al., 2011b). It has been shown that in situations where ruptures have been resolved, clients reported that they had a good relationship with their therapist prior to the rupture; however, in cases where ruptures have not been resolved, clients did not report a good bond with their therapist (Hill & Knox, 2009; Rhodes et al., 1994). The takeaway is that when the bond is strong, there is a greater potential for repair.

Hill and Knox (2009) suggest that clients and therapists address their present feelings about one another and the difficulties that may evolve in the relationship. They explain that if they can do that, feelings can be asserted and accepted, misunderstandings can be resolved, and not only will the therapeutic relationship be enriched, but clients will learn to use their new skills in relationships beyond therapy. For relational therapists, relational work in therapy is critical, and both clients and therapists contribute to the relationship (Hill & Knox, 2009).

Developing a framework in therapy where, for example, therapists and clients such as Tabatha, Eric, and Heather speak explicitly about their therapeutic relationship can provide a template for discussions about ruptures. The focus on the dynamics of their relationship requires that the clients, Tabatha, Eric, and Heather, and their therapists process their therapeutic relationship throughout the course of their work together. Their ability to do so is an essential tool when ruptures or disagreements occur between them. The process of communication between clients and therapists prior to, during, and after a rupture is important, yet hard to do. The extent of this discussion may vary depending upon the therapeutic perspective of therapists and the current state of patients.

The working alliance refers to the extent to which the therapist and the patient accept that they are on the same wavelength. The patient and the therapist may, at times, disagree with each other when there is a positive working alliance; however, for the most part, they feel that they work well together, that they trust each other, that they are receptive to each other, and that they are able to disclose important information to each other. The working alliance is positive when the client and therapist resonate with each other, when the patient feels validated and supported by the therapist and knows that the therapist cares, and when the therapist is genuine and open in interacting with the client. The bottom lines for the patient are: "Does this therapist get me, and, if so, does it make a difference in the quality of my life?"

According to Eubanks, Muran, and colleagues (2018), ruptures in the therapeutic relationship refer to incidents of breakdown in the working alliance between a therapist and a patient. They can include disagreements, fall outs, breakups, and estrangements that may occur within the therapeutic alliance (Bordin, 1979; Safran & Muran, 2006; Safran et al., 2011a). Examples that offer the inner experiences of the therapist and patient (how the therapist and patient are thinking and feeling) prior to, during, and after a rupture are included in this chapter. Melton and colleagues (2005, p. 82) note that inner experiences can be thought of as the way in which an individual processes internally and refer to the "language of experiences" that facilitates individuals to reflect and to communicate with other human beings (e.g., Orlinsky & Howard, 1975). Chapter 1 introduces the concept of a therapeutic relationship rupture in the context of the therapeutic process, generally, and in the working alliance, in particular, and addresses the expansion of the term "rupture" to include disagreements that may occur within and beyond the therapeutic alliance.

What Is the Therapeutic Working Alliance, and Why Is It Important?

THE THERAPEUTIC ALLIANCE: GOALS, TASKS, AND BOND

The therapeutic or working alliance is critical for therapists and patients. Flückiger and colleagues (2018, p. 317) note that from the time of its origins in the psychodynamic writings (e.g., Zetzel, 1956), the term (rather than the concept which dates back to Freud, 1927/1961) "alliance" has garnered popularity in psychiatry, social work, counseling, and other helping professions (e.g., Horvath et al., 2014). They acknowledge the suggestion that pantheoretical variables contributing toward the efficiency of therapeutic practices (e.g., Bordin, 1989; Frank, 1961; Horvath & Symonds, 1991; Rosenzweig, 1936; Wampold & Imel, 2015) has an effect on discussions about the collaborative features of the therapeutic alliance (e.g., Freud, 1912/1958; Rogers & Wood, 1974; Zetzel, 1956).

First, what is the therapeutic alliance? Bordin (1979) refers to the therapeutic alliance as a working alliance between individuals who wish to change (the patients) and their therapists. He explains that the therapeutic alliance consists of an agreement between patients and therapists on goals, on tasks, and on the formation of a bond. For example, behavioral therapists may view the goals of therapy as symptom removal; gestalt therapists may view the tasks for clients to engage in a discussion between two aspects of the self (Safran & Muran, 2000). The bond is composed of the emotional component of the relationship between the therapist and the client (Safran & Muran, 2000). What do clients think about when they consider the bond? They may think about the quality of the therapeutic relationship, or they may have a sense of whether the therapist is on the same wavelength as them. The emotional bond between the therapist and the patient seems to develop from the beginning session and tends to stay stable throughout therapy; however, agreements about tasks and goals tend to change during the course of therapy (Negri et al., 2019). Wampold and Flückiger (2023, p. 27) point out that the therapeutic alliance has been considered from many different perspectives, for example, its client-centered relational side, its origins in a psychodynamic framework, its social influence construct, and a pantheoretical approach (e.g., Bordin, 1979; Horvath, 2018; Horvath & Luborsky, 1993; Luborsky, 1976).

The Therapeutic Alliance: Examples of Different Theoretical Perspectives

Today, the therapeutic alliance has become grounded empirically and is considered a construct that is transtheoretical, an integrative concept shared across various theoretical orientations, (e.g., humanistic, psychodynamic, cognitive-behavioral) (Koole & Tschacher, 2016). The therapeutic alliance has a history. Koole and Tschacher (2016) point out that its origin can be attributed to Freud (1912, 1913) who promoted the idea that a positive attachment to a therapist can assist patients to continue in therapy (see Horvath & Luborsky, 1993). They note that the alliance continues to be a central point in contemporary psychoanalytic circles, where the bond of the dyad tends to be meaningful (e.g., Shedler, 2010). They explain that humanistic approaches hold that the therapist is responsible for the therapeutic alliance, and ideas about the alliance have emanated in the 1950s from the philosophic concepts of philosophers such as Husserl and Kierkegaaard (e.g., Cain, 2002; Van Deurzen, 2012; Yalom, 2002). The humanistic position of Rogers (1951, 1957), the father of client-centered therapy, claims that for therapy to be beneficial for the patient, the therapist needs to be empathic, authentic, and accepting (Koole & Tschacher, 2016). Many cognitive-behavioral therapists understand the therapeutic alliance to be a prerequisite for therapy, but do not consider it to be essentially curative (Koole & Tschacher, 2016).

Whereas the concept of the alliance evolved from psychodynamic views, it is a universally accepted construct no matter which theoretical orientation is considered, a critical factor that has a considerable effect on any intervention's outcome (Swift & Greenberg, 2015). What are the similarities and differences between psychodynamic/psychoanalytic, cognitive-behavioral, and humanistic theories with respect to the therapeutic relationship, the goals, and the tasks of therapy? Hill and Knox (2009) outline the importance of the therapy relationship to the therapy work based upon different theoretical perspectives. They explain that the similarity between the different theories is that most theories delve into the therapy work necessary to address impasses that emerge in the working relationship; however, the difference is one of emphasis. Theories of a relational nature, for example, view work in the relational arena as primary to change in therapy; however, behavioral therapists tend to regard relational work only if the relational issue impedes the therapy (Hill & Knox, 2009). Another difference is that unlike the relationship process in psychoanalysis and cognitive therapy, the emphasis of humanistic, relational, and interpersonal therapists is on clients as equal participants in the working relationship (Hill & Knox, 2009). For example, Hill and Knox (2009) point out that the goal of psychoanalytic models is to assist the patient to develop insight into dysfunctional interpersonal cycles by interpreting the transference; for psychodynamic/object relations therapists (e.g., Cashdan, 1988), the goal in therapy is for the patient to integrate the therapist as a good object. Consider the following examples that are similar to but different from the examples provided by Hill and Knox (2009) that highlight differences between therapists with various theoretical approaches with respect to the therapeutic relationship, the goals, and the tasks of therapy. See Table 1.1.

Suppose a psychoanalyst wishes that a patient, Charlotte, reveals more information about herself. The patient wishes to hold back important thoughts from the psychoanalyst. She is often hesitant to speak, and long periods of silence characterize the therapy sessions. Charlotte is thinking: *Why should I bother telling this therapist my thoughts? No good will come from this anyway just like it never has. I'm not feeling good about talking anyway. It's best if I stay silent and see what she says. I may not wish to involve myself here.* The psychoanalyst is thinking: *I'm going to offer the client an interpretation so that she may understand how the pattern of her past behavior repeats itself in the present with me.* The patient thus far continues to ignore many of the attempts of the psychoanalyst to elicit information from her. She often dismisses the therapist's ideas. She does, however, mention her mother whom she describes as intrusive. The psychoanalyst might interpret Charlotte's tendencies to withhold

Table 1.1   The Therapeutic Alliance: Charlotte and the Withdrawal Rupture

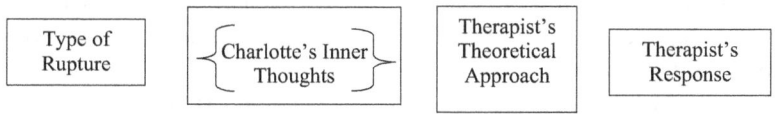

Type of Rupture	Charlotte's Inner Thoughts	Therapist's Theoretical Approach	Therapist's Response
Withdrawal	*No use telling her anything* *(Looks away)*	Psychodynamic	Charlotte, have you considered that you withhold information from me because you are concerned that I will intrude upon you as have others in your past?
Withdrawal	*Why bother disclosing…*	Humanistic	Please feel free to share as much as you wish, whenever you wish.
Withdrawal	*Tell her minimal information*	Cognitive Behavioral	Logically, I am a different person than others, a person with different thoughts and behaviors. I tend to respect other people's boundaries.

Note. The therapeutic alliance is a construct that is shared across different theoretical approaches (Koole & Tschacher, 2016).

information at the right moment and say, "Charlotte, have you considered that you withhold information from me because you are concerned that I will intrude upon you as others have in the past?" The members of the therapeutic dyad are involved in a withdrawal rupture.

The goals and tasks of interpersonal and relational therapists are different from those of psychoanalytic and object relations therapists (Hill & Knox, 2009). For example, for relational therapists (e.g., Safran et al., 2002) the primary goal of therapy is rupture negotiation in the therapeutic alliance, and a primary task of therapy is to develop the capacity to negotiate one's own and others' needs (Hill & Knox, 2009). The focus here is on navigating ruptures and devising creative repairs and resolutions when ruptures occur. This chapter delineates different types of ruptures. Whereas the goal of a humanistic therapist is to assist clients to develop their inner experiences and recognize that this process may lead to ruptures in the working alliance, and in this case, the task of therapy would be to address these impasses, the goal of cognitive therapists is to correct the cognitive distortions of the patient (Hill

& Knox, 2009). The goal of therapists who adopt a behavioral perspective is to focus on particular or limited portions of the patient's life, e.g., symptoms, and to change particular patient behaviors as patients interact with others (Bordin, 1979).

Suppose a humanistic, experiential, or relational therapist wishes that the patient, Charlotte, feel more at ease with revealing information about herself. Again, Charlotte wishes to hold back important thoughts from the humanistic, experiential, or relational therapist. She often looks away from the therapist and moves her chair as far as she can from the therapist. The client is thinking: *Why should I bother telling this therapist anything? No good will come from this anyway just like it never has. Anyway, I don't need her ideas.* The humanistic, experiential, or relational therapist is thinking: *Perhaps, if I share some of my present experiences with the client, she might feel more at ease about sharing hers.* Charlotte, thus far, continues to ignore the therapist's disclosures. She does, however, mention her mother whom she describes as intrusive. The humanistic, experiential, or relational therapist might say the following: "Please feel free to share as much as you wish, whenever you wish." Again, the members of the therapeutic dyad are involved in a withdrawal rupture.

Let us say that a cognitive therapist wishes that the patient, Charlotte, be more at ease with revealing information about herself. Again, Charlotte wishes to hold back important thoughts, this time, from the cognitive therapist. The patient is thinking: *Why should I bother telling this therapist my thoughts? No good will come from this anyway just like it never has. Move back. Stay away.* The cognitive therapist is thinking: *Perhaps, if I correct the distorted thought, she will talk more openly during the session.* Charlotte, thus far, continues to ignore the therapist's attempts to correct her distorted thoughts. She does, however, mention her mother whom she describes as intrusive. The cognitive therapist might make the following statement: "Logically, I am a different person than others, a person with different thoughts and behaviors. I tend to respect other people's boundaries." Again, a withdrawal rupture emerges during the therapy work.

The Formation of a Bond

Many people are familiar with a relationship going well in their lives. For clients, it is being heard and understood that makes the difference in the quality of the therapeutic encounter. Whereas many individuals have experienced that "aha" moment, where someone gets them right, many times people do not feel heard. And that can be hurtful, both in therapy and beyond. It is easy to imagine how a small amount of negativity may impact a relationship, in therapy, or beyond. Feeling connected to a therapist can enhance a client's feelings of progress. The importance of the therapeutic alliance or bond, the human relationship between the therapist and the client, cannot be underestimated. Much has been said with respect to various approaches to psychotherapy, whether psychodynamic, cognitive-behavioral, or existential. Nevertheless, it is the therapeutic alliance that predicts success in therapy outcome, regardless of the theoretical approach employed (Castonguay et al., 1996; Castonguay et al., 2004).

The Importance of the Therapeutic Alliance

Much has been written on the therapeutic alliance, and it may be considered a common or shared factor across various therapy orientations, e.g., psychodynamic, cognitive-behavioral, humanistic. Richards (2011, p. 57) cites the importance of the therapeutic bond or alliance in promoting change during therapy across therapeutic orientations and points out that Freud's (1912) psychoanalytic theory focuses on transference and countertransference, that Rogers' (1965) humanistic perspective focuses on the necessary conditions for effective psychotherapy and includes congruence, unconditional positive regard, and accurate empathy, and that Bordin's (1979) explanation of a tripartite model includes his conceptual frame for a strong alliance between therapists and patients, a positive connection between therapists and patients, consensus about goals, and task agreement. Leibovich and Zilcha-Mano (2017, p. 94) point out that Freud (1912) conceived the alliance to be important for success in treatment and emphasized that the curative part of therapy was dependent upon the alliance. They note that a common denominator of therapy research is concerned with the quality of the alliance, which is related to outcome, with a more robust bond being related to a better outcome in therapy (e.g., Horvath et al., 2011). Impala and colleagues (2023, p. 121) point out that the therapeutic alliance from the cognitive-behavioral perspective has garnered empirical support in its capacity to predict outcome by showing a connection between a decrease in symptoms and the alliance (e.g., Constantino et al., 2020; Rubel et al., 2019). A later section in this chapter describes ruptures and discusses what can happen when the therapeutic alliance falters.

Therapists recognize the therapeutic alliance as a necessary ingredient for change. Castonguay and colleagues (2019) assert that the differences in the ways that therapists focus on the therapeutic relationship can be described, for example, in the way in which CBT therapists and interpersonal/emotional processing (IEP) therapists (e.g., Newman et al., 2004) view the therapy relationship. They explain that a positive therapeutic relationship is viewed in both CBT and IEP therapies as an important ingredient for a patient's engagement in therapy; however, in IEP therapy, the goal is to deepen emotions and alter interpersonal practices as well.

Castonguay and colleagues (2019) develop an integrative psychotherapy framework, the cognitive-behavioral assimilative integration model, where they view the portion of the therapeutic relationship as a precondition to change. They explain that during the CBT segment, therapists are supportive primarily in order to build the patient's trust in the intervention and to facilitate the patient's will to develop adequate coping. They assert that the assumption is that if a solid therapeutic relationship is developed, the patient will more likely be able to face situations that were previously avoided and, during therapy and between therapy sessions, to problem solve new ways of responding to cues that provoke anxiety. Castonguay and colleagues (2019) indicate that the previous assumption holds for the IEP portion of the intervention where a solid bond between patients and therapists is considered to be important so that patients can engage in the difficult tasks of therapy; however, in this portion of the therapy, the relationship between patients and therapists is utilized as a change process as well. They suggest that during therapy, therapists assist patients to change their dysfunctional interpersonal interactions and work with the therapeutic relationship to facilitate the depth of genuine affect and to change previously impaired interpersonal patterns.

Ruptures

How often do individuals go through a year without experiencing some type of rupture, impasse, or tension in daily communication? Probably not as often as they would like. Sometimes ruptures or tensions can occur several times a day, at times only once every few months, or once or twice a year. This section illustrates some common ruptures that occur in daily life, e.g., at work, at home, in social settings. It aims to help the reader recognize the nature of a rupture or a tension in a relationship, and the scenarios are personal rather than examples that take place in the therapeutic encounter.

A Rupture in a Professional Work Setting

Chad has been performing orthopedic surgery at a medium size hospital for 30 years. His case load has not decreased over the last few years, and today he can see that he is scheduled for four surgeries. Chad feels fortunate to be working with a team of surgeons, residents, and interns who have known him for many years. He has grown accustomed to the interns and residents offering him his morning coffee while he prepares for his first case. This morning, however, his head is throbbing, and he can feel the same splitting headache that began during the night. Chad is aware that his first case is complex, and he is looking forward to beginning the procedure. Today, a young surgeon, Emily, relatively new to the team, will be observing, and, at times, pitching in, during the surgery. Chad needs his coffee, and he is thinking: *I need to do some prep work prior to my first case. Why hasn't anybody brought my cup thus far...* Chad turns to Emily and says, "Please bring me a cup of coffee. I like it black." Emily is thinking: *I haven't signed up for waitress service. Who does Chad think he is?* With some sarcasm, Emily responds, "I'm not sure that serving coffee is in my job description." Chad is thinking: *What! What! In all my years, this is a new one on me.* He storms out of the room muttering, "With all this politically correct jargon, a surgeon can't even get his morning cup of coffee." A rupture or misunderstanding has taken place in a professional work setting between a seasoned male surgeon and a third-year female surgeon. Unfortunately, tensions and misattunements such as these are not uncommon in the workplace.

A Rupture in a Family Setting: Siblings

In the following scenario, a brother and a sister are trying to get ready for school in the morning. Charles, while looking for the toothpaste, says to Savannah, "I need a few more minutes. Can you wait up?" Savannah replies, "Okay. I'm downstairs. Let me know when you're ready." Charles is having trouble locating the toothpaste and calls downstairs to Savannah, "Can I borrow your toothpaste? Mine seems to have disappeared." Savannah is trying to finish her homework from last night and feels distracted and somewhat pressured by Charles. She says, "You're always asking for favors. Can't you get your act together?" A minor rupture involving confrontation has occurred. How Charles responds to his sister's confrontation may affect the pattern of their present and future relationship.

A Rupture in a Family Setting: Parents and Children

The following example of a rupture or breakup in the context of a real-life scenario begins at a high school graduation. Thomas is graduating from high school. He hears his name being called, but he has difficulty moving. The dean calls his name again. Thomas knows that he needs to ascend the steps and receive his diploma, but he does not feel able to take another step. Two weeks ago, his father promised that he would be here. Thomas hesitates and glances backward at the rows of parents watching their adolescents graduate. Maybe his father is there. Thomas begins to walk slowly, head down, toward the stage to receive his diploma. He has planned this day for a period of six months. Thomas rapidly checks again to see if his father is occupying one of the seats. Thomas sees his friend, Haley, sitting a few rows back next to his brother, George, and they are trying to catch his eye and encourage him forward. His father is not there. It is the last glance that Thomas will remember. Thomas is beside himself. *I knew he wouldn't be here.* Haley says nothing. The disappointment, one of many through the years, washes over him. He is embarrassed in front of his friends who are taking graduation photos with their families. *How could his father do this to him?* His cell lights up. It is his father. Thomas hears, "Hey, Tom. I had an important meeting at the office. Couldn't make it today. Pick up some dinner, would you." Thomas hangs up. He and George go over to Haley's house after the festivities. Rather than return home, Thomas decides to stay at a friend's house for the next week. A rupture, fall-out, or minor estrangement has occurred within the context of a small family.

A Rupture in a Social Setting

In the next real-life scenario, two friends are at lunch. Athena and Ellen have been friends for five years. They seem to be enjoying their lunch in an outdoor garden when Christina approaches their table and engages Ellen in conversation. Ellen invites Christina to sit down at the table and have a bite to eat with them. Athena knows Christina but is disturbed that Ellen has invited Christina to sit down at their table. Athena is thinking: *How could Ellen do this to me... She knows that I have something on my mind now and that I invited her to lunch so that I can discuss something that's bothering me.* Ellen continues her conversation with Christina throughout lunch and does not notice that Athena has stopped speaking. Athena excuses herself to go to the restroom. Although nothing has been stated explicitly by Athena, a rupture has occurred. The course that the withdrawal rupture takes if and when Athena returns to the table will depend on many variables.

The aforementioned ruptures take place in real life or in life outside of or beyond the therapy setting. Whether individuals like it or not, in life beyond therapy, disagreements happen, presenting a continuous challenge in relationships, and, at times, will not disappear for long periods of time. The next section turns to ruptures that occur during therapy, in the context of the therapeutic alliance.

Ruptures During Therapy: Ruptures in the Therapeutic Alliance

Ruptures in the therapeutic relationship refer to incidents of breakdown in the working alliance between a therapist and a patient (Safran & Muran, 2006; Safran et al., 2011a). They can be thought of as empathic failures (Kohut, 1984) or as tensions (Safran & Muran, 2006), and they relate to outcome in therapy (Safran et al., 2011a). Patients and therapists can contribute to the development of a rupture, that is, they are co-constructed (Muran et al., 2023). Do you consider ruptures in relationships to be the final word, a setback that lasts until the end of time, or do you see them as a challenge for a relationship to improve though time? Stiles and Horvarth (2017, p. 75) point out that although tensions in the therapeutic relationship are negative, they can provide a chance for the client to work out interpersonal difficulties (e.g., Safran et al., 2014). Sometimes ruptures occur between therapy sessions rather than during therapy sessions (Zlotnick et al., 2020). Hill and Knox (2009) point out that it is the rupture in the relationship and its resolution that strengthens the alliance and results in lasting change (e.g., Bordin, 1979, 1994).

What Are the Causes of Ruptures in the Therapeutic Alliance?

How do ruptures or tensions emerge in the therapeutic relationship? Richards (2011) explains that there are many reasons that the therapeutic relationship may be disrupted or for ruptures to occur. She points out that ruptures may occur because of differences in the frame of reference between a therapist and a patient. For example, if a therapist and a patient have a good affective bond, but then begin to disagree on a therapeutic task, without resolution of the task disagreement, the positive alliance might be disrupted by the task disagreement, and an alliance rupture could ensue (Richards, 2011).

Another reason that a rupture can occur is because of strict adherence to a specific intervention framework (Richards, 2011). A therapist who focuses on method to the exclusion of the relational dimension of therapists and patients can cause a rupture in the alliance, e.g., strict adherence to the technical side of cognitive-behavioral therapy (Castonguay et al., 1996; Richards, 2011).

Richards (2011) further attributes ruptures to other causes. These causes can include the patient's style of attachment, a lack of willingness to disclose on the part of the client, a third party who may be interfering in the therapeutic process, a client who has different expectations about the therapy, and clients' feelings that they are not being understood (Richards, 2011). In summary, there are a myriad of reasons that ruptures may occur.

Types of Ruptures

An earlier section discussed Bordin's (1979) concept of the therapeutic alliance as composed of an agreement between patients and therapists on goals, on tasks, and on the formation of a bond. Researchers have delineated different types of ruptures in the therapeutic relationship. Safran and colleagues (2011a, p. 81) point out that there are ruptures or impasses that entail disagreements about goals, those that pertain to the tasks of therapy, or those that stress the alliance between patient and therapist (e.g., Bordin, 1979). These disagreements may result in the occurrence of different types of ruptures, for example, withdrawal (as in the example of Tabatha and Eric) and confrontation (as in the example of Heather) in previous sections.

Withdrawal and Confrontation Ruptures

Researchers classify two types of ruptures, withdrawal and confrontation, and note different resolutions to ruptures depending upon the type of the rupture (Safran & Muran, 1996, 2000; Samstag & Muran, 2019). A withdrawal rupture refers to the process of a client separating, pulling back, or pulling away from the therapist, the self, or from some part of the therapeutic work (Safran & Muran, 1996, 2000; Samstag & Muran, 2019). Ruptures can range from minor incidents or disconnection to major deteriorations (Okamoto et al., 2019). For example, a minor disconnection is depicted in the example of the withdrawal rupture in the introduction section of this chapter. In this example of a with-drawal rupture, the patient, Eric, feels slighted because the therapist did not stop and speak longer with him as she was riding her bicycle after hours. He is wondering: *She's always so friendly. I know that I have a good relationship with her. Why did she avoid me now? Especially since she knows that I recently was turned down for the job that I wanted, and I'm feeling down. This is a hard time in my life. Why did she barely say hello, barely acknowledge me? I wasn't expecting this from my very own therapist. I thought we had a good relationship. I feel somewhat hurt and rejected.* In this example, where Eric has a positive relationship with his therapist, but felt slighted when he met up with the therapist during off hours and the therapist did not spend time to interact much with him, the therapeutic alliance is intact, and the withdrawal rupture is not a major one. The therapist may select to discuss with Eric how he felt when the two, unexpectedly, met outside of the therapy setting and how Eric would want to be greeted if he and the therapist were to inadvertently meet again in the future outside of the therapy setting.

A confrontation rupture occurs when a client conveys a lack of satisfaction with the practitioner or with the treatment itself (Safran & Muran, 1996, 2000; Samstag & Muran, 2019). Okamoto and colleagues (2019, p. 117) point out that some research suggests that confrontation ruptures are associated with premature termination (e.g., Coutinho et al., 2014). Eubanks and colleagues (2021, p. 90) note that ruptures can involve mixtures of the aforementioned two types; one rupture can result in another (e.g., Safran & Muran, 2000), and therapists need to be open to respond to the moment in a flexible way. An example of a confrontation rupture earlier in the chapter involved the situation of Heather. This rupture involved a more than minimal deterioration where the patient, Heather, accuses the therapist of not caring about her and focusing only on being paid. In this example where Heather angrily informs the therapist that she has a headache, the therapeutic alliance is not as solid, the patient is well behind in bill payments, and the confrontation rupture that takes place during the session is more than minimal. The therapist may select to continue in the same manner and assert once again that Heather needs to pay her bill, or she might first select to empathize with the client's complaints about her headache, or she can point out what is occurring and how she feels about what is happening, e.g., may be feeling manipulated by Heather when she does not pay for therapy. Chapter 2 revisits this confrontation rupture with a rupture repair.

The following vignettes focus on confrontation ruptures. Here is a con-frontation rupture that involves the client, Hendrix, who canceled without giving the therapist 24-hours notice.

Vignette of an Example of a Confrontation Rupture

INTRODUCTION

At present, Hendrix, a 33-year-old client, works as a mechanic at a small shop near his apartment. On the weekends, he gets together with his friends to play cards and gamble. A few months ago, Hendrix was forced to file for bankruptcy because he lost his money. This is Hendrix's eighth session. During the session, a confrontation rupture ensues, and Hendrix displays anger toward the therapist.

DIALOGUE

Therapist's statement: I feel that I need to discuss something related to scheduling and cancellations with you. Your therapy appointment was scheduled for four days ago, and an hour prior to your appointment, you called to cancel. This is the fourth time in the last six months that you notified me of a cancellation one or two hours prior to your session. I have a copy of our agreement that we spoke about last session, and it says that you agreed that you would notify me 24 hours in advance if you would be unable to attend a therapy session. I would like you to read a copy of our agreement and sign it.

Patient's inner thoughts: He's such a stickler for rules. He's a darn pain. I don't need no more of this.

Patient's statement: [Sarcastically] Oh yeah. Sure!

Therapist's inner thoughts: I want to be firm.

Therapist's statement: We need to stick to our...

Patient's statement: [Signing in the air with a sarcastic motion] As a future Nobel Prize Winner, my John Hancock costs... And if you ask me sweetly, maybe I can provide it. [Laughs sarcastically] Ha, ha, ha.

Therapist's inner thoughts: Wow! What a sarcastic comment. I am now in a bind. I want to hold the line. Should I address his sarcasm?

Therapist's statement: On the one hand, it seems that I was being inflexible by requesting that you sign a copy of our agreement. It doesn't seem important to you. At times, you need to cancel a previously scheduled appointment, and I understand. From my perspective, late cancellations interfere with therapy. What are your ideas for how we can resolve this issue in the future?

Patient's inner thoughts: Uh-oh... I'm not sure what to say. Maybe I overdid it... I feel bad that I was in such a fighting spirit, but can anyone blame me, ugh, the family I grew up with... What do I do now? Oh no...

Patient's statement: [With some hesitation]. Thank you for asking. I got a lot of responsibilities. I got stuff on my mind. I'm not feeling that well today. Maybe I'm kind of shaky now. I'm gonna take a drink. I don't feel that well...

Therapist's inner thoughts: His outwardly hostile demeanor doesn't seem to match his inner crumbling self. He seems quite distraught.

Therapist's statement: When I began to talk about this issue, I thought I was sounding inflexible. That's not what I wanted to convey.

Patient's inner thoughts: Yeah.

Patient's statement: [Hands shaking] It felt like you were yelling at me. I don't like judgmental people. I grew up with parents who rejected every thin' I did. I can't take it no more. I don't want no more judgment from people. That's it for me.

Therapist's inner thoughts: He is feeling defenseless. It may not be a good idea for me to try to talk to him about this further at present. Given the severe criticism that has endured from his family, he may not be adept at discussing this issue further at this time. He seems fearful that I will judge him. Maybe wait for a better time when conversation between us is less disrupted.

SUMMARY

In this vignette, the therapist grew frustrated by Hendrix's repeated failures to notify him 24 hours in advance of a canceled appointment and wanted to hold firm; however, a confrontation rupture occurred. Hendrix, to a minimal degree, was able to accept the therapist's attempt to compromise by saying thank you, and then the therapist observed Hendrix's fear of judgment and began to better understand the rejection that Hendrix faced earlier in his life along with his present struggles.

The following vignette focuses on a rupture with the client, Russell, who is experiencing difficulty in his marital relationship. This is Russell's fifth session. During the session, a confrontation rupture ensues in the therapeutic alliance, and Russell displays anger toward the therapist.

Vignette of an Example of Another Confrontation Rupture

INTRODUCTION

Russell is a 38-year-old marketing advertiser. He has been feeling some tension at work and much difficulty at home with his wife. He begins the session by sharing with the therapist that he feels somewhat better at work.

DIALOGUE

Patient's inner thoughts: Lately, I've been feeling a bit better at work.

Patient's statement: I am really enjoying my work now. It's a pleasure getting up in the morning, knowing that I will be participating on this new advertising team.

Therapist's inner thoughts: Maybe I'll point out to him how his team is run by that couple who work well together, and that their positive energy impacts the work of their team members.

Therapist's statement: It seems that the married couple who is running your team is providing a positive role model and is giving you leeway to go with your project, the way you wish. It's nice when a married couple can work together like that and have an influence on the team members. It would be productive if other couple teams could lead together for the benefit of the group.

Patient's inner thoughts: Gee whiz! He knows how lousy I feel about separating from my wife. Why is he bringing up how well other couples are doing? Is he trying to stab me? Yet another person who doesn't care about me...

Therapist's inner thoughts: He looks angry. Because he seemed so pleased about his work, I forgot about his failing marriage and the effect it has on him.

Therapist's statement: I may have said something that offended you.

Patient's statement: [Explosively] You therapists are all the same. You say something stupid, and then you expect me to talk more. I was okay when I walked in here today, but now I feel awful.

Therapist's inner thoughts: I need to let him know that I've been insensitive to his current marital situation.

Therapist's statement: I'm sorry. I know that I've missed your situation here, that you are separated from your wife and feel bad about how things are going in your marriage. What I said was insensitive. Please feel free to let me know, in the future, if I'm insensitive.

SUMMARY

Russel shared his good feeling with the therapist, but then the therapist said something that annoyed him and a confrontation rupture ensued. The therapist admits that it would have been preferable to have shown more sensitivity to Russel's circumstances.

Withdrawal and confrontation ruptures have different features that are connected to them. Escudero and colleagues (2012, p., 27) note that that the disagreements that relate directly to the therapeutic alliance, such as the ruptures between the therapist and the patient that concern tasks or goals, or the strain in the affective bond between the therapist and the patient, are, perhaps, the easiest ruptures to detect (e.g., Safran et al., 2011a). Specifically, whereas withdrawal ruptures tend to be more subtle and more difficult for psychotherapists and clients to identify, confrontation ruptures tend to be less subtle and more explicit (Eubanks, Burckell, et al., 2018; Eubanks, Lubitz, et al., 2019). It has been found that psychotherapists tend to self-report confrontation ruptures more than they do withdrawal ruptures (Eubanks, Burckell, et al., 2018; Eubanks, Lubitz, et al., 2019).

The takeaway is that human interactions in therapy consists of delicate and not so delicate moments between the patient and the therapist, and it is the therapist's responsibility, first and foremost, to attune to the moment-to-moment states of the patient. Chapter 2 illustrates how to repair a rupture. Chapter 5 develops a transtheoretical psycholinguistic model that can help therapists to recognize the development of ruptures and to consider strategies for repair or resolution.

Some ruptures can last for a long period of time, some are more intense, and some appear more frequently than others (Escudero et al., 2012). Escudero and colleagues (2012, p. 26) point out that whereas some ruptures reflect a significant issue between the therapist and the patient, expressed in hostile remarks or in resistance to the therapist's efforts to influence, clients' less explicit expressions of discomfort may not be observed during therapy or may require a therapist's astute observation (e.g., Safran et al., 1990, 1994). The transtheoretical model proposed in Chapters 5 and 6 describes how ruptures, breaks, or strains may be reflected in a subtle shift in tone or body position, and speaks to the relevance of verbal synchrony and nonverbal, such as movement synchrony, to the therapy process.

Escudero and colleagues (2012, p. 27) note that some therapeutic relationships are marked by disagreements or ruptures and reflect the interpersonal style of the patient (e.g., Safran & Muran, 1996). According to Escudero and colleagues (2012), it is critical that therapists facilitate a feeling of safety for clients as they navigate the therapeutic endeavor. The duration of a rupture can vary with some lasting only minutes, while others can continue over some sessions; however, there is a risk that if a rupture is extended the patient may end the treatment (Escudero et al., 2012; Safran et al., 1990, 1994). Premature termination, unilateral termination, or dropout from therapy by a client is discussed in later chapters. Some relationships are marked by continuous ruptures, and yet the patient returns, for example, Heather in a previous section where she confronts the therapist and accuses the therapist of caring only about money while not paying her bill for a couple of months.

Ruptures in the Therapeutic Alliance for Therapists With Different Theoretical Perspectives

Although many patients understand the working alliance to be a safe space where they can disclose their inner thoughts, and therapists tend to back the therapeutic alliance, at times, breaks in the therapeutic relationship occur, and when the alliance is threatened, one and/or both members of the dyad may feel bad. With what frequency do therapists with different theoretical orientations report these ruptures or deteriorations? Therapists and clients involved with CBT reported fewer ruptures than therapists and patients involved with short-term dynamic therapy (STDP) and brief relational therapy (BRT), and this finding suggests that more ruptures occurred in STDP and BRT relative to CBT (Muran et al., 2009). How or why is it that therapists who use cognitive-behavioral strategies report a lower number of ruptures than therapists who use other therapeutic approaches? Muran and colleagues (2009) explain that brief relational therapists are specifically taught to discern ruptures, tend to speak freely about them to patients and view them as a potential to delve into patients' impaired relational issues. They suggest that just as brief relational therapists openly recognize ruptures, so too do short-term dynamic therapists who are taught about interpretations of the transference, which tend to facilitate their recognition of tensions in the therapeutic bond. The tendency of brief relational and short-term dynamic therapists to bring ruptures into awareness during therapy sessions may result in more ruptures because when patients become aware of the strains, they may become more anxious, which could lead to further tension (Muran et al., 2009). On the other hand, cognitive-behavioral therapists tend to underscore agreement and smoothness during therapy sessions rather than ruptures (Messer & Winokur, 1980; Muran et al.. 2009).

Therapists, in general, tend to perceive the frequency of ruptures differently than their patients. For example, Aspland and colleagues (2008, p. 699) point out that the report of ruptures by therapists occurred in approximately 50% of sessions; however, clients' report of ruptures was found to be lower than 20% of the time (e.g., Eames & Roth, 2000). The aforementioned results are not inconsistent with the more recent study of Rubel and colleagues (2018) that suggests that therapists tend to perceive a greater number of ruptures than do their clients. Again, when CBT is used, fewer ruptures are reported than when therapists used other therapeutic interventions (Muran et al., 2009).

Ruptures That Test the Therapist

Leibovich & Zilcha-Mano (2017, p.101) note that some research views ruptures as a client's test of a therapist; a test that aims to ascertain whether a therapist would introduce distress in the client and whether a therapist can handle the already existing distress of the patient (e.g., Silberschatz, 2012). According to Leibovich & Zilcha-Mano (2017, p. 101), if a therapist can "pass" the patient's tests, the symptoms of the patient will decrease; however, if the therapist fails to "pass" a patient's tests, there will be no decrease in symptoms, and the patient's symptoms may increase (e.g., Silberschatz, 2012). The aforementioned view pertains to a client's feeling of safety in the therapeutic relationship.

RUPTURES: RACIAL MICROAGGRESSIONS

There are some specific types of ruptures or disagreements that include microaggressions. What are microaggressions, and what is the effect of racial microaggressions in the therapeutic setting? Patients test therapists in a myriad of ways. They test to see if the therapist has the capacity to understand their cultural background and if the therapist is biased. Biases can manifest themselves in the form of racial microaggressions. According to Sue and colleagues (2007, p. 273), microaggressions refer to short interactions that communicate negative meanings to people of color solely because these individuals are part of a racial minority community. There are many themes that are associated with racial microaggressions, for example, criminality, ascription of intelligence (Sue et al., 2007). Here is an example that includes a rupture with a microaggression involving the theme of criminality.

Vignette of an Example of a Rupture with a Racial Microaggression

Last week, the patient, Craig, an African American medical student, age 25, spoke to a Caucasian psychologist over the phone for about 20 minutes, and decided that he would like to try out a therapy session with her. On the designated day, he traveled an hour and a half to reach the psychologist's office.

The patient, Craig, slowly walks into the therapist's office. At the office, the therapist's Caucasian secretary is in the middle of a transaction over the phone, and her purse and wallet are lying on the desk. As soon as Craig approaches the desk, the secretary flings her wallet into her purse and scoops the purse off the desk. She says to Craig, "You need to sit down, and wait until I call you." The secretary is thinking: *He's young, and he's Black. He's going to steal from me.* Craig says, "I'm not after your wallet, but I may need a pen to fill out the paperwork that the therapist described over the phone. When I left the medical school, I was in a rush, and I may have forgotten mine." Craig thinks: *How prejudiced is she. Because I'm Black, she already thinks I'm a criminal. I know that my therapist is White, and that I got along well with her on the phone. But I may not stand a chance here. More of the same... More stress on a daily basis for me. Another slap in a White world....* The therapist emerges from her office, greets Craig, and asks him to follow her. Craig follows the therapist to her office. Prior to sitting down, Craig says, "Your office staff has been rude to me. I demand an apology from her and from you who failed to train her." In this example, Craig encounters racism from the therapist's secretary prior to his first session with the psychologist. A microaggression with the theme of criminality has occurred prior to the therapist emerging from her office to greet Craig. When Craig enters the therapist's office, Craig confronts the therapist.

It is critical that therapists take care not to commit microaggressions, not to enable them, not to dismiss them, and to educate their office staff to be sensitive so that they do not commit microaggressions. Therapists need to be humble in their recognition that they do not have full access to their patient's subjective world (Eubanks et al., 2023). If therapists maintain an attitude of humility (e.g., Eubanks et al., 2023), pay attention to their inner thoughts, and empathize with the position of the patient, they may be able to become aware of and navigate ruptures more easily. In the following vignette, a rupture ensues in the first therapy session because of the therapist's microaggression that occurs at the beginning of the session.

Vignette of an Example of a Rupture that Begins With a Microaggression

Can a therapist's recognition of the effects of racial microaggressions on members of racial minority groups effect a more decisive and lasting change for patients? There are different types of microaggressions. According to Sue and colleagues (2007, p. 276), the type of microaggression that is illustrated in the following vignette is called "alien in own land." It communicates to members of a minority group that they are foreigners despite the fact that they may have been born or have lived for many years in the same country as members of the majority group. Mental health practitioners need to understand that microaggressions are debilitating for patients, convey their understanding to their patients, and assist patients to formulate strategies for coping with the debilitating effects of microaggressions (Ross-Sheriff, 2012). The following vignette is an example of a rupture where a therapist commits a microaggression at the beginning of the session.

INTRODUCTION

In this particular scenario, the therapist meets a 15-year-old client in the first session, who has been referred to the therapist by the client's school psychologist. The client is somewhat depressed and suffering from stress. From the beginning, the therapist observes that the patient, Amelia, looks different than other patients. The therapist is wondering where she was born and where she currently lives and feels somewhat uncomfortable with the new client.

DIALOGUE

Therapist's inner thoughts: She looks different than the rest of my clients. Most of my clients are long term. Is she from the United States, or how long is she going to be around?

Patient's inner thoughts: Oh no. A White therapist. I have enough to deal with. Why didn't the school psychologist refer me to someone in my own culture!

Therapist's statement: Hi. Are you from around here originally?

Patient's statement: [Looks depressed, but answers sarcastically and loudly spells out the letters] LOS ANGELOS, dude. You don't get it!

Therapist's statement: I mean, are you from the United States originally?

Patient's inner thoughts: Oh, give me a break. What do I need this for… I have this abuse all day long from the White teachers at school. White kids telling me to go back to Mexico and that students from Mexico are dumb. They assume that I don't live here when I was born in Los Angelos, like them. He's not gonna get me. He's not gonna understand my cultural background stuff.

[Patient is silent. No speech for eight minutes. Turns her head away from the therapist. Looks like she's going to leave]

Therapist's inner thoughts: How insensitive of me. I'm going to try to start over again.

Therapist's statement: [Said in a straightforward, genuine way] What I said before was a no-no! I feel bad that I said what I did to you. I don't usually start off like that. Perhaps I was a bit distracted. I apologize. Can we start over?

Patient's statement: I was born in Los Angelos, not Mexico, if that's what's important for you to know.

Patient's inner thoughts: He's trying to recover. He looks like he feels bad. I'll give him one more chance, but I hope if I do, he won't tell me that I'm imagining all the racial slurs that I endure every darn day.

Therapist's statement: I want to know what you want to tell me, whatever matters for you.

Patient's statement: Are you sure you're not wanting to keep the same opinion of me as my White school psychologist and the White kids at school? I don't need any more from them.

Patient's inner thoughts: I feel weary, like I'm in a war, forever fending off these kinds of remarks, all day long. I don't need more of this stuff from a therapist. I'm tired. Doesn't this White dude realize that I hear this all day long. Apparently not.

Therapist's inner thoughts: Oh no. I haven't had much experience with clients like this one. I made a faux pas. I wonder if I can redo it. She feels slighted.

How can I build the alliance? How can I be authentic? I'm a caring person, but what to do? I'll try again.

Therapist's statement: It sounds like they're not helpful to you. Other matters are important for you, and I want to learn more about these matters. It's important for me to understand your concerns. Please correct me in the future if I'm insensitive.

Patient's statement: [A tear forms in her eye]: Are you sure? Not many White guys want to know about Latina culture.

SUMMARY

At the beginning of the first session, the therapist committed a microaggression, observed the effect upon the patient, maintained humility, and attempted to recover. The aforementioned interchange included a mixed rupture. Amelia confronted the therapist, but, at another time, withdrew from the therapist and was silent for a long period of time. This client, although understandably put off at the beginning, has allowed the therapist to recover, perhaps because she picked up on his caring and empathetic manner. Therapists need to recognize that other clients may not be as forgiving. Rupture repair is described more fully in Chapter 2.

The Therapeutic Alliance and Teletherapy During COVID-19 and its Aftermath

The previous sections of the chapter underscored the importance of the therapeutic alliance. During the COVID-19 pandemic, many practitioners who were seeing patients in an in-person setting rapidly switched over to a telepsychology format.

How does teletherapy interact with the therapeutic alliance? Simpson and colleagues (2021) explore the way in which technology, e.g., video therapy, can shape the alliance. Practitioners viewed video therapy, the offer of synchronous therapy by way of videoconferencing, as a necessity during the COVID-19 pandemic (Knopf, 2020; Simpson et al., 2021; Torous et al., 2020). Simpson and colleagues (2021) point out that other teletherapy forms that mental health practitioners use include virtual reality, apps, online forums, audio phone calls, and text-chat (e.g., Stubbings et al., 2013). During the pandemic and beyond, the need to integrate videoconferencing and other teletherapy modalities challenges psychotherapists to develop a video therapy framework aimed at developing a strong therapeutic alliance (Simpson et al., 2021).

Simpson and colleagues (2021) note that psychotherapists have adopted technology more slowly than their patients (e.g., Simpson & Reid, 2014). Nevertheless, after the pandemic's onset, there has been a quick increase in teletherapy services among more than 3,000 psychotherapists in the United States (Sammons et al., 2020, Simpson et al., 2021).

What is the effect of teletherapy on the therapeutic alliance? The research is mixed with respect to the interaction between the development of the therapeutic alliance, satisfaction with it, and the use of a telepsychology format. For example, research on telepsychology and the therapeutic alliance shows that teletherapy does not impede the working alliance for patients who were diagnosed with generalized anxiety disorder (GAD) (Inchausti et al., 2020; Watts et al., 2020). In fact, these patients show a more robust alliance via videoconferencing than during in-person therapy (Inchausti et al., 2020; Watts et al., 2020). Similar to the aforementioned results is the research that shows that several patients and therapists perceive the setting of telepsychology to be less threatening than an in-person environment (e.g., Reynolds et al., 2013) and the findings (e.g., Simpson & Reid, 2014) that demonstrate that clients and therapists rate a high degree of the alliance in the setting of video therapy (Simpson et al., 2021). Békés and Aafjes-van Doorn (2020, p. 238) note that despite the benefits of teletherapy, many practitioners who use this format are concerned about their ability to convey empathy to their clients in order to develop the alliance (e.g., Roesler, 2017).

Simpson and colleagues (2021) note that, in contrast to research that cites positive results for teletherapy, other researchers found that psychologists rate the alliance higher for an in-person session than for a videoconferencing session (e.g., Rees & Stone, 2005), and it is suggested that practitioners' concerns about the therapeutic alliance during video therapy may increase because the move to video therapy occurred quickly and during a period in which the lack of in-person therapy was not by choice (e.g., Sammons et al., 2020).

The next section describes a brief vignette that includes a therapeutic dyad's switch from in-person therapy to video therapy, and then to phone therapy, during the pandemic and the interaction between the new modality of videoconferencing and the therapeutic alliance. In order to recognize the importance of interactions between different therapeutic modalities and the working alliance, it is important to include the notion of ruptures, presented in previous sections.

Vignette of an Example of a Rupture that Ensues When a Patient Switches to a Videoconferencing Format During the COVID-19 Pandemic

INTRODUCTION

The following vignette describes the first videoconferencing session of a 61-year-old man, Conrad. Conrad began videoconferencing toward the beginning of the COVID-19 pandemic, in March 2020, after six months of in-person therapy. During a few months prior to the pandemic, the therapeutic work with Conrad addressed his concerns about others overhearing his confidential conversations with the therapist. At times, Conrad feels concerned that others will overhear what he is saying and that his information will be compromised. At this time, he is concerned that somebody may be in the therapist's house during the videoconferencing session. At the same time, he relates well to and has a good relationship with the therapist. In this vignette, the dyad is beginning a switch from in-person therapy to a videoconferencing modality because the therapist's in-person practice closed at the beginning of the pandemic, and a rupture forms when the therapist encourages Conrad to continue videoconferencing.

DIALOGUE

Patient's inner thoughts: Gee, I've never done this before. I'm really not willing to have others in my therapist's house hear my dirty laundry. I don't want to use videoconferencing. I don't feel comfortable with technology. Other people in his house may sway my relationship with my therapist if they hear me, and I don't like this technology stuff.

Patient's statement: [At mid-session] I don't think this videoconferencing is going to work out. I know that sometimes people can hear from room to room.

Therapist's inner thoughts: I'm not sure that he can let go of some of his ideation about being overheard. As much as I've reassured him, these tendencies, in general, seem to be a challenge.

Therapist's statement: I want to reassure you that my equipment is confidential, and I am alone in the house. I can see that you may not prefer this new way of communicating with me. It may take some time for you to become accustomed to using the new technology.

Patient's inner thoughts: How the heck do I know whether he lives with somebody who will walk into his house, and, just at the wrong moment, will see me on...

Patient's statement: You're not getting what I'm saying. I just want to talk on the phone to you without any cameras instead of this videoconferencing which opens up a whole can of worms for me. This whole COVID thing is really on my mind right now. I don't need something else, something new, right now. The phone feels more right for me than the camera.

Therapist's inner thoughts: Maybe I can encourage him once more to use this format. I'll try to reassure him that there's nobody in my house when I speak to him.

Therapist's statement: You're concerned about interception; however, my system is encrypted, and there's nobody in my house when I speak to you. I'm the only one who lives here.

Patient's inner thoughts: Just when I feel I was making some progress. Now he's saying to switch to videoconferencing, and I feel that it's too much for me. He keeps telling me about confidentiality, but he doesn't know it's too much for me now. I have too many other things on my mind right now. He's been asking to switch for some time to videoconferencing. I would much rather speak on the phone. Period. There's no confidentiality with this videoconferencing stuff.

Patient's statement: No. You don't understand what I'm saying. Maybe I want to try only the phone for short periods of time. I don't want what you want.

Therapist's statement: Wait. Of course. I get it. Right now, you feel that talking on the phone is enough and that's what we'll do. In the future, we'll speak on the phone, period, until we can resume sessions that are in-person, and, if you feel up to it in the future, we can also play it by ear and explore other modalities further, if you wish. Would you like to schedule a phone session instead of a videoconferencing session for next week?

Patient's statement: Okay. If it'll be only the phone. Absolutely no videoconferencing, but if it's only the phone, maybe I can do it.

Therapist's statement: It's a deal. Only the phone next time. I want you to feel comfortable. Only the phone.

SUMMARY

In this vignette where the therapeutic dyad was in the process of switching to videoconferencing because of the pandemic, the therapist thought that the patient might agree to videoconferencing if he could reassure the patient that his software was confidential and that there was nobody in his house; however, a confrontation rupture ensued because the patient who, in general, does not like technology did not feel that he could become comfortable with the new format of videoconferencing. Toward the end of the session, the therapist preserved the therapeutic alliance and agreed to speak with Conrad over the phone rather than continue with the videoconferencing format.

Chapter Summary

This chapter, "What Are Therapeutic Relationship Ruptures?" describes the centrality of the therapeutic alliance, the need for therapists to recognize its importance throughout the course of therapy, and the way in which ruptures or strains in the therapeutic relationship present therapists with unique opportunities to develop and maintain the therapeutic alliance. Withdrawal ruptures involve movement away from the other, e.g., becoming silent (Muran et al., 2023). Confrontation ruptures refer to movement against the other, e.g., manipulation (Muran et al., 2023). Examples of the aforementioned types of ruptures with the inner thoughts of therapists are discussed in the chapter. See Table 1.2. Therapists with different theoretical approaches consider the alliance to be important but tend to it differently.

Chapter 1, "What Are Therapeutic Relationship Ruptures?" and Chapter 2, "Ruptures and Repairs in the Therapeutic Process: Diagnostic and Theoretical

Table 1.2 Vignettes: Ruptures Directed Toward and/or Away From The Therapist

Confrontation Rupture	Withdrawal Rupture	Mixed Rupture
Heather	Tabatha	Amelia (microaggression)
Hendrix	Eric	
Russell		
Craig (microaggression)		
Conrad (teletherapy)		

Considerations" address the part that both therapists and patients play in the development of ruptures and their effects on outcome, emphasize the critical role of therapists in the rupture resolution or repair process, look at how to repair ruptures, delve into how the repair of ruptures in the therapeutic relationship differs based on the patient's attachment style and diagnosis, and discuss how therapists with different theoretical perspectives navigate or respond to ruptures. Whereas Chapter 1, "What Are Therapeutic Relationship Ruptures?" is concerned with the constitution of ruptures that occur in and outside of therapy, Chapter 2, "Ruptures and Repairs in the Therapeutic Process: Diagnostic and Theoretical Considerations" describes repairs or resolutions to ruptures and therapists' responses to ruptures.

References

Abbass, A., & Town, J. M. (2023). Alliance rupture and repair in short-term psychodynamic psychotherapy. In C. F. Eubanks, L. W. Samstag, & J. C. Muran, J. C. (Eds.), *Rupture and repair in psychotherapy: A critical process for change* (pp. 221–252). American Psychological Association. https://doi.org/10.1037/0000306-010

Aspland, H., Llewelyn, S., Hardy, G. E., Barkham, M., & Stiles, W. (2008). Alliance ruptures and rupture resolution in cognitive–behavior therapy: A preliminary task analysis. *Psychotherapy Research, 18*(6), 699–710. https://doi.org/10.1080/10503300802291463

Békés, V., & Aafjes-van Doorn, K. (2020). Psychotherapists' attitudes toward online therapy during the COVID-19 pandemic. *Journal of Psychotherapy Integration, 30*(2), 238–247. https://doi.org/10.1037/int0000214

Bordin, E. S. (1979). The generalizability of the psychoanalytic concept of the working alliance. *Psychotherapy: Theory, Research & Practice, 16*(3), 252–260. https://doi.org/10.1037/h0085885

Bordin, E. S. (1989, June). *Building therapeutic alliances: The base for integration.* Paper presented at the Society for Psychotherapy Research, Berkley, CA.

Bordin, E. S. (1994). Theory and research on the therapeutic working alliance: New directions. In A. O. Horvath & L. S. Greenberg (Eds.), *The working alliance: Theory, research, and practice* (pp. 13–37). New York: Wiley.

Borelli, J. L., Sohn, L., Wang, B. A., Hong, K., DeCoste, C., & Suchman, N. E. (2019). Therapist–client language matching: Initial promise as a measure of therapist–client relationship quality. *Psychoanalytic Psychology, 36*(1), 9–18. https://doi.org/10.1037/pap0000177

Cain, D. J., & Seeman, J. (Eds.) (2002). *Humanistic psychotherapies: Handbook of research and practice.* American Psychological Association.

Cashdan, S. (1988). Object relations therapy: Using the relationship. Norton.

Castonguay, L. G., Goldfried, M. R., Wiser, S., Raue, P. J., & Hayes, A. M. (1996). Predicting the effect of cognitive therapy for depression: A study of unique and common factors. *Journal of Consulting and Clinical Psychology, 64*(3), 497–504. https://doi.org/10.1037/0022-006X.64.3.497

Castonguay, L. G., Newman, M. G., & Holtforth, M. G. (2019). Cognitive-behavioral assimilative integration. In J. C. Norcross & M. R. Goldfried (Eds.), *Handbook of psychotherapy integration* (pp. 228–251). Oxford University Press. https://doi.org/10.1093/med-psych/9780190690465.003.0011

Castonguay, L. G., Schut, A. J., Aikens, D. E., Constantino, M. J., Laurenceau, J.-P., Bologh, L., & Burns, D. D. (2004). Integrative cognitive therapy for depression: A preliminary investigation. *Journal of Psychotherapy Integration, 14*(1), 4–20. https://doi.org/10.1037/1053-0479.14.1.4

Constantino, M. J., Aviram, A., Coyne, A. E., Newkirk, K., Greenberg, R. P., Westra, H. A., & Antony, M. M. (2020). Dyadic, longitudinal associations among outcome expectation and alliance, and their indirect effects on patient outcome. *Journal of Counseling Psychology, 67*(1), 40–50. https://doi.org/10.1037/cou0000364

Coutinho, J., Ribeiro, E., Fernandes, C., Sousa, I., & Safran, J. D. (2014). The development of the therapeutic alliance and the emergence of alliance ruptures. *Anales de Psicología, 30*(3), 985–994. https://doi.org/10.6018/analesps.30.3.168911

Eames, V., & Roth, A. (2000). Patient attachment orientation and the early working alliance: A study of patient and therapist reports of alliance quality and ruptures. *Psychotherapy Research, 10*(4), 421–434. https://doi.org/10.1093/ptr/10.4.421

Escudero, V., Boogmans, E., Loots, G., & Friedlander, M. L. (2012). Alliance rupture and repair in conjoint family therapy: An exploratory study. *Psychotherapy, 49*(1), 26–37. https://doi.org/10.1037/a0026747

Eubanks, C. F., Burckell, L. A., & Goldfried, M. R. (2018). Clinical consensus strategies to repair ruptures in the therapeutic alliance. *Journal of Psychotherapy Integration, 28*(1), 60–76. https://doi.org/10.1037/int0000097

Eubanks, C. F., Lubitz, J., Muran, J. C., & Safran, J. D. (2019). Rupture resolution rating system (3RS): Development and validation. *Psychotherapy Research, 29*(3), 306–319. https://doi.org/10.1080/10503307.2018.1552034

Eubanks, C. F., Muran, J. C., & Safran, J. D. (2018). Alliance rupture repair: A meta-analysis. *Psychotherapy, 55*(4), 508–519. https://doi.org/10.1037/pst0000185

Eubanks, C. F., Muran, J. C., & Safran, J. D. (2019). Repairing alliance ruptures. In J. C. Norcross & M. J. Lambert (Eds.), *Psychotherapy relationships that work: Evidence-based therapist contributions* (pp. 549–579). Oxford University Press. https://doi.org/10.1093/med-psych/9780190843953.003.0016

Eubanks, C. F., Samstag, L. W., & Muran, J. C. (2023). Conclusion: Don't be afraid to get messy – Points of convergence in rupture and repair. In C. F. Eubanks, L. W. Samstag, & J. C. Muran (Eds.), *Rupture and repair in psychotherapy: A critical process for change* (pp. 305–317). American Psychological Association. https://doi.org/10.1037/0000306-013

Eubanks, C. F., Sergi, J., & Muran, J. C. (2021). Responsiveness to ruptures and repairs in psychotherapy. In J. C. Watson & H. Wiseman (Eds.), *The responsive psychotherapist: Attuning to clients in the moment* (pp. 83–103). American Psychological Association. https://doi.org/10.1037/0000240-005

Flückiger, C., Del Re, A. C., Wampold, B. E., & Horvath, A. O. (2018). The alliance in adult psychotherapy: A meta-analytic synthesis. *Psychotherapy, 55*(4), 316–340. https://doi.org/10.1037/pst0000172

Flückiger, C., Del Re, A. C., Wampold, B. E., Symonds, D., & Horvath, A. O. (2012). How central is the alliance in psychotherapy? A multilevel longitudinal meta-analysis. *Journal of Counseling Psychology, 59*, 10–17. https://doi.org/10.1037/a0025749

Frank, J. D. (1961). *Persuasion and healing.* John Hopkins Press.

Freud, S. (1912/1958). The dynamics of transference. In J. Strachey (Ed.), *The standard edition of the complete psychological works of Sigmund Freud* (Vol. 12, pp. 99–108). Hogarth Press.

Freud, S. (1912/2001). The dynamics of transference. In J. Strachey (Ed. and Trans.), *The standard edition of the complete psychological works of Sigmund Freud* (Vol. 12, pp. 97–108). Hogarth Press.

Freud, S. (1913). On the beginning of treatment: Further recommendations on the technique of psychoanalysis. In J. Strachey (Ed.), *The standard edition of the complete psychological works of Sigmund Freud* (Vol. 12, pp. 122–144). Hogarth Press.

Freud, S. (1927/1961). The future of an illusion, civilization and its discontents, and other works. In J. Strachey (Ed.), *The standard edition of the complete psychological works of Sigmund Freud* (Vol. 21, pp. 5–58). Hogarth Press.

Gaston, L., Marmar, C. R., Gallagher, D., & Thompson, L. W. (1991). Alliance prediction of outcome beyond in-treatment symptomatic change as psychotherapy processes. *Psychotherapy Research, 1*(2), 104–112. https://doi.org/10.1080/1050330911233 1335531

Gaston, L., Thompson, L., Gallagher, D., Cournoyer, L.-G., & Gagnon, R. (1998). Alliance, technique, and their interactions in predicting outcome of behavioral, cognitive, and brief dynamic therapy. *Psychotherapy Research, 8*(2), 190–209. https://psycnet.apa.org/record/1998-04139-006

Gelso, C. J., & Hayes, J. A. (2007). *Countertransference and the therapist's inner experience: Perils and possibilities.* Lawrence Erlbaum Associates Publishers.

Gersh, E., Hulbert, C. A., McKechnie, B., Ramadan, R., Worotniuk, T., & Chanen, A. M. (2017). Alliance rupture and repair processes and therapeutic change in youth with borderline personality disorder. *Psychology and Psychotherapy: Theory, Research and Practice, 90*(1), 84–104. https://doi.org/10.1111/papt.12097

Hatcher, R. L., & Barends, A. W. (2006). How a return to theory could help alliance research. *Psychotherapy: Theory, Research, Practice, Training, 43*(3), 292–299. https://doi.org/10.1037/0033-3204.43.3.292

Hill, C. E., & Knox, S. (2009). Processing the therapeutic relationship. *Psychotherapy Research, 19*(1), 13–29. https://doi.org/10.1080/10503300802621206

Horvath, A. O. (2006). The alliance in context: Accomplishments, challenges, and future directions. *Psychotherapy: Theory, Research, Practice, Training, 43*(3), 258–263. https://doi.org/10.1037/0033-3204.43.3.258

Horvath, A. O. (2018). Research on the alliance: Knowledge in search of a theory. *Psychotherapy Research, 28*(4), 499–516. https://doi.org/10.1080/10503307.2017.1373204

Horvath, A. O., Del Re, A. C., Flückiger, C., & Symonds, D. (2011). Alliance in individual psychotherapy. *Psychotherapy, 48*(1), 9–16. https://doi.org/10.1037/a0022186

Horvath, A. O., Flückiger, C., Symonds, D., Lee, E., Jafari, H., & Del Re, A. C. (2014, June). *The relationship between helper and client: Looking beyond psychotherapy.* Paper presented at the Society for Psychotherapy Research, Copenhagen, Netherlands.

Horvath, A. O., & Luborsky, L. (1993). The role of the therapeutic alliance in psychotherapy. *Journal of Consulting and Clinical Psychology, 61*(4), 561–573. https://doi.org/10.1037/0022-006X.61.4.561

Horvath, A. O., & Symonds, B. D. (1991). Relation between working alliance and outcome in psychotherapy: A meta-analysis. *Journal of Counseling Psychology, 38*(2), 139–149. https://doi.org/10.1037/0022-0167.38.2.139

Impala, A., Okamoto, A., & Kazantzis, N. (2023). Alliance rupture and repair in cognitive behavior therapy. In C. F. Eubanks, L. W. Samstag, & J. C. Muran (Eds.), *Rupture and repair in psychotherapy: A critical process for change* (pp. 119–139). American Psychological Association. https://doi.org/10.1037/0000306-006

Inchausti, F., MacBeth, A., Hasson-Ohayon, I., & Dimaggio, G. (2020). Telepsychotherapy in the age of COVID-19: A commentary. *Journal of Psychotherapy Integration, 30*(2), 394–405. https://doi.org/10.1037/int0000222

Kline, K. V., Hill, C. E., Morris, T., O'Connor, S., Sappington, R., Vernay, C., Arrazola, G., Dagne, M., & Okuno, H. (2019). Ruptures in psychotherapy: Experiences of therapist trainees. *Psychotherapy Research, 29*(8), 1086–1098. https://doi.org/10.1080/10503307.2018.1492164

Knopf, A. (2020). Telemental health comes into its own with social distancing. *The Brown University Child and Adolescent Behavior Letter, 36*(5), 7–7. https://doi.org/10.1002/cbl.30463

Kohut, H. (1984). How does analysis cure? University of Chicago Press.

Koole, S. L., & Tschacher, W. (2016). Synchrony in psychotherapy: A review and an integrative framework for the therapeutic alliance. *Frontiers in Psychology, 7*, Article 862. https://doi.org/10.3389/fpsyg.2016.00862

Leibovich, L., & Zilcha-Mano, S. (2017). Integration and clinical demonstration of active ingredients of short-term psychodynamic therapy for depression. *Journal of Psychotherapy Integration, 27*(1), 93–106. https://doi.org/10.1037/int0000043

Luborsky, L. (1976). Helping alliance in psychotherapy. In J. L. Cleghhorn (Ed.), *Successful psychotherapy* (pp. 92–116). Brunner/Mazel.

Luo, X., Liu, S., Levendosky, A. A., Good, E. W., Turchan, J. E., & Hopwood, C. J. (2022). Idiographic and nomothetic relationships between momentary interpersonal behaviors, interpersonal complementarity, and alliance ruptures in psychotherapy. *Journal of Counseling Psychology, 69*(5), 642–655. https://doi.org/10.1037/cou0000619

Melton, J. L., Nofzinger-Collins, D., Wynne, M. E., & Susman, M. (2005). Exploring the affective inner experiences of therapists in training: The qualitative interaction between session experience and session content. *Counselor Education and Supervision, 45*(2), 82–96. https://doi.org/10.1002/j.1556-6978.2005.tb00132.x

Messer, S. B., & Winokur, M. (1980). Some limits to the integration of psychoanalytic and behavior therapy. *American Psychologist, 35*(9), 818–827. https://doi.org/10.1037/0003-066X.35.9.818

Muran, J. C., Eubanks, C. F., & Samstag, L. W. (2023). Introduction: Rupture in a wicked and wonderful world. In C. F. Eubanks, L. W. Samstag, & J. C. Muran (Eds.), *Rupture and repair in psychotherapy: A critical process for change* (pp. 3–20). American Psychological Association. https://doi.org/10.1037/0000306-001

Muran, J. C., Safran, J. D., Gorman, B. S., Samstag, L. W., Eubanks-Carter, C., & Winston, A. (2009). The relationship of early alliance ruptures and their resolution to process and outcome in three time-limited psychotherapies for personality disorders. *Psychotherapy: Theory, Research, Practice, Training, 46*(2), 233–248. https://doi.org/10.1037/a0016085

Mylona, A., & Avdi, E. (2021). Alliance ruptures and embodied arousal in psychodynamic psychotherapy: An exploratory study. *Hellenic Journal of Psychology, 18*(2), 226–248. https://doi.org/10.26262/hjp.v18i2.8193

Negri, A., Christian, C., Mariani, R., Belotti, L., Andreoli, G., & Danskin, K. (2019). Linguistic features of the therapeutic alliance in the first session: A psychotherapy process study. *Research in Psychotherapy: Psychopathology, Process and Outcome, 22*(1), 374, 71–82. https://doi.org/10.4081/ripppo.2019.374

Newman, M. G., Castonguay, L. G., Borkovec, T. D., & Molnar, C. (2004). Integrative psychotherapy. In R. G. Heimberg, C. L. Turk, & D. S. Mennin (Eds.), *Generalized anxiety disorder: Advances in research and practice* (pp. 320–350). The Guilford Press.

Okamoto, A., Dattilio, F. M., Dobson, K. S., & Kazantzis, N. (2019). The therapeutic relationship in cognitive–behavioral therapy: Essential features and common challenges. *Practice Innovations, 4*(2), 112–133. https://doi.org/10.1037/pri0000088

Orlinsky, D. O., & Howard, K. I. (1975). *Varieties of psychotherapeutic experience*. Teachers College Press.

Rees, C. S., & Stone, S. (2005). Therapeutic alliance in face-to-face versus videoconferenced psychotherapy. *Professional Psychology: Research and Practice, 36*(6), 649–653. https://doi.org/10.1037/0735-7028.36.6.649

Reich A. (1951). On countertransference. *The International Journal of Psychoanalysis, 32*, 25–31.

Reich, A. (1960). Further remarks on countertransference. *International Journal of Psychoanalysis, 41*, 389–395.

Reynolds, D. J., Stiles, W. B., Bailer, A. J., & Hughes, M. R. (2013). Impact of exchanges and client–therapist alliance in online-text psychotherapy. *Cyberpsychology, Behavior, and Social Networking, 16*(5), 370–377. https://doi.org/10.1089/cyber.2012.0195

Rhodes, R. H., Hill, C. E., Thompson, B. J., & Elliott, R. (1994). Client retrospective recall of resolved and unresolved misunderstanding events. *Journal of Counseling Psychology, 41*(4), 473–483. https://doi.org/10.1037/0022-0167.41.4.473

Richards, C. (2011). Alliance ruptures: Etiology and resolution. Counselling Psychology Review, 26(3), 56–62.

Roesler, C. (2017). Tele-analysis: The use of media technology in psychotherapy and its impact on the therapeutic relationship. *The Journal of Analytical Psychology, 62*(3), 372–394. https://doi.org/10.1111/1468-5922.12317

Rogers, C. R. (1951). *Client-centered therapy: Its current practice, implications, and theory.* Constable.

Rogers, C. R. (1957). The necessary and sufficient conditions of therapeutic personality change. *Journal of Consulting Psychology, 21*(2), 95–103. https://doi.org/10.1037/h0045357

Rogers, C. R. (1965). *Client-centered therapy: Its current practice, implications, and theory.* Houghton Mifflin.

Rogers, C. R., & Wood, J. K. (1974). Client-centered theory: Carl R. Rogers. In A. Burton (Ed.), *Operational theories of personality* (pp. 211–258). Bruner/Mazel.

Rosenzweig, S. (1936). Some implicit common factors in diverse methods of psychotherapy. *American Journal of Orthopsychiatry, 6*(3), 412–415. https://doi.org/10.1111/j.1939-0025.1936.tb05248.x

Ross-Sheriff, F. (2012). Microaggression, women, and social work. *Affilia: Journal of Women and Social Work, 27*(3) 233–236. https://doi.org/10.1177/0886109912454366

Rubel, J. A., Hilpert, P., Wolfer, C., Held, J., Vîslă, A., & Flückiger, C. (2019). The working alliance in manualized CBT for generalized anxiety disorder: Does it lead to change and does the effect vary depending on manual implementation flexibility? *Journal of Consulting and Clinical Psychology*, *87*(11), 989–1002. https://doi.org/10.1037/ccp 0000433

Rubel, J. A., Zilcha-Mano, S., Feils-Klaus, V., & Lutz, W. (2018). Session-to-session effects of alliance ruptures in outpatient CBT: Within- and between-patient associations. *Journal of Consulting and Clinical Psychology*, *86*(4), 354–366. https://doi.org/10.1037/ ccp0000286

Safran, J. D., Crocker, P., McMain, S., & Murray, P. (1990). Therapeutic alliance rupture as a therapy event for empirical investigation. *Psychotherapy: Theory, Research, Practice, Training*, *27*(2), 154–165. https://doi.org/10.1037/0033-3204.27.2.154

Safran, J. D., & Kraus, J. (2014). Alliance ruptures, impasses, and enactments: A relational perspective. *Psychotherapy*, *51*(3), 381–387. https://doi.org/10.1037/a0036815

Safran J. D., & Muran J. C. (1996). The resolution of ruptures in the therapeutic alliance. *Journal of Consulting and Clinical Psychology*, *64*(3), 447–458. https://doi.org/10.1037/ 0022-006x.64.3.447

Safran, J. D., & Muran, J. C. (2000). *Negotiating the therapeutic alliance: A relational treatment guide*. Guilford Press.

Safran, J. D., & Muran, J. C. (2006). Has the concept of the therapeutic alliance outlived its usefulness? *Psychotherapy: Theory, Research, Practice, Training*, *43*(3), 286–291. https:// doi.org/10.1037/0033-3204.43.3.286

Safran, J., Muran, J. C., Demaria, A., Boutwell, C., Eubanks-Carter, C., & Winston, A. (2014). Investigating the impact of alliance-focused training on interpersonal process and therapists' capacity for experiential reflection. *Psychotherapy Research*, *24*(3), 269–285. https://doi.org/10.1080/10503307.2013.874054

Safran, J., Muran, J. C., & Eubanks-Carter, C. (2011a). Repairing alliance ruptures. *Psychotherapy: Theory, Research, Practice, Training*, *48*(1), 80–87. https://doi.org/ 10.1037/a0022140

Safran, J., Muran, C., & Eubanks-Carter, C. (2011b). Repairing alliance ruptures. In J. C. Norcross (Ed.), *Psychotherapy relationships that work: Evidence-based responsiveness* (2nd ed., pp. 224–238). Oxford University Press. https://doi.org/10.1093/acprof:oso/ 9780199737208.003.0011

Safran, J. D., Muran, J. C., & Samstag, L. W. (1994). Resolving therapeutic alliance ruptures: A task analytic investigation. In A. O. Horvath & L. S. Greenberg (Eds.), *The working alliance: Theory, research and practice* (pp. 225–255). Wiley.

Safran, J. D., Muran, J. C., Samstag, L. W., & Stevens, C. (2002). Repairing alliance ruptures. In J. C. Norcross (Ed.), *Psychotherapy relationships that work: Therapist contributions and responsiveness to patients* (pp. 235–255). Oxford University Press.

Sammons, M. T., VandenBos, G. R., & Martin, J. N. (2020). Psychological practice and the COVID-19 crisis: A rapid response survey. *Journal of Health Service Psychology*, *46*, 51–57. https://doi.org/10.1007/s42843-020-00013-2

Samstag, L. W., & Muran, J. C. (2019). Ruptures, repairs, and reflections: Contributions of Jeremy Safran. *Research in Psychotherapy: Psychopathology, Process and Outcome*, *22*(1), 7–14. https://doi.org/10.4081/ripppo.2019.376

Shedler, J. (2010). The efficacy of psychodynamic psychotherapy. *American Psychologist*, *65*(2), 98–109. https://doi.org/10.1037/a0018378

Silberschatz, G. (2012). Transformative processes in psychotherapy: How patients work in therapy to overcome their problems. *Psychotherapy in Australia, 18*(4), 30–35. https://search.informit.org/doi/10.3316/informit.736513696662220

Simpson, S., & Reid, C. (2014). Therapeutic alliance in videoconferencing psychotherapy: A review. *The Australian Journal of Rural Health, 22*(6), 280–299. https://doi.org/10.1111/ajr.12149

Simpson, S., Richardson, L., Pietrabissa, G., Castelnuovo, G., & Reid, C. (2021). Videotherapy and therapeutic alliance in the age of COVID-19. *Clinical Psychology & Psychotherapy, 28*(2), 409–421. https://doi.org/10.1002/cpp.2521

Stiles, W. B., & Horvath, A. O. (2017). Appropriate responsiveness as a contribution to therapist effects. In L. G. Castonguay & C. E. Hill (Eds.), *How and why are some therapists better than others?: Understanding therapist effects* (pp. 71–84). American Psychological Association. https://doi.org/10.1037/0000034-005

Stubbings, D. R., Rees, C. S., Roberts, L. D., & Kane, R. T. (2013). Comparing in-person to videoconference-based cognitive behavioral therapy for mood and anxiety disorders: Randomized controlled trial. *Journal of Medical Internet Research, 15*(11), 169–184. https://doi.org/10.2196/jmir.2564

Sue, D. W., Capodilupo, C. M., Torino, G. C., Bucceri, J. M., Holder, A. M. B., Nadal, K. L., & Esquilin, M. (2007). Racial microaggressions in everyday life: Implications for clinical practice. *American Psychologist, 62*(4), 271–286. https://doi.org/10.1037/0003-066X.62.4.271

Swift, J. K., & Greenberg, R. P. (2015). Premature termination in psychotherapy: Strategies for engaging clients and improving outcomes. American Psychological Association. https://doi.org/10.1037/14469-000

Torous, J., Myrick, K. J., Rauseo-Ricupero, N., & Firth, J. (2020). Digital mental health and COVID-19: Using technology today to accelerate the curve on access and quality tomorrow. *JMIR Mental Health, 7*(3), e18848. https://doi.org/10.2196/18848

Van Deurzen, E. (2012). *Existential Counselling & Psychotherapy in Practice*. Sage.

Wampold, B. E., Baldwin, S. A., Holtforth, M. G., & Imel, Z. E. (2017). What characterizes effective therapists? In L. G. Castonguay & C. E. Hill (Eds.), *How and why are some therapists better than others?: Understanding therapist effects* (pp. 37–53). American Psychological Association. https://doi.org/10.1037/0000034-003

Wampold, B. E., & Flückiger (2023) The alliance in mental health care: conceptualization, evidence and clinical applications. *World Psychiatry, 22*(1), 25–41. https://doi.org/10.1002/wps.21035

Wampold, B. E., & Imel, Z. E. (2015). *The great psychotherapy debate – The evidence for what makes psychotherapy work*. Routledge.

Watts, S., Marchand, A., Bouchard, S., Gosselin, P., Langlois, F., Belleville, G., & Dugas, M. J. (2020). Telepsychotherapy for generalized anxiety disorder: Impact on the working alliance. *Journal of Psychotherapy Integration, 30*(2), 208–225. https://doi.org/10.1037/int0000223

Wolfe, B. E., & Goldfried, M. R. (1988). Research on psychotherapy integration: Recommendations and conclusions from an NIMH workshop. *Journal of Consulting and Clinical Psychology, 56*(3), 448–451. https://doi.org/10.1037/0022-006X.56.3.448

Yalom, I. D. (2002). *The gift of therapy. An open letter to a new generation of therapists and their patients*. HarperCollins Publishers.

Zetzel, E. R. (1956). Current concepts of transference. *The International Journal of Psychoanalysis, 37,* 369–376.

Zlotnick, E., Strauss, A. Y., Ellis, P., Abargil, M., Tishby, O., & Huppert, J. D. (2020). Reevaluating ruptures and repairs in alliance: Between- and within-session processes in cognitive–behavioral therapy and short-term psychodynamic psychotherapy. *Journal of Consulting and Clinical Psychology, 88*(9), 859–869. https://doi.org/10.1037/ccp0000598

Ruptures and Repairs in the Therapeutic Process
Diagnostic and Theoretical Considerations

2

Introduction

It can be humbling for us to acknowledge that our relationships are more fragile than we care to admit, that tensions in a relationship in and beyond therapy may occur regardless of how we think or what we do. Chapter 1, "What Are Therapeutic Relationship Ruptures," discussed the importance of one such relationship, the therapeutic alliance, and the need for therapists to recognize the critical nature of the alliance throughout the course of therapy. Ruptures or impasses that occur early in therapy are linked with poor outcomes, and it is suggested that therapists attend to potential ruptures early in therapy (Gersh et al., 2017). Macdonald and colleagues (2023) assert that ruptures or breaks in the alliance may not be a one-time occurrence, that these strains or breaks in the alliance are often cyclical in nature, revisited throughout the therapy rather than resolved permanently.

Ruptures refer to negative turns in the quality of the therapeutic alliance, or difficulties in developing a therapeutic alliance, and these nuanced misattunements can cumulatively influence the alliance and outcome in therapy (Eames & Roth, 2000; Eubanks, Sergi et al., 2021).

Chapter 1 addressed withdrawal and confrontation ruptures (e.g., Safran et al., 1990; Safran & Kraus, 2014; Safran & Muran, 1996, 2000a; Safran et al.,

DOI: 10.4324/9781003128489-3

1994). When a withdrawal rupture occurs, clients tend to respond minimally, become silent, shift to a different topic, or act in a compliant way, and to repair a withdrawal rupture, a therapist may need to help patients explore the obstacles that prevent them from expressing their negative feelings and encourage them to express their need (Safran & Kraus, 2014). When a confrontation rupture takes place, clients tend to show dissatisfaction with the therapist or the therapy itself, by demanding or blaming, and to repair a confrontation rupture, a therapist may need to show empathy in order to help the patient express disowned feelings of hurt and disappointment (Safran & Kraus, 2014; Safran & Muran, 1996, 2000a).

Chapter 1 illustrated how ruptures or strains in the therapeutic alliance challenge therapists and patients, described the different types of ruptures or impasses, and explored how ruptures in the dyadic relationship present therapists with unique opportunities to develop and maintain the therapeutic alliance and create opportunities for change and growth. Ruptures or strains in relationships are problematic in therapy and beyond. Chapter 1, "What Are Therapeutic Relationship Ruptures," described how these misattunements may evoke strong feelings for the parties involved and discussed how after a disagreement in therapy or outside of therapy, some individuals may feel hurt, discouraged, angry, or worried, or others may move on with little awareness or care about what transpires at the moment of the impasse. It explained that during these delicate and not so delicate moments in therapy, clients may realize that the relationship is in jeopardy, that it could deteriorate further, and showed how clients may be at a loss about how to proceed. The examples included in the previous chapter illustrated that whereas some therapists or clients may reflect on, ruminate, or overanalyze the situation, other individuals may tell themselves that they could care less. The bottom line is that unlike times when a relationship is smooth and feels flowing, during a rupture, the members of the therapeutic dyad may feel stressed.

Rudenstine and colleagues (2023, p. 279) point out that regardless of theoretical perspective, therapists need to attend to ruptures in order for clients to progress in therapy (e.g., Boritz et al., 2018; Zilcha-Mano et al., 2020). Chapter 2, "Ruptures and Repairs in the Therapeutic Relationship: Diagnostic and Theoretical Considerations," focuses on the repair of ruptures. Prior to repairing a rupture, a therapist needs to acknowledge the rupture (Muran et al., 2023). Muran and colleagues (2023) suggest routes or steps for repairing a rupture, and these routes or pathways may interact. They explain that, at the outset of a rupture, therapists need to use immediate strategies such as reattunement to feelings, which can be followed by a renegotiation of therapy tasks and goals, and finally, therapists need to employ expressive strategies such as the exploration of the misattunement experience.

The book, *Navigating Ruptures, Repairs, and Termination Within the Therapeutic Process*, is about more than the development of ruptures in therapy and beyond. Chapter 2, "Ruptures and Repairs in the Therapeutic Relationship: Diagnostic and Theoretical Considerations," expands on the concept of ruptures and covers repairs or resolutions to ruptures, therapists' responses to ruptures, how to repair ruptures, how the repair of ruptures in the therapeutic relationship differs based on the patient's attachment style and diagnosis, and how therapists with different theoretical approaches, for example, cognitive-behavioral, psychodynamic, or existential/humanistic, may navigate or respond to ruptures. The chapter presents case examples in the form of vignettes. These vignettes include the dialogue between the patient and the therapist as well as their inner thoughts.

What Are Rupture Repairs or Resolutions?

Ruptures will occur and need not be considered obstacles in therapy (Safran & Kraus, 2014). Rather, therapists and clients may view ruptures as opportunities for growth (Safran & Kraus, 2014). A repair or resolution of a rupture in the alliance refers to a scenario where a therapist and a patient, subsequent to a rupture, continue to work together in therapy at an increased level of alliance or at the same level of alliance that they had prior to the rupture (Zlotnick et al., 2020). Similar to ruptures, both the therapist and the patient can contribute to the repair of a rupture, that is, the repair of ruptures is co-constructed (Muran et al., 2023). What can happen when ruptures are not resolved? Whereas ruptures that have not been repaired have been shown to lead to unsuccessful outcomes where the patient does not progress or ends therapy, ruptures that have been resolved tend to have outcomes that lead to growth and change (Eubanks, Muran, et al., 2018; Safran et al., 2011; Zlotnick et al., 2020). If the rupture is not that intense and the rupture resolution is high, then therapeutic alliance ratings and the overall quality of the therapy session will be higher (Muran et al., 2009).

Many would agree that for therapy to be meaningful for clients, it is critical that therapists focus on repairing the rupture. A novice therapist who begins to think about ruptures first needs to learn how to identify them. The takeaway is that therapists need to pay attention to ruptures, that if a rupture does take place, and it is likely that it will at some point during therapy, the therapist needs to focus on repairing it with as much finesse as possible so that the quality of the therapeutic alliance is preserved. Repairing ruptures can be a delicate matter and requires fine interpersonal skills at the moment of the rupture. Repairs may require attendance to the inner thoughts of therapists and patients. When repairing ruptures, novice therapists need to learn to attend to nonverbal cues as well as to the verbal responses of their clients, to what the client says, and perhaps, more importantly, to what the client does not say, to the conscious as well as to the unconscious, and to the client's ability and willingness to share information during the therapy session. Therapists who think about repairing ruptures need to learn to become aware of their own inner thoughts and to elicit the inner cognitions of their clients. Luo et al. (2022, p. 652) point out that therapists need to adjust their interventions based on what transpires on a moment-to-moment basis with clients, specifically during tense moments (e.g., Constantino et al., 2020; Stiles, 2009). Ruptures, although difficult to navigate, have the potential to facilitate an opportunity for the patient and the therapist to get to know each other better, and their repair is related to successful therapy outcomes (Eubanks, Muran, et al., 2018; Eubanks et al., 2023). In short, what goes wrong during a therapy session may be as instructive, if not more important, than what goes right, and things that go wrong in therapy may turn out right when therapists are intentional in their responses.

Chapter 1 described different types of ruptures: Withdrawal, confrontation, and mixed. It set the stage for a discussion of different resolutions to ruptures depending upon the type. Although there are similarities in the process that therapists use for repairing ruptures, i.e., empathy, self-disclosure, authenticity, care, a toolbox of relational skills, therapists may approach the process of repairing ruptures in different ways. Safran and Muran (1996) suggest that therapists offer different repairs for ruptures depending upon the rupture type (withdrawal or confrontation), and the focus of a resolution is on facilitating a patient's access to unarticulated feelings. They offer the following example: If a patient's rupture includes confrontation or hostility, the therapist needs to be careful not to react with anger or aggression, but rather to facilitate access to the patient's unexpressed feeling, which will tend to be vulnerability. If, on the other hand, the rupture includes withdrawal or submissiveness, the therapist needs to take care to refrain from responding in a complementary way by controlling the patient or ignoring the withdrawal rupture, but rather to facilitate the patient's access to a primary wish, which is likely to be self-assertion. According to Safran and Muran (1996), at times it is difficult to discern the different types of ruptures, and they explain that a patient, in the beginning, may express what appears to be a confrontation rupture, an expression of hostility toward the therapist, but then at a later time,

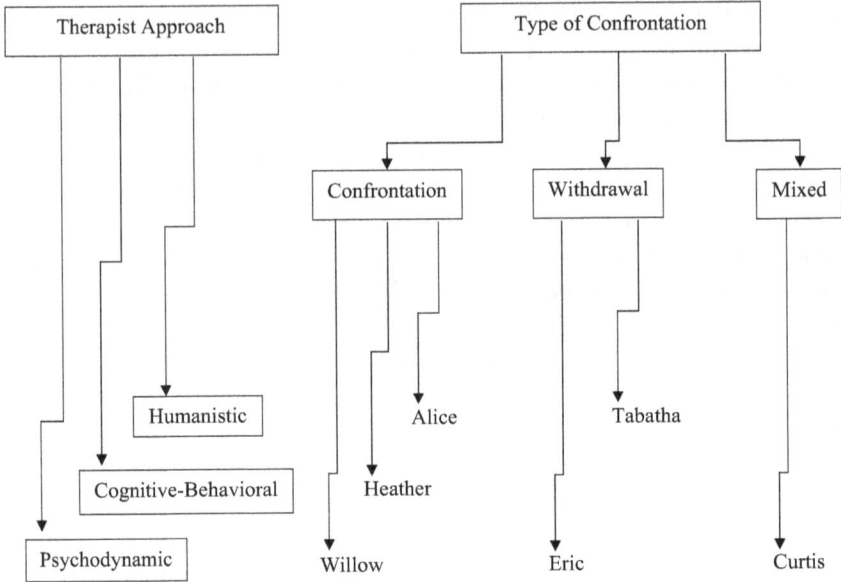

Figure 2.1   Vignettes: Rupture, Repairs or Resolutions

Note. This figure illustrates examples of the repair of different types of ruptures by therapists with different treatment approaches.

may feel anxious about expressing aggression, and then will withdraw from the unexpressed feeling of vulnerability. Chapter 2, "Ruptures and Repairs in the Therapeutic Relationship: Diagnostic and Theoretical Considerations," provides vignettes of the process of ruptures and specific resolutions or repairs along with the inner thoughts of therapists and patients. See Figure 2.1.

Responding To Ruptures

In order to repair a rupture, therapists need to recognize that a rupture has occurred, and the recognition of withdrawal ruptures may particularly challenge therapists because they are difficult to discern (Eubanks et al., 2023). Therapists need to be self-aware, to regulate emotion, and to cultivate interpersonal sensitivity if they are to repair ruptures (Chang et al., 2023). There is more that is needed than just awareness of ruptures and rupture identification. Therapists need to take responsibility for their contribution to the rupture (Eubanks et al., 2021). How to respond to a rupture or impasse and engage in the process of repair is an essential part of the therapeutic process (Samstag & Muran, 2019), and therapists need to show respect for clients along with a willingness to be authentic, non-defensive, and open. Therapists who are authentic and self-aware explore the specific parts of their patients, for example, personal history and personality style, while seeking to understand the patients' covert or inner thoughts and attuning themselves to patients' moment-to-moment communications. Eubanks, Muran, and colleagues (2018) suggest that there are strategies for the repair of ruptures that are direct and indirect. They explain that direct strategies for rupture repairs involve focusing on the rupture and asking clients to offer thoughts about the rupture, and indirect strategies refer to a process where the therapist is able to resolve the impasse without focusing attention on it, for example, modifying a requested task when the patient finds it annoying.

Therapists' mistakes, disagreements over tasks and goals, and difficulties related to patients' transference and therapists' countertransference, or therapists' own issues, such as therapists' anxiety that impedes their ability to fulfill their therapeutic functions are cited as reasons for dropout from therapy during a rupture or an impasse (Hill et al., 1996). Although therapists aim to be attuned to the nuances of clients' moment-to moment communications, sometimes their own difficulties related to patients' transference and their own countertransference may be reasons that patients end therapy. Gelso and Hayes (2007) define countertransference as the external or internal responses of therapists that develop given the past or present vulnerabilities or conflicts of therapists. They assert that although countertransference, the unconscious or the conflicted reactions of therapists to the transference of their patients, is a concept that has its origin in psychoanalysis, it is a universal notion, a concept that is present in other therapies, for example, experiential, cognitive-behavioral, and psychodynamic, as well. According to these authors, countertransference includes more than the transference of the therapist to the transference of the patient; it can include the therapist's non-transference responses to the non-transference material of the patient. A behavior therapist's countertransference, for example, may impede the therapist's ability to identify the patient's behaviors that need change, to recognize how the patient's behaviors have been previously reinforced, and to discern the interventions necessary for the patient to change the behaviors (Gelso & Hayes, 2007). According to Gelso and Hayes (2007) when therapists do not manage their countertransference well, the therapy is not serviced; however, when therapists do manage their countertransference in an effective way, the countertransference itself can benefit the therapy.

At times, therapists' vulnerabilities connected to regulating or managing negative emotion may contribute to an impasse, disagreement, or a rupture that is difficult to resolve (Bachelor & Horvath, 1999). Therapists need to be able to manage the vulnerabilities related to their own countertransference in order to promote patients' progress in therapy (Bimont & Werbart, 2018). The next section presents a vignette that illustrates an example of a humanistic therapist's countertransference response that interferes with the therapeutic process. In this vignette, the therapist's response led to a rupture, and then the therapist repaired the rupture. Specifically, the vignette illustrates how a rupture can unfold in the face of a therapist's countertransference and what it takes to repair the impasse.

Vignette of an Example of a Humanistic Therapist's Countertransference Response Followed by a Repair of a Rupture

INTRODUCTION

In the following vignette, a novice therapist with a humanistic theoretical approach interacts with her client, Alice, who relates her story about a shared day with her sister at a museum. Alice, a 38-year-old policewoman, begins to speak during her fifth session of therapy. She expresses annoyance over what happened when she arrived at her sister's house yesterday.

DIALOGUE

> **Patient's statement:** You've been encouraging me to develop my interpersonal relationships. My sister and I planned a day at the museum. I drove to the house at 9 A.M., but she wasn't ready. I sat around for over an hour again until she was ready. After you encouraged me to set aside time for her, I set up a time last week, and we agreed that Sunday at 9 A.M. would be our day. But she was on the phone for over an hour until we finally left. She does this kind of thing all of the time. We've spoken about it in the past. A total waste of my time. I really don't enjoy her company anyway. [Speaking loudly] Once we got to the museum, she was so critical of me. It was hard to get her off my back.
>
> *Therapist's inner thoughts: I was hoping that Alice could have a nice day with her sister. I treasure the days that I was able to spend with my sister before the accident. Maybe I was being too idealistic. My older sister suffered a debilitating illness after her accident, and because of her many operations and*

treatments, she's in a wheelchair and needs daily care, and we aren't able to share the activities that we enjoyed as much as I had hoped.

Therapist's statement: I understand how frustrating it can be, but perhaps you can…

Patient's inner thoughts: She's starting to act like an attorney for my sister.

Patient's statement: [With irritation, raising her voice] I don't need you to be a lawyer for my sister.

Therapist's inner thoughts: I'm not quite sure what to say now. I turned her off. I'm anxious about turning her off.

Therapist's statement: Maybe you can try… Begin with…

Patient's inner thoughts: She does not hear me. I don't need advice. And I'm not sure that I want to give up a day off waiting around for my sister. I feel like walking out of here.

Patient's statement: [Loudly] I SAID that I don't need you to be a lawyer for my sister. You're not getting it.

Therapist's inner thoughts: I made another mistake. I turned her off further. Ah… I may have some thoughts that can help me recover.

Therapist's statement: You were looking forward to this day with her. You planned it three weeks ago, called her to remind her about it, and took time off from your work. You would have, at least, wanted her to try to be on time rather than sit around waiting for her for over an hour. And then, you didn't enjoy yourself at the museum either.

Patient's inner thoughts: [Smiling. Feeling relief] Now my therapist is on the right track.

Patient's statement: Yeah. Exactly.

Summary

The therapist's own ideas about her relationship with her older sister (her countertransference) began to interfere with her responses to Alice. The therapist feels sorry that after her sister's accident she was not able to spend more time with her sister sharing the activities that they mutually enjoyed. The therapist's countertransference related to her own sister interfered with her ability to respond to Alice in a way that was therapeutic for Alice, and Alice became irritated with the therapist. In this vignette, the therapist was not aware of her own countertransference.

Initial attempts to repair tensions in the alliance may not succeed, and at times, attempts at resolutions may lead to other ruptures (Eubanks et al., 2023). In this vignette, a confrontation rupture occurred. The therapist is aware that there is tension in the alliance. How can the therapist repair this rupture? She thinks about what she can do to repair the rupture and to offer Alice a corrective emotional experience. The following continuation of the session where the humanistic therapist discloses to Alice in a genuine way some personal history helps to repair the rupture in the alliance.

Dialogue

Therapist's thoughts: Alice is irritated. I am encouraging her to increase her opportunities for interpersonal relationships by engaging with her sister. I wish that my sister had not had the accident and that we could spend more time sharing the activities that we enjoy together.

Therapist's statement: Your situation is quite different from mine. My sister had an accident, and I regret that we are unable to spend more time with each other. It's hard for me to think about the time that I miss with her today. It may not be productive for me to compare your sister with mine. Your situation is a whole different ball game. Your life events are not the same as mine.

Patient's inner thoughts: She's upfront and honest about what happened here. I really respect that.

Patient's statement: You and I are different people.

Therapist's inner thoughts: Yes.

Therapist's statement: Exactly. I apologize that my own life experiences did not allow me to recognize the difficulties that you had when you went to the museum with your sister yesterday, and how the last incident with her was yet another time where she kept you waiting, on hold, while you catered to her schedule, and she didn't recognize that you were around. You have discussed with her how she treats you several times.

Patient's inner thoughts: So helpful for me to hear that my stuff is not being dismissed, at last.

Patient's statement: Exactly. My sister is focused on her own needs without recognizing that anyone else is around. She has been used to being the center of attention, while everybody else's needs are on hold.

This is not the first time with her. These kinds of incidents where she acts like she's the only one around have happened many, many times. Maybe in the past, I kept going in for another round because I wanted her approval, some recognition, maybe some interaction, like a friend, but at this time, I don't really think I need her approval anymore.

Therapist's inner thoughts: The tension has dissipated. The therapy can continue.

Therapist's statement: There's a history of your sister considering herself without paying much attention to your needs, and in the past, you have been hurt by her behavior. I understand. I can see how, at this point, you may want to limit your exposure to some of her inconsiderate behaviors given that the two of you have spoken a few times about her actions in the past.

Summary

In this vignette, the therapist managed her countertransference by using it in her work with Alice. Here, the therapist realized her own contribution to the confrontation rupture. Then, by being upfront, the therapist was able to engage in a meaningful way with Alice. In this vignette, by self-disclosing in an authentic way, the humanistic therapist facilitated an opportunity to visit the interpersonal tension in a new way. The confrontation rupture that was created because of the therapist's countertransference was overcome, and the repair strategy of the therapist's sharing her own experience in an authentic way facilitated a corrective experience for Alice.

How To Repair Ruptures

This section explores the way in which therapists can work to repair ruptures. Mahoney and Marquis (2002) suggest that an integral approach to psychotherapy includes a therapist's invitation to utilize the therapeutic bond as a safe space for the patient to learn to explore. They explain that when therapists attend to impasses in the therapeutic relationship, which patients feel disturb their experience of cohesion, patients have a chance to integrate ruptured emotional states.

Chapter 1 offered an example of a withdrawal rupture or breach that occurred in the therapeutic alliance where a therapist and a patient, Eric, have a solid relationship. In this example, Eric has been in psychodynamic therapy for about three months. One morning, the therapist who was riding along on her bike greeted Eric who was out for a walk. During a subsequent therapy session, the therapist noticed that the patient entered the room and pouted, and she could not figure out why Eric was withdrawing from her. In the example, the therapist asked Eric about his week, but he did not seem to open up further. She then asked if she had done something to upset him while empathizing with Eric's unwillingness to speak. The patient turned away, and meekly replied, "You barely noticed me this morning." A withdrawal rupture occurred in an otherwise solid therapeutic relationship. The following vignette is a continuation of the dialogue with the inner thoughts of the therapist and the patient that take place during the session with Eric as the therapist pays careful attention to the rupture and attempts to repair it.

Vignette of an Example of a Psychodynamic Therapist's Repair of a Withdrawal Rupture (Eric of Chapter 1)

DIALOGUE

> *Therapist's inner thoughts: He seems put off by the encounter we had this morning. It might benefit Eric if we could explore this morning's occurrence further.*
>
> **Therapist's statement:** You felt slighted this morning when we accidentally bumped into each other, and I didn't speak further.
>
> *Patient's inner thoughts: Oh. She acts like she cares so much, but barely says hello to me outside the session. Like the rest of my friends, but they don't make believe that they care.*
>
> **Patient's statement:** [A bit more assertive] Yes. I felt bad.
>
> *Therapist's inner thoughts: He's expressing his feelings directly rather than pouting. I want to empathize further with his disappointment.*
>
> **Therapist's statement:** My response this morning was disappointing to you.
>
> *Patient' inner thoughts: Maybe some people in this world do care.*
>
> **Patient's statement:** Yeah, it was.
>
> *Therapist's inner thoughts: Here it may be possible to explore and learn about Eric's inner experiences.*

Therapist's statement: Can you tell me more?

Patient's statement: I wished you would have stopped and talked to me this morning. I felt like I wasn't important enough. Like I've often felt with my friends who ignore my needs. They make like I'm not around.

Therapist's statement: Thank you for letting me know your experiences. You've been overlooked and dismissed and made to feel irrelevant by some of your friends. This morning, I was in a rush, time pressed. I'm wondering, how would you like me to respond in the future if we accidentally bump into each other again?

Patient's inner thoughts: I feel like a human being again. Somebody is listening to me, like I'm a person who matters. Finally, not being dismissed.

Patient's statement: I would like you to talk to me for a few minutes so that I don't feel ignored, so I don't feel again like I'm like some object to just pass by.

Therapist's inner thoughts: He seems to be feeling better now. His boundaries and understanding of our relationship are fine, and so it would be okay for me to do as he wishes if, by chance, I were to bump into him again in the future.

Therapist's statement: It would be my pleasure to do so.

Summary

In this vignette, the therapist pays careful attention to the rupture, responds to the rupture, and the rupture is repaired. The therapist knows that her patient has good boundaries, and the two have had a solid relationship up until this point where there is a minor withdrawal rupture. The therapist takes the opportunity to explore Eric's past experiences with his friends further while responding to the moment and repairing the rupture. In a safe space, as his therapist attends to a withdrawal rupture, Eric begins to integrate fragmented parts of his painful emotional being and to feel more whole within himself and in the therapeutic relationship.

The therapist and patient evolve as they interact dynamically, verbally, and nonverbally throughout the therapeutic process. Ruptures and their resolutions are important components of this process. Attunement, finesse, and care throughout the therapeutic process help the therapist to avoid ruptures. Nevertheless, as illustrated in the aforementioned vignettes, therapists and patients cannot stop ruptures from taking place regardless of whether therapists attune to patient's moment-to-moment communications. At the same time, in these examples, patients' progress in therapy and the repair of ruptures seem to go hand in hand.

Therapists often wonder about repairing ruptures. They wonder whether rupture-repair training results in increased progress in therapy. Why is it important to repair ruptures? It has been shown that repairing ruptures that occur in the working alliance is associated with positive outcome and increased retention in therapy (Muran et al., 2009; Safran et al., 2011). Misattunements will inevitably take place, and when practitioners become aware of a rupture, it is critical to empathize with what the patient is feeling and to validate the patient for confronting a divisive issue during therapy (Safran et al., 2011). Empathy, a purpose toward which the therapeutic dyad works, is a process that continuously evolves (Lipner et al., 2019). A rupture can be viewed as a break in empathy, and a repair of a rupture or a reattunement can restore the dyad's mutual empathy (Lipner et al., 2019). When therapists become aware of ruptures and repair them, the therapy may facilitate a corrective affective experience for patients, and after experiencing the repair of a rupture, patients may learn how to cope better with interpersonal conflicts that are distressing and to adapt in a more meaningful and relational way (Lipner et al., 2019). The therapist in the previous example of a withdrawal rupture showed empathy for Eric's feelings about being dismissed earlier that morning and succeeded in helping Eric to feel less ignored. Generally, it is easier to show empathy to patients who share their inner thoughts, and empathy predicts outcome for patients in therapy regardless of the problems of patients and the theoretical perspectives of therapists (Elliott et al., 2018). Such was the empathic scenario of Eric and his therapist in the previous vignette of a repair of a withdrawal rupture. With minimal difficulty, the therapist repaired the rupture that took place in the morning.

A calm therapeutic environment aids in rupture repair, offers space to the patient, and helps restore the positive parts of the therapeutic alliance. Chapter 1 presented an example that included a scenario where a withdrawal rupture or impasse in the therapeutic alliance took place between an existential therapist and a client, Tabatha. During the seventh therapy session, the therapist disclosed a personal piece of information about himself to Tabatha. His intention for self-disclosure was to encourage Tabatha to open up about herself, but the opposite took place. Tabatha looked down for several minutes and no longer seemed engaged in the conversation. A withdrawal rupture occurred. The following is a continuation of the dialogue with the inner thoughts of the therapist and the patient that take place during the session as the therapist observes Tabatha's communications, recognizes the withdrawal rupture, and attempts to repair it.

Vignette of an Example of a Humanistic Therapist's Repair of a Withdrawal Rupture (Tabatha of Chapter 1)

Dialogue

Therapist's inner thoughts: I need to tread lightly. She may not be ready to re-engage.

Therapist's statement: You seem put off by what I disclosed.

Patient's inner thoughts: [Looking down, somewhat disinterested] I thought he said this therapy is about me. Why then would I want to know about his personal problems? I'm feeling uncomfortable knowing them. It distracts from my problems. Why couldn't my therapist at least have realized how burdened I feel about my own problems?

Patient's statement: [Looking down, but a bit more engaged] Yup.

Therapist's inner thoughts: I meant for her to speak more. But my disclosure may have been ill-timed and seemed to have the opposite effect. Not sure what to do, but I will try to stay more silent until I learn what's up.

Therapist's statement: My disclosure may have invaded your space.

Patient' inner thoughts: Maybe he gets it. If he doesn't intrude on my space, I may continue.

Patient's statement: [Looking away, with some hesitancy] Yea. I wished you would have been more in touch with what I need… [silence, then looks away] … rather than disclosing your stuff. [Low voice] I'm really not up to hearing your disclosures right now with all the problems that I have on my list.

Therapist's inner thoughts: My self-disclosure was ill-timed.

Therapist's statement: I'm sorry for not considering your needs. I now understand that my self-disclosure was ill-timed and unnecessary. Thank you for letting me know. Take your time, and proceed with what you need first.

Patient's inner thoughts: A breath of fresh air and quiet. He's giving me space so that I don't need to be elsewhere.

Patient's statement: [More engaged. Looks toward therapist] In general, I like when people don't assume things with me. I like when they ask first.

Therapist's inner thoughts: She's letting me know what she needs.

Therapist's statement: Thank you for letting me know what you need. If I misstep in the future, please let me know.

Patient's statement: [Smiling] It's a deal.

Summary

Withdrawal ruptures tend to be subtle, and therapists need to learn how to discern them (Eubanks, Burckell, et al., 2018). In this vignette, the humanistic therapist observes the effect of his self-disclosure on the patient, Tabatha, responds to the withdrawal rupture, and the rupture is repaired with some ease. The therapist understands that Tabatha needs space to be able to develop her own presence. The therapist stands back so that Tabatha feels that she has more space and comfort for herself. In this vignette, it seems that the therapist's repair of the rupture provided the patient with a corrective emotional experience.

As illustrated in the aforementioned examples, the process of repairing ruptures can be a challenge for therapists. The therapists in situations such as the ones in previous sections may not be sure about what to say or do during a rupture, and, sometimes, they may become defensive or annoyed; responses that may not be in the service of patients. Rather, responding in a manner that is not defensive when a rupture unfolds is part and parcel of the way in which a therapist can help to develop a successful therapeutic milieu for patients who may not be willing to tell a therapist when they experience a rupture (Safran et al., 2011). Such was the scenario with Tabatha, who seemed, initially, hesitant to tell the therapist what she was experiencing. In this example, Tabatha's therapist repaired the rupture and developed a safe space where Tabatha was able to discuss her need to lead the conversation at her own pace.

While observing patients' emotional states during a therapy session, therapists make minute-to-minute decisions about communications during the therapeutic process. These moment-to-moment decisions during interventions are, for the most part, intuitive rather than guided by a particular psychotherapy perspective, and the therapy entails a fluid process where therapists' different interventions match the changes in the affective states of patients (Marquis & Elliott, 2015). The decisions can be intuitive, and there are ways that therapists check their intuition against their understanding of the client and their theoretical viewpoint. Sometimes the inner thoughts of therapists are negative when they are confronted with challenging clients. They may be thinking thoughts such as the following:

> *I'm so bored. I've heard about her hurt over and over. I hope she doesn't repeat it. It's becoming oppressive.*
>
> *He thinks the world of himself. He's so blown up. No wonder he cannot land a job.*
>
> *He's forever in a negative cycle with his friends. The heated arguments spill over in here on a weekly schedule… I'm not sure how much more I can take of it.*

Therapists need to become aware of and regulate their inner expressions, and when these emotions are negative, therapists need to work toward an empathic understanding of the patient's inner world (Gelso & Perez-Rojas, 2017; Wolf et al., 2013). When the therapist empathizes with and reframes the patient's perspective, the patient can experience calm. This process may be similar to a parent who mirrors and soothes a young child. Through the experience of a therapeutic relationship, patients can begin to recognize and share their emotional states, an experience which can lead to renewed security and openness in evolving friendships that can take place beyond therapy (Fosha, 2001). Through empathy and an awareness of their own inner experiences as well as the inner views of their clients, novice therapists may learn to assist patients during delicate moments, to repair ruptures, and to facilitate corrective emotional experiences.

Can therapists discern ruptures so that they can repair them? How aware are therapists and patients of ruptures, and is there a distinction between the report of ruptures depending upon type, for example, withdrawal or confrontation, and who reports ruptures? Muran and colleagues (2023, p. 12) point to research (e.g., Eubanks, Muran, et al., 2018; Muran, 2019; Safran et al., 2011) that studies ruptures and repair, that defines the aforementioned process in terms of indirect assessments (in how clients rate the therapeutic alliance after the session), and that suggests that ruptures take place in 25% to 68% of cases and that repairs take place in 16% to 81% of cases. They note studies that examine ruptures in terms of direct assessment (during the session) that show that confrontation markers vary from 43% to 91% of the sessions, and withdrawal markers during 100% of the sessions (e.g., Colli et al., 2019; Eubanks et al., 2019). Therapists tend to perceive more ruptures than do their clients (Rubel et al., 2018). According to Aspland and colleagues (2008, p. 699), in one study, therapists' reports of ruptures take place in approximately 50%

of sessions and patients' reports of ruptures is less than 20% of the time (e.g., Eames & Roth, 2000).

Sometimes therapists will focus the work on repairing the ruptures that are task or goal oriented; however, other times, they will concentrate on repairing ruptures that relate to the working alliance itself (Safran et al., 2011). For therapists who wish to know how to repair ruptures, it is important to be aware of how they develop, to recognize the delicate moments of the rupture, and to strive to use these impasses to enhance the therapeutic dyad rather than to derail the therapy's purpose. In thinking about the development of ruptures, it is important for therapists to become familiar with their patients' points of view. In part, therapists can observe the subtle nuances of their patients' refined communications that may emerge as an ongoing or repetitive pattern.

Patient and therapist variables can affect the emergence of ruptures. The next sections discuss how these variables influence the therapeutic alliance, ruptures, their repair, and therapy outcome.

Ruptures, Repairs, and Patient Variables: Patients' Attachment Styles and Ruptures and Repairs

How secure is your patient's attachment style? The example included in this section's vignette illustrates the need for therapists to recognize the patient variables that contribute to ruptures and their resolutions, and to assess their responses to patients based on their patients' attachment styles. Patient factors such as style of attachment have an important impact on the nature of the therapeutic bond (Lingiardi et al., 2016). Style of attachment refers to a variety of ways that patients communicate about internal feelings during therapy (Miller-Bottome et al., 2019; Talia et al., 2017). This section explores the relationship between patients' attachment styles and ruptures or impasses in the therapeutic alliance. It describes how the repair of ruptures in the therapeutic relationship can differ based on the patient's attachment style. Depending upon different patient attachment orientations, for example, secure, preoccupied, fearful, or dismissing, the frequency of the reports of ruptures can vary, and therapists' response styles can vary (Eames & Roth, 2000; Hardy et al., 1998). Borelli and colleagues (2019, p. 11) point out that patients with secure attachments tend to develop more robust therapeutic alliances with their psychotherapists (Eames & Roth, 2000; Sauer et al., 2010).

Individuals with a secure attachment style have positive views of themselves and others, are not concerned about abandonment and do not avoid intimacy, and individuals with a preoccupied attachment style hold negative views of themselves, but positive views of others, are worried about their own attachment needs, but wish for intimacy (Bartholomew & Horowitz, 1991; Eames & Roth, 2000). Therapists may anticipate that it would be easier to repair a rupture or tension with individuals who have a secure attachment style because these clients tend to develop alliances that are more positive (Bartholomew & Horowitz, 1991; Eames & Roth, 2000, Miller-Bottome et al., 2019). Whereas individuals with a fearful attachment style hold a negative view of themselves and others, are worried about abandonment, and tend to avoid intimacy, individuals with a dismissive attachment style hold a positive view of themselves and a negative view of others, are not concerned about abandonment, but tend to avoid intimate relationships (Bartholomew & Horowitz, 1991; Eames & Roth, 2000). Therapists can anticipate that patients with different attachment styles will relate differently to the therapist, and in turn, the therapists' response styles will differ based on patients' attachment styles (Eames & Roth, 2000).

Eames and Roth (2000, p. 422) note that the early stages of the therapeutic relationship cannot be underestimated, and it is these early stages, more than later stages, that can foretell unilateral termination by clients and therapy outcome (e.g., Horvath & Symonds, 1991; Piper, Azim, Joyce, & McCallum, 1991; Piper, Azim, Joyce, McCallum, Nixon, & Segal, 1991) Novice therapists may not know that strains or misattunements in communication between the therapist and the client may likely emerge as the therapeutic relationship begins to develop, and supervisors need to apprise therapists who seek consultation that these unpleasant events may rear their heads suddenly or abruptly, or may evolve more gradually in subtle interactions as the therapy progresses. Eames and Roth (2002) assert that patients have different attachment styles, and these styles affect the way that the patient relates in therapy. They offer the example of a patient with a fearful attachment style, a style that is associated with ratings of a lower therapeutic alliance; the example of a patient with a secure attachment style, a style that is linked to ratings of a higher alliance; the example of a patient with a preoccupied attachment orientation, an orientation that is related to reports of ruptures that occur more frequently; and the example of a patient with a dismissive attachment orientation, an orientation that is linked to a lower number of reports of ruptures. Eames and Roth (2000, p. 431) note that in response to patients with a greater preoccupied attachment style of interpersonal relating, therapists utilize a more emotional and relationship style; however, in response to patients with a dismissive attachment orientation, therapists adopt a more cognitive approach (e.g., Hardy et al., 1998). Miller-Bottome and colleagues (2019) found that secure client attachment during therapy is related to higher ratings (by therapists and clients) of the repair of ruptures, and when ruptures or misattunements are more intense, the connection between a secure attachment during the session and rupture repair becomes greater. They explain that it is possible that clients with a secure attachment style are more likely to develop robust alliances because they are able to relate about the tensions that emerge during therapy. The next segment includes a vignette with a patient who has a dismissive attachment style.

Vignette of an Example of a Psychodynamic Therapist's Repair for a Patient With a Dismissive Attachment Style

The following vignette includes withdrawal ruptures and confrontation ruptures, a mixed pattern of ruptures, during the third therapy session with a 25-year-old patient, Curtis, who has a dismissive attachment style and who recently broke up with his fiancé.

Dialogue

Therapist's inner thoughts: Curtis is having a difficult time and feels unhappy. He tends to dismiss his problems.

Patient's inner thoughts. Nothing much matters to me. Who cares.

Therapist's statement: Last time, you seemed down about the breakup.

Patient's statement: [Shrugs shoulder] No. It's no big deal. I don't know how to focus on it at all. Just want to end therapy early today. I don't like being here.

Therapist's inner thoughts: Curtis seems to be dismissing his experience. I'll stick with it.

Therapist's statement: Last time we spoke, you seemed well able to focus on and express what is disappointing for you. Can you tell me more? I'm interested, and I care.

Patient's inner thoughts: Shrug him off.

Patient's statement: [Silence for a minute, looks down, and then away] May not be able to stick around today. [Looks toward the door]

Therapist's inner thoughts: He's withdrawing.

Therapist's statement: You don't feel well today? Can you describe what you're feeling?

Patient's inner thoughts: Maybe because I'm drained from what happened to me with my broken engagement.

Patient's statement: I'm not with it because of what happened to me.

Therapist's inner thoughts: He's less dismissive and beginning to disclose rather than to dismiss.

Therapist's statement: I'm sorry that you don't feel well. Broken relationships can hurt.

Patient's inner thoughts: That's what they all say, these psychologists, they're all the same.

Patient's statement: [Sarcastic] I don't believe you. You guys are all trained to say that. (Loudly) It's in your canned speech box!

Summary

In this vignette, a mixed pattern of ruptures emerge, and withdrawal and confrontation ruptures occur. In the beginning, Curtis, a patient with a dismissive attachment style, dismisses the therapist, and he withdraws. The therapist tries to repair the rupture by inviting Curtis to express himself. Then, Curtis offers the therapist a window into his sadness when he discloses a reason for it. When the therapist empathizes with him, Curtis, again, dismisses the therapist, this time with a confrontation rupture.

This section described the relationship between ruptures, repairs, and patient variables such as attachment styles. It highlighted the association between patients with different attachment styles or patients with interpersonal difficulties and the development of the therapeutic alliance. Although individuals who have interpersonal problems tend to have difficulty developing a strong bond with therapists, therapists are human, and they, too, play a part in problems that will, at some point, emerge in the therapeutic alliance (Eubanks et al., 2019). Why is a positive interpersonal relationship with a therapist important? Safran and Muran (2000b) suggest that positive interpersonal connections can change patients' dysfunctional patterns of associating with others as they learn to generalize the experience they have with their therapist to their relationships that are external to the therapy setting. They explain that the process of repairing a rupture in the alliance can assist patients to develop interpersonal views about themselves where they can perceive themselves as able to relate to others and where they can understand that others can be emotionally available. This section concludes the material relevant to the link between patient variables and the therapeutic alliance, ruptures, and their repairs. The next section discusses the therapist factors that are related to ruptures and repairs, i.e., how therapists with different theoretical orientations address and repair ruptures.

Ruptures, Repairs, and Therapist Variables: The Association Between Therapists With Different Theoretical Orientations (E.g., Psychodynamic, Cognitive-Behavioral, Humanistic) and Ruptures

Effective Therapists and Strategies for Rupture Repair

Some therapists are more effective than others. Who is an effective therapist? A therapist who adjusts therapeutic methods and the relationship to patients and their specific circumstances can be viewed as an effective one (Norcross & Lambert, 2019, p. 19). The intervention that therapists use and the therapeutic relationship itself, influence the outcome of therapy (Norcross & Lambert, 2019). This section addresses the interaction between therapists' different theoretical approaches, their methods, and ruptures, and it outlines the strategies that therapists use to repair ruptures.

Do therapists agree on the strategies needed to repair ruptures? Eubanks, Burckell, and colleagues (2018) assert that there is some agreement on effective strategies for rupture repair. They explain that practitioners of different theoretical perspectives, to some extent, have been able to agree on effective strategies for repairing ruptures, such as considering the patient's experience of the rupture and validating the patient's viewpoint. According to Eubank, Burckell, and colleagues (2018), strategies that have been shown to be ineffective for repairing ruptures include interpretation and cognitive restructuring. These researchers found that during a session with a rupture, therapists with different theoretical perspectives address the rupture and validate the patient; however, after the session in which the impasse took place, during subsequent sessions, they shift to a promotion of interventions for therapy that are consistent with their own theoretical perspectives. For example, in sessions that took place after the session that included the rupture, humanistic therapists shift to a focus on validation, a key characteristic of an experiential approach; cognitive-behavioral therapists, to a focus on coping tactics; psychodynamic therapists, to a focus on transference interpretations (Eubanks, Burckell et al., 2018).

Ruptures, Repairs, the Therapeutic Alliance, and Therapists With Different Theoretical Approaches

This section compares different theories with respect to their focus on the alliance and specifies the relationship between a therapist's theoretical framework and strategies for rupture repairs. What does it take to repair or resolve a rupture if you are a cognitive behavioral therapist, a psychodynamic therapist, an integrative cognitive therapist, or an emotion-focused therapist? The following theories or frameworks that consider the relationship between the therapist and the client are but a few examples of how rupture processes can be conceptualized and how dyads in therapy work through ruptures.

Ruptures, Repairs, and CBT

Is there a relationship between ruptures, repairs, and the therapeutic relationship in CBT? Impala and colleagues (2023, p. 122) point out that therapists use relational components present in other therapies, for example, validation of the client, exploration of the relationship and the rupture, to address ruptures in CBT (e.g., Sommerfeld et al., 2008). They note that the process of rupture repair in CBT involves the following steps:

1. Elicit the views of the client.
2. Discuss the process of making decisions with the client.
3. Facilitate the client's opinions.
4. Attend to the replies of the client (e.g., Okamoto & Kazantzis, 2019).

Ruptures, Repairs, and Intensive Short-Term Dynamic Psychotherapy (ISTDP)

What is the relationship between ruptures, repairs, and the therapeutic alliance in psychodynamic therapy? Abbass and Town (2023) conceptualize the rupture and repair process from a psychodynamic perspective, and they view ruptures as defense mechanisms that manifest during therapy sessions because of the emergence of emotions that provoke anxiety. They explain that an essential intervention for repairing ruptures in intensive short-term dynamic psychotherapy (ISTDP) is the clarification of the defense. Therapists who use ISTDP anticipate that ruptures in the therapeutic alliance will occur, and therapists can influence developments whereby patients can experience corrective emotional experiences or sequences of alliance ruptures and resolutions (Abbass & Town, 2023).

Ruptures, Repairs, and Integrative Cognitive Therapy (ICT)

Constantino and colleagues (2008, p. 123) note that in order to repair alliance ruptures, Castonguay (1996) formulated ICT, which includes cognitive therapy as a base with an integration of interpersonal and humanistic interventions. When using ICT, practitioners are trained to take a pause from the cognitive therapy portion when they confront markers that represent an impasse in the alliance (Castonguay, 1996; Constantino et al., 2008). During the pause, therapists use interpersonal methods rather than increase the cognitive therapy portion, and only when the rupture is resolved do they resume the cognitive portion (Constantino et al., 2008).

Ruptures, Repairs, and Emotion-Focused Therapy

How do therapists with an experiential orientation address ruptures? Safran and Muran (2000b, p. 234) note that a key component of Watson and Greenberg's (1995) experiential approach is that difficulties that are associated with the bond part of the therapeutic alliance are represented as impasses in the present interchange between therapist and patient rather than as representative of the patient's past or typical interpersonal exchanges. The nature of the bond and the emerging impasses or difficulties change over time, and require that experiential therapists be continuously responsive to the needs of their clients (Elliott et al., 2004). In order to repair ruptures in the alliance, Elliott and colleagues (2004) suggest six stages that are common to the tasks of emotion-focused therapy. These stages include a confirm marker, task negotiation and initiation, deepening, partial resolution, exploration and solutions, and full resolution. In this model, when the therapist perceives a difficulty during the therapy session, the therapist moves from listening in a manner that is not defensive to a full resolution of the alliance difficulty where the patient feels satisfied with the dialogue and is ready to proceed with the work of therapy (Elliott et al., 2004).

Ruptures, Repairs and a Comparison of Therapists' Theoretical Approaches

A previous section explained that therapists tend to report more ruptures than do patients (e.g., Aspland et al., 2008; Eames & Roth, 2000; Rubel et al., 2018). According to Muran and colleagues (2009), therapists and patients tend to report fewer ruptures during CBT than during STDP and BRT. These researchers explain that for clients in brief relational therapy and cognitive-behavioral therapy, there is a relationship between more elevated therapist ratings of repair and therapist report of greater ease of the session. From a cognitive-behavioral perspective, sometimes it is better to explore the impasses in the alliance; however, sometimes it may not be helpful to focus on them directly (Arnkoff, 1995; Safran & Muran, 2000b).

Therapists may use different repair strategies for ruptures. Eubanks, Sergi, and colleagues (2021) distinguish between immediate rupture repair strategies, which can be direct or indirect, and exploratory rupture repair strategies, and they assert that one strategy has not been shown to be more effective than another. They explain that when therapists use a direct strategy, they explicitly recognize the rupture, and when they use an indirect strategy, they repair the rupture without directly acknowledging it. Eubanks, Sergi, and colleagues (2021, p. 91) point out that task analyses of the repair of ruptures in emotion-focused therapy (e.g., Swank & Wittenborn, 2013), a therapy derived from a humanistic perspective that integrated the gestalt therapy of Perls (1969) and Rogers' (1951) client-centered therapy, included direct acknowledgment of the rupture at the beginning of the rupture repair process. Conversely, task analyses of the repair of ruptures in CBT (Aspland et al., 2008) found that it is not necessary to begin with explicit acknowledgment of the rupture, and practitioners were able to repair ruptures by using an immediate strategy that is indirect such as attending to the issue that was most outstanding for the client at that minute rather than persisting with another item on the therapist's list (Eubanks, Sergi, et al., 2021). When therapists use an exploratory strategy to repair ruptures, they explicitly focus on exploring their and their patients' experience of the rupture in order to understand what is happening between the two members of the dyad, and this exploration is not without its challenges (Eubanks, Sergi, et al., 2021).

Kline and colleagues (2019) explain that the process of resolving ruptures is nuanced in that the consequences of ruptures may be positive and negative. They found that, on the one hand, therapists felt that the rupture strained the dyad's relationship, and on the other hand, therapists found that subsequent to the repair of a rupture, the work in therapy became more meaningful. It seems that the positive effects of a rupture may buffer the negative as the members of the therapeutic dyad work through the rupture so that it is resolved (Kline et al., 2019). The aforementioned findings are different from Coutinho and colleagues' (2011) conclusions that therapists, generally, did not sense that tensions had an effect on the alliance and that there were no changes in the therapy because of ruptures that were confrontational. Kline and colleagues (2019) suggest that the discrepancy in findings may be attributed to the fact that the therapists in their study were interpersonal-psychodynamic and paid more attention to how tensions in the relationship affect the therapy; however, the therapists in the study of Coutinho and colleagues (2011) were cognitive-behavioral. Kline and colleagues (2019) note that in their study most of the impasses were on the way to being repaired; however, Coutinho and colleagues (2011) reported that the breaks in the relationship in their study did not seem to be repaired.

Chapter 1 described different types of ruptures, for example, confrontation, withdrawal, and mixed. Okamoto and colleagues (2019) point out that whereas withdrawal ruptures lead to a lower opportunity for patients to benefit (e.g., Boritz et al., 2018), confrontation ruptures tend to result in premature termination if the therapist does not repair them (e.g., Coutinho et al., 2014). According to Eubanks and colleagues (2019), lower rupture repair or resolution ratings were found to be associated with client dropout from therapy, and ratings of psychotherapists' contributions to these impasses were associated with client dropout from therapy. The following section illustrates a vignette that is an example of a confrontation rupture or impasse between a patient and a therapist with a specific theoretical and therapy perspective, e.g., a psychodynamic approach, that could have led to the client dropping out of therapy had the therapist not repaired the confrontation rupture. It takes time for the therapist with a psychodynamic approach to repair the rupture, for the tension to resolve, before the dyad can continue the work of therapy.

Vignette of an Example of a Rupture Repair of a Therapist With A Psychodynamic Approach

Introduction

The patient, Willow, a 41-year-old woman, recently filed for divorce from her husband and has been negotiating the divorce agreement with him through her lawyer. Willow began therapy a year ago with a psychodynamic therapist. The goals of the therapy were to help her navigate the changes that have ensued since she decided to divorce. In addition, the therapist has explored with the patient her original family issues that may underpin her current crisis. The work has revealed that Willow has a poor relationship with her father, particularly around money issues. The vignette includes both the inner thoughts of the therapist and the client along with their responses during the tenth therapy session.

Dialogue

Patient's inner thoughts: I have a lot to get off my chest today.

Patient's statement: [Angry, almost shouting] Ron is giving me a hard time about money. I'm furious about the deal that he's cutting for me and the kids, and how the MALE judge is leaning his way. Last night, I was so angry that I cut up some of his clothing. I hate him. How can he do this to me and the kids! It is so unsettling. What will we do?

Therapist's inner thoughts: There's a pattern that emerges from her past here.

Therapist's statement: [Sounding sure about his intervention] It seems that you are concerned about your present situation with your finances and feel rage toward Ron just like you felt when your father withheld money from you.

Patient's inner thoughts: Oh, how annoying. My own therapist cannot even hear me or feel what I'm going through. A dude who has it easy.

Patient's statement: [Sarcastic and annoyed] Oh, give me a break. Here we go again with your psychoanalysis when the kids and I are suffering and trying to make ends meet. It's easy for you to say, sitting there comfortably in your therapy chair. I'm not sure that I'm going to be able to pay you for these sessions. I'm sick and tired of hearing this ridiculous stuff about my father time and time again [tears], and I'm suffering so much right now.

Summary

The therapist responded with an approach that relied on his own psychodynamic hypothesis. Willow felt misunderstood, and a confrontation rupture ensued. The therapist proceeded with a psychodynamic, interpretive approach and did not repair the rupture. The therapist insisted on emphasizing the psychodynamic framework from which he was operating at the expense of repairing the relationship.

The session continues with the therapist attempting to promote his psychodynamic interpretation. He does not pick up on the patient's anger and insecurity.

Dialogue

Therapist's inner thoughts. This client is unable to get beyond the moment and reflect on the history of her current response. My interpretation was right on. I will not step back from what I think is a major component in her strong reaction to Ron, to me, and to others.

Patient's inner thoughts. He's not saying anything. I am sick of these men like him who tag the woman will all the fault in the marriage. I was right. How many times does he have to bring up my father? I'm sick of his one-sided approach.

Therapist's statement: You really need to consider what I said. I'll repeat it so that it can sink in a bit. It appears that you are concerned about your present finances and feel rage toward Ron as you felt when you were young, and your father withheld money from you. Now you're expressing anger toward me as well.

Patient's inner thoughts: I have had it!

Patient's statement: [Angry. Gets up from her chair] To heck with you, dude. Once again, your psychobabble rather than you hearing my situation. You're not out for me.

Therapist's inner thoughts: It seems that I erred. I may lose her as a client if I don't change course.

Therapist's statement: Exactly. I understand how difficult your situation is for you, at present. What is on the line is your future and the future of your children. I'm with you.

[Silence]

Summary

The therapist annoyed Willow with his persistent psychodynamic interpretations. When he recognized that a confrontation rupture occurred, he began to hear the pain of the critical moment that Willow felt that she was experiencing, and he shifted gears to a more empathic approach, but the rupture is not yet resolved.

At this time, the therapist begins to integrate a relational strategy when addressing the rupture that occurred in the therapeutic relationship. The following continuation of the vignette describes how the therapist with a psychodynamic approach repaired the rupture by focusing on relational aspects rather than by continuing with an interpretive approach. The therapist did, however, keep in mind, but on hold, the psychodynamic framework from which he was operating.

Dialogue

[During the silence, the therapist and the patient reflect about their disagreement and how they could move from the strain to a smoother plain]

Therapist's inner thoughts: Wow. I am surely off. I thought my psychodynamic interpretation aimed toward the target, but it seems that my timing was not in sync with this patient. How to move forward? I want to be authentic, but not altogether recede from what I think is a key component of her strong reaction to Ron.

Patient's inner thoughts: He's silent, not responding, not saying anything. I am tired of dudes who get out of sort like this. I'm not off. He's out of it. How many times does he have to bring up my father! This is old stuff. I get it. I know. I know. Should I say that I'm sorry, but I'm irritated?

Therapist's statement: I apologize for what I said. I do recognize how concerned you are about your present discussions with Ron. Important events. Your financial situation will have an impact on your life and the life of your family going forward, and your finances need particular consideration at this time. It was not a suitable time for me to talk about past issues, like your father. What is important is your present situation as it will have an effect on your future. What you and I are talking about regarding Ron is critical, in the present and for the future, and I did not need to remind you about your father at this time.

Patient's inner thoughts: Whew! What a relief. A man who can admit that he wasn't right all the time. That means something to me. I don't get support from any of the other members of my family. Maybe I can talk to this therapist further about my stuff that is taking place on a daily basis. I'll try to let him know how I feel, and I'll see from there.

Patient's statement: I know you were trying to help and didn't have bad intentions, but I need you to not bring up my father, and I need you to attend to my difficult time, at present [Apologetic tone].

Therapist's inner thoughts: I'm so attached to my inner point of view and my psychodynamic approach that sometimes I fail to see what's in front of me, the obvious. I may have a chance to salvage the relationship.

Therapist's statement: Exactly. I messed up. There may be a time and a place for my psychodynamic interpretations. It's surely not now, and, during your discussions with Ron about your financial concerns, I won't mention the past. I'm with you, and I recognize how distressed you feel during this time. You need your wits about you to make important decisions, and I understand your anger at Ron and the judge.

Summary

The therapist in this vignette was able to repair the rupture by focusing on relational components rather than by continuing with his usual psychodynamic theoretical approach. Had the therapist not been able to switch gears, it seems that the client may have dropped out of therapy. In this vignette, the therapist was slow to get in touch with the deteriorating break that was occurring in their communication. He was intent on making the point that Willow needs to see the connection between her current situation and her past, and he missed the intensity of her feelings about Ron, the impending divorce, and its ripple effect. In order to repair misunderstandings and misattunements that are at the base of therapeutic ruptures, therapists need to astutely observe moment-to-moment interactions of therapy sessions that contain delicate material. Furthermore, the therapist's capacity to repair ruptures depends upon how aware the therapist is of his own missteps and his ability to shift gears, to be empathic, and to be authentic in the moment.

The next section offers a vignette that is an example of a rupture or impasse between a patient and a therapist with a cognitive-behavioral approach that results in a confrontation rupture. Similar to the therapist with the psychodynamic orientation in the previous vignette, the therapist with the cognitive-behavioral orientation repairs the rupture by shifting from her favored cognitive-behavioral theoretical approach and adopting a relational style. This example revisits the vignette from Chapter 1, a scenario of a confrontation rupture or impasse in the therapeutic alliance with the patient, Heather.

Vignette of an Example of a Rupture Repair of a Therapist with a Cognitive-Behavioral Approach

INTRODUCTION

In the past, the therapeutic relationship with Heather has been characterized by a good deal of contention. Today, the client, Heather, who looks a bit pale, tells a cognitive-behavioral therapist that she is not feeling well. The cognitive-behavioral therapist says, "Last week, we talked about paying your bill on time. You're now two months overdue." Heather is thinking: *I feel physically ill with a headache today. How can I focus on this stuff now? I wish she knew better. I'll put her in her place.* Heather responds angrily, "You care only about being paid. Didn't you hear that I said that I have a headache today?" A confrontation rupture has taken place. The next vignette revisits the scenario with Heather that was included in Chapter 1, but this time with an idea for rupture resolution. In this example, the therapist integrates a relational strategy when addressing the confrontation rupture that occurred in the therapeutic relationship. The vignette describes how the therapist with a cognitive-behavioral approach repaired the rupture by focusing on relational aspects rather than by continuing with a behavioral task-oriented approach. The therapist did, however, keep in mind the framework from which she was operating.

DIALOGUE

> *Therapist's inner thoughts: Wow. She's angry. I thought my cognitive-behavioral, logical plan toward getting Heather on track with her responsibilities such as bill payment and completing homework assignments was right on, but my approach was ill-timed. I want to have a smooth interpersonal session like the sessions that I have with my other patients with whom I use a cognitive-behavioral approach, and not step back from what I think is Heather's general lack of commitment to her responsibilities, in this case, bill payment.*

Therapist's statement: I do understand about your headache today and how bad you feel. It was not the time for me to bring up money without barely saying hello when I see that you look pale and fatigued. I did not need to bring it up before saying hello.

Patient's inner thoughts: I owe her money. I was going to bring it today, but I'm in such turmoil because of the headache. How many times does she have to bring up my responsibilities? I get it. I get it. Should I let her know that I was going to bring the money today? At last, she stopped nagging. I wish all the members of my family would stop nagging at me. Maybe I can tell her that I was going to bring the money today anyway, but simply forgot because of how lousy I am feeling.

Patient's statement: [Apologetic tone] I know you were trying to remind me of my responsibilities, but I am tired of hearing about it so much of the time without you getting what I am going through in the present moment. Why I got paid last week, and I was going to bring most of the payment today, but because I felt so ill with the headache (which was much worse earlier in the morning), I just got into the car without the envelope with the money.

Therapist's inner thoughts: I'm so conditioned and loyal to my cognitive-behavioral strategies that sometimes I fail to see the fabric of the relationship in the moment. I may have missed a chance to teach my model, which includes interpersonal skills, because of my intense focus on Heather's responsibilities.

Therapist's statement: OK. I could have at least said hello, asked how you are doing first, and had a less terse attitude. I understand how bad you feel because of the headache. You have a lot of responsibilities, and, today, because you feel ill, it was particularly hard for you to meet your commitments.

Summary

The cognitive-behavioral therapist was intent on teaching the patient, Heather, to honor her responsibilities by paying her bill, and she missed that Heather was feeling physically ill. The therapist in this vignette was able to repair the confrontation rupture by focusing on relational aspects rather than by continuing with cognitive-behavioral strategies. Had the therapist not been able to shift away from her loyalty to her cognitive-behavioral theoretical position by being more flexible, it seems that the client may have become angrier and dropped out of therapy. In this vignette, the therapist picked up on the impasse that was occurring in the interpersonal communication before the situation deteriorated in its entirety. Therapists, regardless of their theoretical approaches, need to use astute observation to monitor moment-to-moment interactions in order to correct strains that are at the core of therapeutic ruptures. Furthermore, therapists' capacity to repair the rupture is dependent on them being aware of their own missteps and their ability to be flexible and empathic regardless of theoretical orientation.

This concludes the section on ruptures, repairs, and therapist variables, the association between therapists with different theoretical approaches and ruptures. The next portion focuses on an interaction between ruptures, repairs, and therapists' theoretical approach and ruptures, repairs, and patients with different diagnoses.

The Interaction Between Ruptures, Repairs, and Therapists' Theoretical Perspective, and Ruptures, Repairs, and Patients With Different Diagnoses

Novice therapists may be curious about the frequency of ruptures in patients with certain characterological issues. This portion explores the interaction between therapist variables such as theoretical perspective, patient variables such as diagnosis, the therapeutic alliance, and ruptures. Specifically, it explores the interaction for patients who have been diagnosed with personality disorders. The concept of a therapeutic alliance has been extensively studied for existential and psychodynamic therapeutic orientations; however, it has been found to be critical for cognitive-behavioral and cognitive perspectives as well (Strauss et al., 2006; Waddington, 2002). The alliance has been investigated less for individuals with personality disorders (disorders that include chronic interpersonal difficulties) than for individuals with an Axis I diagnosis (disorders that include, for example, mood, anxiety), has been shown to be hard to develop with individuals who have personality disorders, and the client dropout rates for individuals with personality disorders have been reported to range from 38% to 57% (with means that extend from 15% to 22%) (Leichsenring & Leibing, 2003; Perry et al., 1999; Strauss et al., 2006). The bottom line is that therapists tend to encounter difficulties in the alliance with patients diagnosed with personality disorders, and this finding may be attributed to the fact that therapists may have a greater problem showing empathy to individuals who are more labile or constricted (Muran et al., 2009).

Is there a connection between clients with different personality disorders and rupture profiles in the therapeutic alliance? Personality disorders are persistent patterns of behaviors and experiences that diverge considerably from the expectations of one's culture and that result in distress or dysfunction (American Psychiatric Association [APA], 2022). According to the fifth edition of the Diagnostic and Statistical Manual of Mental Disorders (DSM-5-TR) (APA, 2022), the three groups or clusters of personality disorders include cluster A (e.g., schizotypal, paranoid, or schizoid), cluster B (e.g., narcissistic, borderline, anti-social, or histrionic), and cluster C (e.g., obsessive-compulsive, dependent, or avoidant). Lipsitz-Odess and colleagues (2022) assert that individuals with personality disorders have specific profiles of ruptures. They explain that clients with cluster A and B characteristics have a higher likelihood of displaying withdrawal and confrontation ruptures than clients with cluster C characteristics; however, as therapy progresses, clients with elevated levels of cluster A characteristics tend to display fewer confrontation ruptures, clients with elevated levels of cluster B characteristics tend to display fewer withdrawal ruptures, and clients with elevated levels of cluster C characteristics tend to display more withdrawal and confrontation ruptures.

There are a myriad of examples that depict the association between ruptures and patients with personality disorders; however, this section, by no means comprehensive, briefly reviews only a few instances of this relationship. For example, Borelli and colleagues (2019) note that patients with diagnoses such as borderline personality disorder have been associated with a poor therapeutic alliance (e.g., Gunderson et al., 1989; Pereira et al., 2006). Zalman and colleagues (2019) illustrate the difficulty that therapists have in working with patients who are severely narcissistic. They use language analysis (number of words and linguistic inquiry) to show the unconscious elements of the therapeutic alliance that begin to decline prior to the emergence of a rupture for a patient diagnosed with severe narcissistic tendencies. It is suggested that therapists recognize the vulnerabilities of patients with narcissistic tendencies as they attempt to repair the ruptures in the alliance, and that therapists be aware of the defenses that these patients use to counter interpersonal and inner struggles that manifest as ruptures in the therapeutic alliance (Zalman et al., 2019). For individuals with avoidant and obsessive-compulsive personality disorders, it was found that strong alliances that occurred in the early stages of therapy and the occurrence of ruptures followed by repairs effected positive change in depressive and personality symptoms for these patients (Strauss et al., 2006).

What Contributes to a Rupture, and What Does It Take to Repair It?

Can ruptures be repaired in most circumstances? It may or may not be possible to repair a rupture. It depends on a variety of variables. Kline and colleagues (2019) explain that sometimes therapists feel that it would not help to repair a rupture, or therapists try to resolve the rupture, but the exploration of the break does not proceed because of a variety of reasons, and sometimes a surface attempt to resolve a rupture does not lead to a positive outcome. They suggest that sometimes therapists do not have the skill to resolve a rupture, or their countertransference blocks the resolution. The focus of this section is on the variety of reasons that ruptures occur, the complexity of the contributors, and what it takes to repair ruptures. Sometimes therapists feel that the interpersonal difficulties of patients contribute to the rupture (Kline et al., 2019; Sommerfeld et al., 2008). Kline and colleagues (2019) assert that therapist trainees were able to recognize that patients' interpersonal difficulties surfaced at the time of a rupture; however, the therapists did not use their understanding to facilitate the insight of patients about the impasse in the relationship. They explain that the therapists understood that they contributed to impasses by failing to manage their own responses and by their lack of attunement with patients. Kline and colleagues (2019, p. 1096) point out that the management of countertransference may contribute to repairing ruptures (e.g., Gelso & Hayes, 2007).

What does it take to repair a rupture? Lipner and colleagues (2019) suggest that ruptures represent important moments that offer the therapeutic dyad a chance for cooperation between patients and therapists, and these moments can enhance the striving toward empathy in a mutual relationship. The point is that these moments are delicate ones that can make or break relationships in therapy and beyond, and often they evolve when least anticipated.

A rupture that relates to the alliance may facilitate integration in therapy as it encourages therapists to be open and to integrate an alliance type of strategy when addressing an impasse in the therapeutic relationship (Eubanks, Burckell, et al., 2018). Friedlander (2015) claims that it takes more than technical acumen on the part of therapists to repair a rupture and explains that it requires that therapists genuinely want to discuss their role in the relational rupture. For early career therapists, the willingness to review errors is made difficult by their recognition that they will be evaluated by their supervisors (Friedlander, 2015). Eubanks, Burckell, and colleagues (2018) note that it was found that when compared to STDP, BRT was more likely to increase retention in therapy (e.g., Muran et al., 2005), and this finding suggests that the use of strategies for repairing ruptures can positively influence variables such as premature termination. Luo and colleagues (2022, p. 643) note that the process of repairing ruptures can help clients gain experience with their interpersonal issues during therapy sessions and outside the therapy milieu (e.g., Safran et al., 2011).

Alliance Training

A robust, positive relationship is shown to exist between the therapeutic or working alliance and treatment outcome (Flückiger et al., 2018). This chapter focuses on the importance for therapists to learn how to recognize and work with ruptures in the therapeutic or helping alliance, how to repair them, and suggests that therapists seek alliance training. A program that offers alliance-focused training (AFT), a supervision framework (e.g., Eubanks-Carter et al., 2015; Muran et al., 2010), emphasizes responsiveness that can help supervisees to enhance their interpersonal skills, particularly with patients with personality disorders with whom they find it difficult to work (Muran et al., 2018; Eubanks, Sergi, et al., 2021). Themes that are underscored in the context of AFT include the concepts of nuanced ruptures and metacommunication (Eubanks, Warren, et al., 2021). The art of metacommunication is discussed in Chapter 5 within the context of a transtheoretical model of ruptures and repair.

Repairing Ruptures and a Mode or Format of Therapy: Teletherapy

Therapists, regardless of their particular theoretical perspective, sought to accommodate their clients during the pandemic by inviting them to join teletherapy sessions. Chapter 1 explored the effect of teletherapy upon the therapeutic alliance during the COVID-19 pandemic, discussed different types of teletherapy, and presented a vignette that illustrates the interaction between the therapeutic alliance, a rupture, and teletherapy.

Dolev-Amit and colleagues (2021) describe the use of a supportive telepsychotherapy approach for resolving ruptures in the therapeutic alliance specifically targeted to the pandemic period. They explain the critical nature of these supportive methods during a pandemic when anxiety, depression, isolation, and powerlessness tend to increase. The unfamiliarity of many therapists with different modes of telepsychotherapy makes it hard for them to discern alliance ruptures, which may include tensions that derive from the teletherapy milieu itself (Dolev-Amit et al., 2021; Safran & Muran, 2000a; Safran et al., 2011). The vignette in Chapter 1 illustrated the example that showed the tension that emerged and the rupture that ensued when the client, Conrad, switched from in-person therapy to videoconferencing during the COVID-19 pandemic.

Chapter Summary

In therapy and beyond, we discover new ways to attend to the unfolding turns of our relationships. Sometimes, no matter how we proceed, a rupture or strain in the relationship may occur. Chapter 2, "Ruptures and Repairs in the Therapeutic Process: Diagnostic and Theoretical Considerations," explored the repair of ruptures for patients' with different attachment styles, investigated the interaction between therapists' theoretical perspective and ruptures, and discussed the connection between therapists' theoretical approach, patients' diagnosis, and ruptures along with their resolutions. Immediate rupture repair strategies aim to quickly focus on the rupture; exploratory strategies to explore the rupture with the client (Eubanks et al., 2023). Do therapists and clients think that rupture repair is paradoxical or perplexing? Rupture resolution necessitates collaboration with the individual against whom or away from whom one is moving, and efforts to resolve may create yet another rupture (Eubanks et al., 2023). Chapters 1 and 2 discussed how many therapists recognized that they needed, at times, to change their therapy delivery modes from in-person sessions to variations of teletherapy during the pandemic, and addressed the relationship between a teletherapy approach and ruptures in the therapeutic alliance and their repair during the pandemic period.

The next chapter defines the termination process or ending stage of therapy and examines different types of terminations, for example, mutual or premature. The connection between rupture repair, the focus of this chapter, and the termination or ending of therapy, to be explored in Chapter 3, is reflected in the findings of an association between the reduced ratings of rupture resolution and dropout from therapy (e.g., Eubanks et al., 2019; Gersh et al., 2017). The aforementioned chapters and the connection between them underscore the importance for therapists to pay attention to potential ruptures that are sources of stress for patients and therapists and to resolve emerging ruptures with finesse while navigating delicate and not so delicate moment-to-moment exchanges during therapy.

References

Abbass, A., & Town, J. M. (2023). Alliance rupture and repair in short-term psychodynamic therapy. In C. F. Eubanks, L. W. Samstag, & J. C. Muran (Eds.), *Rupture and repair in psychotherapy: A critical process for change* (pp. 221–252). American Psychological Association. https://doi.org/10.1037/0000306-010

American Psychiatric Association. (2022). Diagnostic and statistical manual of mental disorders (5th ed., text rev.). American Psychiatric Association Publishing. https://doi.org/10.1176/appi.books.9780890425787

Arnkoff, D. B. (1995). Two examples of strains in the therapeutic alliance in an integrative cognitive therapy. *In Session:* Psychotherapy in Practice, 1(1), 33–46. Reprinted (2000) in *Journal of Clinical Psychology, 56*(2), 187–200. https://doi.org/10.1002/(sici)1097-4679(200002)56:2<187::aid-jclp5>3.0.co;2-y

Aspland, H., Llewelyn, S., Hardy, G. E., Barkham, M., & Stiles, W. (2008). Alliance ruptures and rupture resolution in cognitive-behavior therapy: A preliminary task analysis. *Psychotherapy Research, 18*(6), 699–710. https://doi.org/10.1080/10503300802291463

Bachelor, A., & Horvath, A. (1999). The therapeutic relationship. In M. A. Hubble, B. L. Duncan, & S. D. Miller (Eds.), *The heart and soul of change: What works in therapy* (pp. 133–178). American Psychological Association. https://doi.org/10.1037/11132-004

Bartholomew, K., & Horowitz, L. M. (1991). Attachment styles among young adults: A test of a four-category model. *Journal of Personality and Social Psychology, 61*(2), 226–244. https://doi.org/10.1037//0022-3514.61.2.226

Bimont, D., & Werbart, A. (2018). "I've got you under my skin": Relational therapists' experiences of patients who occupy their inner world. *Counselling Psychology Quarterly, 31*(2), 243–268. https://doi.org/10.1080/09515070.2017.1300135

Borelli, J. L., Sohn, L., Wang, B. A., Hong, K., DeCoste, C., & Suchman, N. E. (2019). Therapist–client language matching: Initial promise as a measure of therapist–client relationship quality. *Psychoanalytic Psychology, 36*(1), 9–18. https://doi.org/10.1037/pap0000177

Boritz, T., Barnhart, R., Eubanks, C. F., & McMain, S. (2018). Alliance rupture and resolution in dialectical behavior therapy for borderline personality disorder. *Journal of Personality Disorders, 32*(Supplement), 115–128. https://doi.org/10.1521/pedi.2018.32.supp.115

Castonguay, L. G. (1996). Integrative cognitive therapy for depression treatment manual. Unpublished manuscript, The Pennsylvania State University.

Chang, D. F., Omidi, M., & Dunn, J. J. (2023). Antioppressive approaches to alliance rupture and repair: A critical-cultural-relational model of rupture resolution. In C. F. Eubanks, L. W., Samstag, & J. C. Muran (Eds.), (2023). *Rupture and repair in psychotherapy: A critical process for change* (pp. 21–52). American Psychological Association. https://doi.org/10.1037/0000306-002

Colli, A., Gentile, D., Condino, V., & Lingiardi, V. (2019). Assessing alliance ruptures and resolutions: Reliability and validity of the Collaborative Interactions Scale-revised version. *Psychotherapy Research, 29*(3), 279–292. https://doi.org/10.1080/10503307.2017.1414331

Constantino, M. J., Coyne, A. E., & Muir, H. J. (2020). Evidence-based therapist responsivity to disruptive clinical process. *Cognitive and Behavioral Practice, 27*(4), 405–416. https://doi.org/10.1016/j.cbpra.2020.01.003

Constantino, M. J., Marnell, M. E., Haile, A. J., Kanther-Sista, S. N., Wolman, K., Zappert, L., & Arnow, B. A. (2008). Integrative cognitive therapy for depression: A randomized pilot comparison. *Psychotherapy: Theory, Research, Practice, Training, 45*(2), 122–134. https://doi.org/10.1037/0033-3204.45.2.122

Coutinho, J., Ribeiro, E., Fernandes, C., Sousa, I., & Safran, J. D. (2014). The development of the therapeutic alliance and the emergence of alliance ruptures. *Anales de Psicología, 30*(3), 985–994. https://doi.org/10.6018/analesps.30.3.168911

Coutinho, J., Ribeiro, E., Hill, C., & Safran, J. (2011). Therapists' and clients' experiences of alliance ruptures: A qualitative study. *Psychotherapy Research, 21*(5), 525–540. https://doi.org/10.1080/10503307.2011.587469

Dolev-Amit, T., Leibovich, L., & Zilcha-Mano, S. (2021). Repairing alliance ruptures using supportive techniques in telepsychotherapy during the COVID-19 pandemic. *Counselling Psychology Quarterly, 34*(3–4), 485–498. https://doi.org/10.1080/09515070.2020.1777089

Eames, V., & Roth, A. (2000). Patient attachment orientation and the early working alliance-A study of patient and therapist reports of alliance quality and ruptures. *Psychotherapy Research, 10*(4), 421–434. https://doi.org/10.1093/ptr/10.4.421

Elliott, R., Bohart, A. C., Watson, J. C., & Murphy, D. (2018). Therapist empathy and client outcome: An updated meta-analysis. *Psychotherapy, 55*(4), 399–410. https://doi.org/10.1037/pst0000175

Elliott, R., Watson, J. C., Goldman, R. N., & Greenberg, L. S. (2004). Learning emotion focused therapy: The process-experiential approach to change. American Psychological Association. https://doi.org/10.1037/10725-000

Eubanks, C. F., Burckell, L. A., & Goldfried, M. R. (2018). Clinical consensus strategies to repair ruptures in the therapeutic alliance. *Journal of Psychotherapy Integration, 28*(1), 60–76. https://doi.org/10.1037/int0000097

Eubanks, C. F., Lubitz, J., Muran, J. C., & Safran, J. D. (2019). Rupture resolution rating system (3RS): Development and validation. *Psychotherapy Research, 29*(3), 306–319. https://doi.org/10.1080/10503307.2018.1552034

Eubanks, C. F., Muran, J. C., Safran, J. D. (2018). Alliance rupture repair: A meta-analysis. *Psychotherapy, 55*(4), 508–519. https://doi.org/10.1037/pst0000185

Eubanks, C. F., Samstag, L. W., & Muran, J. C. (2023). Conclusion: Don't be afraid to get messy – Points of convergence in rupture and repair. In C. F. Eubanks, L. W. Samstag, & J. C. Muran (Eds.), *Rupture and repair in psychotherapy: A critical process for change* (pp. 305–317). American Psychological Association.

Eubanks, C. F., Sergi, J., & Muran, J. C. (2021). Responsiveness to ruptures and repairs in psychotherapy. In J. C. Watson & H. Wiseman (Eds.), *The responsive psychotherapist: Attuning to clients in the moment* (pp. 83–103). American Psychological Association. https://doi.org/10.1037/0000240-005

Eubanks, C. F., Warren, J. T., & Muran, J. C. (2021). Identifying ruptures and repairs in alliance-focused training group supervision. *International Journal of Group Psychotherapy, 71*(2), 275–309. https://doi.org/10.1080/00207284.2020.1805618

Eubanks-Carter, C., Muran, J. C., & Safran, J. D. (2015). Alliance-focused training. *Psychotherapy: Theory, Research, & Practice, 52*(2), 169–173. https://doi.org/10.1037/a0037596

Flückiger, C., Del Re, A. C., Wampold, B. E., & Horvath, A. O. (2018). The alliance in adult psychotherapy: A meta-analytic synthesis. *Psychotherapy, 55*(4), 316–340. https://doi.org/10.1037/pst0000172

Fosha, D. (2001). The dyadic regulation of affect. *Journal of Clinical Psychology, 57*(2), 227–242. https://doi.org/10.1002/1097-4679(200102)57:2<227::aid-jclp8>3.0.co;2-1

Friedlander, M. L. (2015). Use of relational strategies to repair alliance ruptures: How responsive supervisors train responsive psychotherapists. *Psychotherapy, 52*(2), 174–179. https://doi.org/10.1037/a0037044

Gelso, C. J., & Hayes, J. A. (2007). *Countertransference and the therapist's inner experience: Perils and possibilities.* Lawrence Erlbaum Associates Publishers.

Gelso, C. J., & Perez-Rojas, A. E. (2017). Inner experience and the good therapist. In L. G. Castonguay & C. E. Hill (Eds.), *How and why are some therapists better than others?: Understanding therapist effects* (pp. 101–115). American Psychological Association. https://doi.org/10.1037/0000034-007

Gersh, E., Hulbert, C. A., McKechnie, B., Ramadan, R., Worotniuk, T., & Chanen, A. M. (2017). Alliance rupture and repair processes and therapeutic change in youth with borderline personality disorder. *Psychology and Psychotherapy: Theory, Research and Practice, 90*(1), 84–104. https://doi.org/10.1111/papt.12097

Gunderson, J. G., Prank, A. F., Ronningstam, E. F., Wachter, S., Lynch, V. J., & Wolf, P. J. (1989). Early discontinuance of borderline patients from psychotherapy. *The Journal of Nervous and Mental Disease, 177*(1), 38–42. https://doi.org/10.1097/00005053-198901000-00006

Hardy, G. E., Stiles, W. B., Barkham, M., & Startup, M. (1998). Therapist responsiveness to client interpersonal styles during time-limited treatments for depression. *Journal of Consulting and Clinical Psychology, 66*(2), 304–312. https://doi.org/10.1037/0022-006x.66.2.304

Hill, C. E., Nutt-Williams, E., Heaton, K. J., Thompson, B. J., & Rhodes, R. H. (1996). Therapist retrospective recall of impasses in long-term psychotherapy: A qualitative analysis. *Journal of Counseling Psychology, 43*(2), 207–217. https://doi.org/10.1037/0022-0167.43.2.207

Horvath, A. O., & Symonds, B. D. (1991). Relation between working alliance and outcome in psychotherapy: A meta-analysis. *Journal of Counseling Psychology, 38*(2), 139–149. https://doi.org/10.1037/0022-0167.38.2.139

Impala, T., Okomoto, A., & Kazantzis, N. (2023). Alliance rupture and repair in cognitive-behavior therapy. In C. F. Eubanks, L. W. Samstag, & J. C. Muran (Eds.), *Rupture and repair in psychotherapy: A critical process for change* (pp. 119–139). American Psychological Association.

Kline, K. V., Hill, C. E., Morris, T., O'Connor, S., Sappington, R., Vernay, C., Arrazola, G., Dagne, M., & Okuno, H. (2019). Ruptures in psychotherapy: Experiences of therapist trainees. *Psychotherapy Research, 29*(8), 1086–1098. https://doi.org/10.1080/10503307.2018.1492164

Leichsenring, F., & Leibing, E. (2003). The effectiveness of psychodynamic therapy and cognitive behavior therapy in the treatment of personality disorders: A meta-analysis. *The American Journal of Psychiatry, 160*(7), 1223–1232. https://doi.org/10.1176/appi.ajp.160.7.1223

Lingiardi, V., Holmqvist, R., & Safran, J. D. (2016). Relational turn and psychotherapy research. *Contemporary Psychoanalysis, 52*(2), 275–312. https://doi.org/10.1080/00107530.2015.1137177

Lipner, L. M., Liu, D., & Muran, J. C. (2019). Getting on the same page: Introducing alliance rupture as a path to mutual empathy and change in psychotherapy. In A. E. Foster & Z. S. Yaseen (Eds.), *Teaching empathy in healthcare: Building a new core competency* (pp. 117–126). Springer. https://doi.org/10.1007/978-3-030-29876-0_7

Lipsitz-Odess, I., Benisty, H., Dolev-Amit, T., & Zilcha-Mano, S. (2022). Alliance rupture profiles by personality disorder pathology in psychotherapy for depression: Tendencies, development, and timing. *Clinical Psychology & Psychotherapy, 29*(3), 1125–1134.https://doi.org/10.1002/cpp.2700

Luo, X., Liu, S., Levendosky, A. A., Good, E. W., Turchan, J. E., & Hopwood, C. J. (2022). Idiographic and nomothetic relationships between momentary interpersonal behaviors, interpersonal complementarity, and alliance ruptures in psychotherapy. *Journal of Counseling Psychology, 69*(5), 642–655. https://doi.org/10.1037/cou0000619

Macdonald, J., Elliott, R., & Couto, A. B. (2023). Relational dialogue in emotion-focused therapy: Process analysis and comparison with the alliance-focused training model. In C. F. Eubanks, L. W. Samstag, & J. C. Muran (Eds.), *Rupture and repair in psychotherapy: A critical process for change* (pp. 187–220). American Psychological Association. https://doi.org/10.1037/0000306-009

Mahoney, M. J., & Marquis, A. (2002). Integral constructivism and dynamic systems in psychotherapy processes. *Psychoanalytic Inquiry, 22*(5), 794–813. https://doi.org/10.1080/07351692209349018

Marquis, A., & Elliot, A. (2015). Integral psychotherapy in practice, Part 2: Revisions to the metatheory of Integral Psychotherapy based on therapeutic practice. *Journal of Unified Psychotherapy and Clinical Science, 3*(1), 1–40.

Miller-Bottome, M., Talia, A., Eubanks, C. F., Safran, J. D., & Muran, J. C. (2019). Secure in-session attachment predicts rupture resolution: Negotiating a secure base. *Psychoanalytic Psychology, 36*(2), 132–138. https://doi.org/10.1037/pap0000232

Muran, J. C. (2019). Confessions of a New York rupture researcher: An insider's guide and critique. *Psychotherapy Research, 29*(1), 1–14. https://doi.org/10.1080/10503307.2017.1413261

Muran, J. C., Eubanks, C. F., & Samstag, L. W. (2023). Introduction: Rupture in a wicked and wonderful world. In C. F. Eubanks, L. W. Samstag, & J. C. Muran (Eds.), *Rupture and repair in psychotherapy: A critical process for change* (pp. 3–20). American Psychological Association. https://doi.org/10.1037/0000306-001

Muran, J. C., Safran, J. D., Eubanks, C. F., & Gorman, B. S. (2018). The effect of alliance-focused training on a cognitive-behavioral therapy for personality disorders. *Journal of Consulting and Clinical Psychology, 86*(4), 384–397. https://doi.org/10.1037/ccp0000284

Muran, J. C., Safran, J. D., & Eubanks-Carter, C. (2010). Developing therapist abilities to negotiate alliance ruptures. In J. C. Muran & J. P. Barber (Eds.), *The therapeutic alliance: An evidence-based guide to practice* (pp. 320–340). The Guilford Press.

Muran, J. C., Safran, J. D., Gorman, B. S., Samstag, L. W., Eubanks-Carter, C., & Winston, A. (2009). The relationship of early alliance ruptures and their resolution to process and outcome in three time-limited psychotherapies for personality disorders. *Psychotherapy: Theory, Research, Practice, Training, 46*(2), 233–248. https://doi.org/10.1037/a0016085

Muran, J. C., Safran, J. D., Samstag, L. W., & Winston, A. (2005). Evaluating an alliance-focused treatment for personality disorders. *Psychotherapy: Theory, Research, Practice, Training, 42*(4), 532–545. https://doi.org/10.1037/0033-3204.42.4.532

Norcross, J. C., & Lambert, M. J. (2019). Evidence-based psychotherapy relationships: The third task force. In J. C. Norcross & M. J. Lambert (Eds.), *Psychotherapy relationships that work: Evidence-based therapist contributions* (pp. 1–23). Oxford University Press. https://doi.org/10.1093/med-psych/9780190843953.003.0001

Okamoto, A., Dattilio, F. M., Dobson, K. S., & Kazantzis, N. (2019). The therapeutic relationship in cognitive–behavioral therapy: Essential features and common challenges. *Practice Innovations, 4*(2), 112–123. https://doi.org/10.1037/pri0000088

Okamoto, A., & Kazantzis, N. (2021). Alliance ruptures in cognitive-behavioral therapy: A cognitive conceptualization. *Journal of Clinical Psychology, 77*(2), 384–397. https://doi.org/10.1002/jclp.23116

Pereira, T., Lock, J., & Oggins, J. (2006). Role of therapeutic alliance in family therapy for adolescent anorexia nervosa. *International Journal of Eating Disorders, 39*(8), 677–684. https://doi.org/10.1002/eat.20303

Perls, F. S. (1969). *Gestalt therapy verbatim*. Real People Press.

Perry, J. C., Banon, E., & Ianni, F. (1999). Effectiveness of psychotherapy for personality disorders. *The American Journal of Psychiatry, 156*(9), 1312–1321. https://doi.org/10.1176/ajp.156.9.1312

Piper, W. E., Azim, H. F., Joyce, A. S., & McCallum, M. (1991). Transference interpretations, therapeutic alliance, and outcome in short-term individual psychotherapy. *Archives of General Psychiatry, 48*(10), 946–953. https://doi.org/10.1001/archpsyc.1991.01810340078010

Piper, W. E., Azim, H. F., Joyce, A. S., McCallum, M., Nixon, G. W., & Segal, P. S. (1991). Quality of object relations versus interpersonal functioning as predictors of therapeutic alliance and psychotherapy outcome. *The Journal of Nervous and Mental Disease, 170*(7), 432–438. https://doi.org/10.1097/00005053-199107000-00008

Rogers, C. R. (1951). *Client-centered therapy*. Houghton Mifflin.

Rubel, J. A., Zilcha-Mano, S., Feils-Klaus, V., & Lutz, W. (2018). Session-to-session effects of alliance ruptures in outpatient CBT: Within- and between-patient associations. *Journal of Consulting and Clinical Psychology, 86*(4), 354–366. https://doi.org/10.1037/ccp0000286

Rudenstine, S., Wachtel, P. L., Schulder, T., & Bernstein, B. (2023). Expanding the rupture resolution paradigm: An integrative perspective. In C. F. Eubanks, L. W. Samstag, & J. C. Muran (Eds.), *Rupture and repair in psychotherapy: A critical process for change* (pp. 277–304). American Psychological Association.

Safran, J. D., Crocker, P., McMain, S., & Murray, P. (1990). Therapeutic alliance rupture as a therapy event for empirical investigation. *Psychotherapy: Theory, Research, Practice, Training, 27*(2), 154–165. https://doi.org/10.1037/0033-3204.27.2.154

Safran, J. D., & Kraus, J. (2014). Alliance ruptures, impasses, and enactments: A relational perspective. *Psychotherapy, 51*(3), 381–387. https://doi.org/10.1037/a0036815

Safran J. D., & Muran J. C. (1996). The resolution of ruptures in the therapeutic alliance. *Journal of Consulting and Clinical Psychology, 64*(3), 447–458. https://doi.org/10.1037/0022-006x.64.3.447

Safran, J. D., & Muran, J. C. (2000a). *Negotiating the therapeutic alliance: A relational treatment guide*. Guilford Press.

Safran, J. D., & Muran, J. C. (2000b). Resolving therapeutic alliance ruptures: Diversity and integration. *Journal of Clinical Psychology, 56*(2), 233–243. https://doi.org/10.1002/(SICI)1097-4679(200002)56:2<233::AID-JCLP9>3.0.CO;2-3

Safran, J. D., Muran, J. C., & Eubanks-Carter, C. (2011). Repairing alliance ruptures. *Psychotherapy: Theory, Research, Practice, Training*, 48(1), 80–87. https://doi.org/10.1037/a0022140

Safran, J. D., Muran, J. C., & Samstag, L. W. (1994). Resolving therapeutic alliance ruptures: A task analytic investigation. In A. O. Horvath & L. S. Greenberg (Eds.), *The working alliance: Theory, research and practice* (pp. 225–255). Wiley.

Samstag, L. W., & Muran, J. C. (2019). Ruptures, repairs, and reflections: Contributions of Jeremy Safran. *Research in Psychotherapy: Psychopathology, Process and Outcome*, 22(1), 7–14. https://doi.org/10.4081/ripppo.2019.376

Sauer, E. M., Anderson, M. Z., Gormley, B., Richmond, C. J., & Preacco, L. (2010). Client attachment orientations, working alliances, and responses to therapy: A psychology training clinic study. *Psychotherapy Research*, 20(6), 702–711. https://doi.org/10.1080/10503307.2010.518635

Sommerfeld, E., Orbach, I., Zim, S., & Mikulincer, M. (2008). An in-session exploration of ruptures in working alliance and their associations with clients' core conflictual relationship themes, alliance-related discourse, and clients' postsession evaluations. *Psychotherapy Research*, 18(4), 377–388. https://doi.org/10.1080/10503300701675873

Stiles, W. B. (2009). Responsiveness as an obstacle for psychotherapy outcome research: It's worse than you think. *Clinical Psychology: Science and Practice*, 16(1), 86–91. https://doi.org/10.1111/j.1468-2850.2009.01148.x

Strauss, J. L., Hayes, A. M., Johnson, S. L., Newman, C. F., Brown, G. K., Barber, J. P., Laurenceau, J.-P., & Beck, A. T. (2006). Early alliance, alliance ruptures, and symptom change in a nonrandomized trial of cognitive therapy for avoidant and obsessive-compulsive personality disorders. *Journal of Consulting and Clinical Psychology*, 74(2), 337–345. https://doi.org/10.1037/0022-006X.74.2.337

Swank, L. E., & Wittenborn, A. K. (2013). Repairing alliance ruptures in emotionally focused couple therapy: A preliminary task analysis. *The American Journal of Family*, 41(5), 389–402. https://doi.org/10.1080/01926187.2012.726595

Talia, A., Miller-Bottome, M., & Daniel, S. I. F. (2017). Assessing attachment in psychotherapy: Validation of the patient attachment coding system (PACS). *Clinical Psychology & Psychotherapy*, 24(1), 149–161. https://doi.org/10.1002/cpp.1990

Waddington, L. (2002). The therapy relationship in cognitive therapy: A review. *Behavioural and Cognitive Psychotherapy*, 30(2), 179–192. https://doi.org/10.1017/S1352465802002059

Watson, J. C., & Greenberg, L. S. (1995). Alliance ruptures and repairs in experiential therapy. *In Session: Psychotherapy in Practice*, 1(1), 19–31.

Wolf, A. W., Goldfried, M. R., & Muran, J. C. (Eds.). (2013). Transforming negative reactions to clients: From frustration to compassion. American Psychological Association. https://doi.org/10.1037/13940-000

Zalman, H., Aafjes-van Doorn, K., & Eubanks, C. F. (2019). Alliance challenges in the treatment of a narcissistic patient: The case of Alex. *Research in Psychotherapy: Psychopathology, Process and Outcome*, 22(2), 212–223. https://doi.org/10.4081/ripppo.2019.351

Zilcha-Mano, S., Eubanks, C. F., Bloch-Elkouby, S., & Muran, J. C. (2020). Can we agree we just had a rupture? Patient-therapist congruence on ruptures and its effects on outcome in brief relational therapy versus cognitive-behavioral therapy. Journal of Counseling Psychology, 67(3), 315–325. https://doi.org/10.1037/cou0000400

Zlotnick, E., Strauss, A. Y., Ellis, P., Abargil, M., Tishby, O., & Huppert, J. D. (2020). Reevaluating ruptures and repairs in alliance: Between- and within-session processes in cognitive–behavioral therapy and short-term psychodynamic psychotherapy. *Journal of Consulting and Clinical Psychology*, 88(9), 859–869. https://doi.org/10.1037ccp0000598

Part II

Termination

The patient, Calvin, shows up for his seventh therapy session and proceeds to answer a phone call during the first ten minutes of the session. The therapist sits quietly. Then Calvin says, "I am so sick of coming here. I don't see much improvement in my life, and you don't really understand what I'm going through. Your therapy is a hoax." The therapist feels tired of Calvin's chronic complaints, and he lets the patient know that maybe if he focused on the therapy rather than his phone he would feel more progress. Calvin gets up to leave, and shouts, "You couldn't care less about me and my problems. As long as you collect your fee. I'm ready to leave now." The therapist understands that his patient's outburst may signal a critical point in the therapy, and that a premature termination is at hand. He calmly says, "It was not my place to reprimand you. You can do what you wish during your time, but it may be helpful if you could tell me the reasons that you feel that the therapy has not benefitted you." Calvin sits down, but is silent for several minutes, before the therapist intervenes again. In the aforementioned example, a confrontation rupture precipitates a potential premature termination. The therapist actively intervenes by seeking to repair the rupture. The patient does not unilaterally end therapy; however, a withdrawal rupture ensues.

What is an ideal psychotherapy termination? Kealy and colleagues (2020) suggest that the process of psychotherapy termination is not a one size fits all. They explain that its complexity varies depending upon the therapist, the therapeutic orientation, and the patient. For example, with respect to patients, some may decide to terminate therapy once their symptoms have decreased; other patients, to practice their new skills that they have learned in

DOI: 10.4324/9781003128489-4

therapy (Kealy et al., 2020). Kealy and colleagues (2020, p. 511) point out that whereas therapists with an interpersonal approach, in preparation for termination, may focus on clients' feelings of loss that emerge as their relationship with the therapist is drawing to its end, therapists with a cognitive-behavioral approach, in preparation for termination, may facilitate a decrease in clients' reliance on support from the therapist and attend to relapse prevention (e.g., Joyce et al., 2007).

Part II, "Termination," includes Chapter 3, "Definition, Types, and Duration of the Termination Process," and Chapter 4, "Termination Across Different Diagnoses and Theories." Chapters 3 and 4 point out the relationship between ruptures, their repairs, and termination. Chapter 3, "Definition, Types, and Duration of the Termination Process," defines the termination process, outlines the different types of terminations, e.g., mutual, premature, patient initiated, initiated by the client, and illustrates the effects of the duration of the termination process. The focus of Chapter 4, "Termination Across Different Diagnoses and Theories," is on the different types of termination that evolve for patients with different emotional and personality disorders and on how therapists and patients of different theoretical orientations navigate the termination process. Vignettes with the examples of the inner thoughts of the therapist and patient during the termination process are included throughout Chapters 3 and 4.

References

Joyce, A. S., Piper, W. E., Ogrodniczuk, J. S., & Klien, R. H. (2007). *Termination in psychotherapy: A psychodynamic model of processes and outcomes.* American Psychological Association. https://doi.org/10.1037/11545-000

Kealy, D., Gazzillo, F., Silberschatz, G., & Curtis, J. T. (2020). Plan-compatible termination in psychotherapy: Perspectives from control-mastery theory. *Psychotherapy, 57*(4), 508–514. https://doi.org/10.1037/pst0000300

Definition, Types, and Duration of the Termination Process

3

Introduction

Have you felt bewildered, disappointed, and confused about the termination of a friendship because you cannot figure out how or why it ended? Athena and Violet have been friends since the beginning of high school. They are seniors and have applied to the same college. Two weeks ago, Athena received word that she had received a scholarship to the college of her choice. Athena's dad served in Afghanistan, and her mother has been planning a surprise get together for Athena's friends to celebrate her daughter's acceptance at the new school. Violet volunteered to bring the desserts and salads and to help Athena's mom on Wednesday to set up for a few hours prior to the celebration. A few days prior to the get together, Violet received a letter informing her that the college which awarded a scholarship to Athena had not accepted her. Violet has, thus far, not been accepted at any other college.

On Wednesday, Athena's mother is joyful that she has the opportunity to plan a surprise celebration for her daughter. She is counting on Violet to bring the salads and desserts a few hours prior to the celebration, which is at 7 P.M. At approximately 3 P.M. that afternoon, Athena's mother looks out the window to see if Violet is on her way. Athena is not in the house. She is with another friend who volunteered to spend the rest of the day with her after school so that Athena can be surprised by the celebration when she returns to her house in the evening. It is almost 4 P.M. and Athena's mother calls Violet. She leaves a voice message. At 5 P.M., Athena's mother becomes concerned and contacts Violet's mother who says that Violet is not in the house. Athens's

DOI: 10.4324/9781003128489-5

mother shares the situation with Violet's mother who becomes concerned. Violet pops up at the get together at approximately 8 P.M. She looks like she has had a bit to drink. Athena has already been briefed by her mom, and approaches Violet who becomes hostile, creates a scene, and storms out. Athena calls Violet the next day but receives no return phone call. She sees Violet at school and attempts to discuss their relationship and what has occurred; however, Violet refuses to speak to her. Violet does not contact Athena again. Their relationship has ended, and Athena feels bewildered. Imagine the sense of bafflement and concern that Athena feels upon experiencing the loss of a friendship with Violet at a joyful time in her life.

An ending to a relationship, whether in therapy or beyond, can come in different sizes and flavors, accompanied by feelings of sadness, bewilderment, anger, or disappointment. It may take place inside the therapy setting or external to therapy, among friends or among family members, or during a therapy session, between a therapist and a patient. Therapists are not perfect, patients are not perfect, and endings in therapy may not be perfect (Gabbard, 2009). Is a live and let live model sufficient for termination, a suggestion for a therapist to respect that patients may need to end therapy in the way that they choose? Gabbard (2009) suggests that endings in therapy be tailored to an individual patient, the situational context, and the process of the dyad. He recommends that psychoanalysts consider different options so that an intervention is tailored to the needs of patients rather than to the theoretical choices of analysts.

Joyce and colleagues (2007) assert that a well-thought-out, mutually agreed termination between members of the therapeutic dyad, therapists and patients, is a desirable ending to a therapeutic relationship that is critical for maintaining the gains made during therapy. They explain that the gains are the first outcome of termination; relationship issues, the second outcome; future planning, the third outcome. Terminations from therapy emerge in different sizes and shapes. When ending therapy, do patients feel that they have received from therapy that which they have set out to obtain? It has been found that 56% of patients who attended their last session were considered not to have fulfilled their goals (Bartholomew et al., 2019). Therapy terminations may be mutual or unilateral; therapist initiated or patient initiated, planned or unplanned (Joyce et al., 2007). The dynamics of different therapy dyads are complex, and members of the therapeutic dyad, clients and therapists, may select to end the relationship for a variety of different reasons. For example, a patient may move out of state and decide to initiate a premature termination, or a patient may decide to drop out of therapy altogether, and may initiate a premature or unilateral termination (Joyce et al., 2007). A patient dropout (without the therapist's agreement) is considered a negative event, an obstacle to the therapeutic process, and therapists may be able to avoid these circumstances (Joyce et al., 2007; Swift & Greenberg, 2015). In these types of situations, invariably, patients' felt advantages of continuing therapy are offset by the projected costs of attending sessions (Swift & Greenberg, 2015). When therapists nurture the alliance, abrupt therapy endings are reduced (Bischoff et al., 2020; Swift, Greenberg, Whipple et al., 2012). Bartholomew and colleagues (2019, p. 84) point out that it has been found that patients who experience mutually agreed terminations tend to display a lower degree of symptom distress when they terminate therapy than do patients who initiate unilateral terminations (e.g., Westmacott et al., 2010). At the same time, it is possible that ending in therapy that underscores only symptoms does not fully portray the value of ending therapy with a patient, and that ending therapy with patients may need to highlight what patients have gained, not only that which they have lost (Bartholomew et al., 2019).

Westmacott and Hunsley (2017, p. 694) note that therapists need to realize that although they may view patients as not motivated for therapy, in reality, patients may drop out because of other reasons, such as the lack of a match between a therapist and a patient or the dissatisfaction with the process of therapy (e.g., Westmacott et al., 2010). They explain that this finding is consistent with previous research that shows therapists' tendencies to attribute unilateral termination by a patient to a patient's problem (e.g., Kendall et al., 1992). Generally, therapists may feel frustrated, sad, guilty, or anxious when patients select to drop out of therapy (da Silva et al., 2022). At times, it may not be possible to avoid premature terminations. The chapter, "Definition, Types, and Duration of the Termination Process," defines the termination process in therapy, outlines the different types of terminations from therapy, e.g., mutual or premature, patient initiated, therapist initiated, planned and unplanned, and explores the duration of the termination process.

Chapter 3 illustrates the different ways in which terminations in therapeutic settings occur, the reason that they may occur, and, as in prior chapters on ruptures, includes vignettes of examples of the therapist's and patient's dialogue along with their inner thoughts. This chapter describes different types of terminations, e.g., mutual terminations, endings that are premature, and planned and unplanned endings. The connection between Chapter 2, "Ruptures and Repairs in the Therapeutic Process: Diagnostic and Theoretical Considerations," and Chapter 3, "Definition, Types, and Duration of the Termination Process," is realized as some premature terminations occur abruptly because of ruptures in the therapeutic alliance. For example, a premature termination can occur when there is a rupture or impasse in the therapeutic relationship with a loss of trust by the client. It is suggested that the process of rupture resolution in the alliance may contribute to retention of clients in therapy and outcome (Muran et al., 2009). Chapter 3 distinguishes between terminations initiated by the patient and endings initiated by the therapist.

What Is Termination in Therapy?

What is termination, and how does termination take place in therapy? How do therapeutic relationships end? Termination, a complex process in therapy, refers to the ending of the psychotherapeutic relationship (da Silva et al., 2022). When considering the ending phase, an essential task in the process of psychotherapy, the therapist hopes to guide the client through the experience of letting go (da Silva et al., 2022). da Silva and colleagues (2022) suggest that the integrative termination model, a paradigmatic complementarity framework where therapy is viewed as a multifactorial concept that can transition between therapy and beyond, proposes that the ending of therapy is a process that can happen at various phases along the way. With respect to the duration of termination in therapy, endings may be abrupt or well-planned (Barnett, 2016; da Silva et al., 2022).

Endings in therapy may happen for a host of reasons. They may be a mutual decision between clients and therapists, or they may happen prematurely or unilaterally, initiated either by therapists or clients. Shahar and Ziv-Beiman (2020) suggest that determining a preset date for termination in psychotherapy helps to facilitate a perception of agency and can serve to extend the recognition of one's schemas (the organization or the plan of one's cognitive perceptions and behaviors). They explain that in this way, the termination planning is part and parcel of the therapeutic experience. Norcross and colleagues (2017, p. 67) point out that when a short-term therapy model, for example, CBT, is used during the termination process, rather than emphasize feelings of loss or underscore a deep exploration of the therapeutic relationship as in long-term therapy models, the therapist involved with a short-term approach focuses on gradually decreasing the number of sessions and facilitates the clients' holding onto the skills that they learned while applying these skills to different situations on their own (e.g., Goldfried, 2002).

During the termination phase of therapy, it is not uncommon for clients to regress and think and/or say the following thoughts:

> *Was I in my right mind when I said that I would discontinue therapy? I really don't want to stop at this time. Also, I don't want to insult him, but I just told him, uh-oh, that I want to be on my own now. How to tell him that I changed my mind? I'll worry about it next time.*
>
> *It's going to be too hard for me to be out there all alone. I'm used to relying on her for support. What am I going to do when nobody's around for me?*

At any point during the therapy and/or during the termination, a leap to health may occur, and clients may think and/or say the following:

> *I'll be fine on my own. I don't need any of this. This therapy is surely too expensive. How did I ever agree to therapy sessions? I'll start getting out now.*
>
> *I didn't need this therapist before, and I don't need him now. I'm ending this as soon as possible. I'll let him know immediately next time, or better yet, I'll call and leave a message on his voicemail.*

This chapter offers examples via vignettes that illustrate how clients' responses to ending therapy emerge as their own inherent styles of coping with difficult situations or losses. The chapter underscores therapists' processing of clients' styles of reacting and referencing their particular coping styles and how these client styles play out during the end phase of therapy as part and parcel of the termination process. The examples included in the vignettes illustrate the need for therapists to consider that during the termination phase clients may feel more at risk than usual. The clients in the vignettes may not be aware that their current struggle is associated with the ending phase of therapy itself, and the termination phase may stir new material or painful feelings that are linked to prior life experiences that have not been addressed during the course of therapy. For a variety of reasons, not all the therapists and clients included in the vignettes have had ample opportunity or have been willing or able to think about the closure or the ending phase of therapy, to discuss thoughts and feelings about the ending, to consider loss, to revisit the goals of therapy, and/or to explore what has taken place during therapy. Chapter 3 illustrates the connection between the termination phase of therapy and shows how during termination it is possible for new material to emerge, themes that include experiences that further illustrate clients' general styles for coping with loss, stress, and/or ruptures, and other kinds of conflicts that may surface during the termination phase.

Types of Termination: Planned and Unplanned

What are the different types of termination that may take place at the end of therapy? See Table 3.1 for a brief sketch of the termination types discussed in this chapter.

The therapeutic milieu affords different opportunities for termination depending upon the theoretical model, e.g., integrative, cognitive-behavioral, humanistic, psychodynamic. For example, as illustrated in a few of the vignettes throughout this book, for therapists with a psychodynamic perspective, the therapeutic encounter is one where patients act out many of their internal conflicts as they engage with their therapists. To build a picture of the struggles experienced by patients, therapists with a psychodynamic or a psychoanalytic perspective focus on the transference and the countertransference along with the subtleties of the real relationship, and, in the aforementioned long-term therapies, it is the mutually agreed termination (as in the example of the client, Melissa, in Chapter 4) that is the sought after therapy ending, a goodbye that is valued by the members of the therapeutic dyad. The terminations portrayed in Chapters 3 and 4 occur because of a planned or an unplanned event, initiated by either patient or therapist. Terminations in therapy can happen because the circumstances of the therapist or the client may change over time.

Table 3.1 Vignettes: Types of Termination From Therapy

Initiated by Client or Therapist	Planned and Unplanned		

	Mutually Agreed	Treatment Refusal	Premature Termination	Forced Termination
Client Initiated	Anthony	Jennifer	Salvadore	
Client Initiated	Darci		Tracy	
Client Initiated			Zoey	
Client Initiated			Miles	
Client Initiated (post microaggression)			Paul	
Client Initiated			Paisley	
Therapist Initiated				Pat

For example, the patient or therapist or a family member of the patient or therapist may experience a temporary physical concern, illness, or diagnosis (e.g., Kirk's therapist), or either may die; one of the members of the therapeutic dyad may move to another state or to another country (e.g., the client, Darren); one may take a sabbatical, another may change jobs (e.g., Pat's therapist); the therapist may retire or complete an internship or a practicum; the client may decide to drop out of therapy (e.g., the client, Miles; the client, Hank), or terminations may have occurred as a result of non-payment of a bill. During times when patients are not able to pay their bill, they may be thinking the following thoughts:

> *Should I ask my therapist to meet with me until I can afford to pay?*
> *Where does this leave me now?*
> *Should I pay my rent or my therapist?*
> *How will I have enough food this month if I pay my therapist?*
> *Is my therapist going to drop me now that my coverage has run out?*
> *Maybe I can see this therapist less frequently so that I can afford it.*
> *Shall I take a break from therapy at this time?*
> *Maybe I don't need therapy anyway.*

Chapters 3 and 4 underscore that no matter the therapeutic treatment approach, for example, existential, cognitive-behavioral, or psychodynamic, preparing for the ending phase of therapy is an essential common theme in the provision of closure of the therapy work, and in some of the aforementioned situations, particularly during forced terminations, careful planning on the part of therapists can mitigate the consequences of a negative event for patients.

The following section begins with an ideal type of termination, a mutually agreed termination; an ending in therapy where the therapist and the patient agree that the goals of therapy have been met. This type of termination, one that therapists and patients desire, contrasts with the unilateral or premature termination or the type of termination where the patient drops out of therapy. In general, therapists, regardless of their theoretical point of view, and patients hope and aim for mutually agreed terminations.

Mutually Agreed Terminations

It is accepted that there are different types of terminations in therapy. The process of endings in therapy may vary across therapists, clients, and types of therapy (Kealy et al., 2020). This section delves into mutually agreed terminations that occur when the members of a therapy dyad, the therapist and the patient, agree that the goals of the therapy have been reached or that a time-limited treatment has ended. Premature terminations, on the other hand, take place when the patient begins therapy, but then ends therapy contrary to a practitioner's suggestions and before recovering from the issue that led the patient to seek therapy initially (Swift & Greenberg, 2012).

A mutually agreed termination between the therapist and the patient can include a therapist's letter to the patient at termination. Gelman and colleagues (2010) view the provision of written materials as a part of therapy where patients can utilize these documents as transitional objects (e.g., Winnicott, 1953) between therapy sessions or upon termination from therapy. They explain that a letter from a therapist to a patient at the end of therapy facilitates a summary of the patients' gains. Similar to a transitional object, the letter offers patients a bridge between having been assisted in therapy to assisting themselves, and it offers therapists the opportunity to assess clearly the therapy work and if any further work is needed (Gelman et al., 2010). It has been shown that patients tend to accept summary letters at termination in a positive way (Gelman et al., 2010; Leibovich & Zilcha-Mano, 2017). The letter can serve as a summary of a successful course of therapy.

Are there tasks that comprise the termination phase? Norcross et al. (2017, p. 71) delineate eight core therapeutic tasks of termination that lead to a successful course of therapy across theoretical approaches. The tasks include the following: 1) focus on the feelings of the members of the therapeutic dyad; 2) plan for ways in the future for patients to deal with new challenges; 3) assist clients to apply their skills outside the therapy milieu; 4) underscore the development of patients as not fully completed; 5) discuss the potential for progress after therapy; 6) focus on planning for ending therapy; 7) review the gains of clients; and 8) convey pride to patients about their growth and their contribution to the therapeutic relationship. The therapist can initiate the aforementioned core pantheoretical principles during the termination process in order to facilitate growth for patients (Norcross et al., 2017).

Are there factors that contribute to the different reactions that patients have during the termination phase of therapy? Marmarosh (2017, p. 4) explains that attachment theory can explain the varying responses that individuals have when ending therapy and how losses experienced earlier in life color a patient's self, capacity to cope with affect, and potential for intimacy (e.g., Bowlby, 1980; Stroebe, 2002; Wayment & Vierthaler, 2002). She notes that patients who are secure are more equipped to face loss, are more skilled in developing intimacy, deal better with termination, feel able to recognize gains and losses at termination, regulate affect better, can better cope with distress, are more skilled at seeking support outside of therapy, and can rely on a greater base of resources at termination when the therapist will no longer be there for them (e.g., Fraley & Shaver, 1999; Holmes, 1997, 2009; Shulman, 1999). According to Marmarosh (2017), patients who are secure have the ability to count on inner memories of attachment objects that facilitate connection in the face of the physical absence of the therapist post termination (e.g., Bowlby, 1980). The following vignette illustrates the therapist's response to a planned, mutually agreed termination initiated by a patient with a secure attachment.

Vignette of an Example of a Mutually Agreed Termination

INTRODUCTION

Here is an example of a mutually agreed termination that illustrates some of the aforementioned therapeutic tasks of termination. The patient, Anthony, has been in therapy for a year and a half, and expresses his wishes to end because he has accomplished his goals and has completed the tasks of therapy. Anthony has a secure attachment to the therapist. The following segment shows how a therapist engaged in the termination process by processing the feelings of the patient, Anthony, as well as his own feelings, began to address Anthony's future coping, planned for termination, and expressed pride in the mutual relationship during a session that took place a few sessions prior to termination.

DIALOGUE

> *Therapist's inner thoughts: Anthony spoke only briefly about ending therapy last week. Today, I wonder how he's thinking about the upcoming ending of therapy. He said that he has accomplished his goals and has completed the tasks involved in these goals.*
>
> **Therapist's statement:** I'm wondering if you have some thoughts about ending therapy that you'd like to share.
>
> *Patient's inner thoughts: I'll miss him. I'm wondering if I should try out being without him for a bit. How to do it?*

Patient's statement: I thought we were on the same wavelength, and I appreciated that. It took me two years to feel satisfied with myself, my new job, and my relationship. I'll miss you, but I think I'll be okay, and I want to know if I can try out being without you for a short time.

Therapist's inner thoughts: He values our positive relationship but wants to check out how he'll do without therapy for a short period of time.

Therapist's statement: We have a positive relationship. I'm proud of the progress that you made. I think that you'll be fine on your own. You want to check out how you'll be on your own prior to your last session.

Patient's inner thoughts: [Relief] Whew! He gets it. I'm relieved that he said that he agrees that I'll be okay. I'm also thinking that I want to try out how I'll be if I have a few more sessions, but every two weeks instead of every week.

Patient's statement: Yes. Good. I was hoping to have a few more sessions, every other week, to see how I do on my own during the alternate week when I'm not going to therapy. Is that okay?

Therapist's statement: That is a good idea. I'm with you here. That way, you'll have a chance to try out how you'll be prior to your last session.

Summary

In this vignette, which took place five sessions prior to the last session, the therapist began to process some of Anthony's feelings about the end of therapy and feelings about how he will be coping in the future. Anthony expressed positive feelings about the current relationship but was somewhat concerned that he needed to check out how it would feel to be on his own prior to his last session, when he would be on his own. Anthony seemed satisfied with how the therapist responded to his feelings by offering the possibility of a smooth transition to his last session and to his life after therapy.

Planned, mutually agreed terminations may be less challenging to patients and therapists than premature, unilateral terminations that are not planned. The following vignette is an example of a planned, mutually agreed termination that was initiated by a patient who was in short-term therapy.

Vignette of an Example of a Planned, Mutually Agreed Termination

INTRODUCTION

The following is a vignette of a planned termination between a cognitive-behavioral therapist and a patient with a phobia. This ending was initiated by a patient and was a mutually agreed termination. The client, Darci, initially contacted the therapist because of a specific phobia, a feeling of intense disgust every time she saw a cat. Darci is happily married with three children and has recently been promoted at work. The therapist treated the phobia with CBT, and the client responded well to the therapy. Darci has been in therapy for four months.

DIALOGUE

> *Patient's inner thoughts: Now that I no longer have my severe reaction to cats, I wonder how he'll take to my wish to end therapy.*
>
> **Patient's statement:** [With a bit of hesitation] You know when I see a cat now, I no longer get nauseous or feel my heart beating loudly, and I, sometimes, think that cats are nice.
>
> *Therapist's inner thoughts: I enjoyed working with this client; however, I agree that it is time for the client to end therapy since the goals of therapy have been met.*
>
> **Therapist's statement:** We went through several step-by-step exercises during the last few sessions, and, indeed, you are correct that you have accomplished your goal in therapy. How about I offer you one more homework assignment today, and then let's schedule another session to discuss how the homework session goes. After that, I would suggest one additional session to process the ending of therapy, and, at that time, if all is well, I would agree you can end therapy, having met your goal.

SUMMARY

The vignette described a termination between a therapist with a cognitive-behavioral approach and a patient with a phobia who initiated termination.

The goals of therapy were accomplished, and Darci and her therapist agreed to a mutual termination.

Whether in short-term therapy, where the goals of therapy are explicit and direct, as in the case of Darci in the prior example, or in long-term treatment, when patients reach a point in their work with the therapist where they feel that they are ready to end therapy, the termination process needs to take place with care; care on the part of therapists and on the part of patients. Perhaps patients have made changes in their life that have increased their confidence and insight, or perhaps clients were depressed, as in the case of Dolores with dysthymia (in Chapter 4), and with the work that they accomplished through therapy have developed ways to cope that allow them to feel more energetic in settings beyond therapy, as in the case of Darren (in Chapter 4). In any case, patients will, at times, question whether they have progressed and no longer need therapy. Some patients in this chapter and in the next will discuss their thoughts and feelings with their therapists. Others such as Salvadore (in a later section) are reluctant to express their feelings about being ready to end for fear that they will hurt their therapists' feelings, that the therapist will not agree that they are ready, or that, in reality, they are not ready to end therapy. As illustrated in the vignettes included in this chapter, thoughts and feelings about termination might create a conflict for patients. Although most therapists discuss the goals of therapy with their patients, particularly psychotherapists with a cognitive-behavioral viewpoint, some practitioners, many from an experiential, relational, and psychodynamic perspective, have a more open-ended process. More long term and in depth, with a focus on extended growth through the life cycle, relationships with therapists with a psychodynamic perspective, as in the case of Melissa and her therapist (in Chapter 4), can continue for many months. Although the members of the therapeutic dyad are aware that therapy will end at some point, they recognize that they will engage in a process of exploration for a long period of time.

The termination initiated by the patient, Darci, in the previous vignette was a mutually agreed termination that took place in short-term therapy. Darci and the therapist agreed that an end to therapy was acceptable. There are other types of termination that are not mutually agreed upon or are unplanned terminations. For example, premature or unilateral terminations or dropouts are unplanned. Some terminations that are unplanned occur as a result of ruptures or disagreements in the therapeutic relationship. Some unplanned terminations can happen because the goals or tasks of therapy are not realistic or are not necessarily the core of the problem. A premature termination that is initiated by a patient is one where the patient decides to terminate therapy contrary to the advice of the therapist and to the initial contract between the therapist and the patient (Ogrodniczuk et al., 2005). Many times, premature terminations may happen early in the therapy, prior to the patient having an opportunity to garner much improvement; however, there are other times when patients initiate a unilateral termination when they have felt that they have benefitted from the therapy (Ogrodniczuk et al., 2005). In cases when a rupture leads to the ending of therapy, unfinished business remains for both the therapist and the client, with the therapist wondering about what she or he did wrong, or if there might have been anything that she or he could have done differently so that the process would not have ended abruptly, without any closure (Garfield,1994; Ogrodniczuk et al., 2005). Sometimes, during abrupt premature terminations (e.g., Zoey in a later section), for example, where the client walks out in the middle of the session because of a serious rupture or the client does not show up for another session and does not call to cancel the next appointment and/or does not return the therapist's call, the client does not think and/or does not care about the effect of the termination on the therapist. Some clients (e.g., Paisley in a later section) who feel that the therapy did not meet their expectations, that their goals were unmet, may be hesitant to seek therapy services in the future, and/or they may become reluctant to build sustaining relationships beyond therapy. Given these scenarios, it is critical for therapists to seek to become aware of unplanned terminations and to explore how to decrease these deleterious events (Swift et al., 2018). Throughout the therapy process, it is useful for therapists to work on building the therapeutic alliance, and to observe verbal and nonverbal minute-to-minute shifts in the therapy relationship.

Why do patient-initiated premature or unilateral terminations happen? Part I described a scenario where a patient, Glen, felt disappointed after trying out several approaches that were recommended by his therapist only to discover that these approaches did not work. A rupture in the therapeutic alliance was occurring, and the patient seemed to be on the verge of initiating a premature termination because he perceived that improvement did not happen quickly enough or was not happening at all. Other reasons for premature terminations initiated by a patient may be that the patient is scared about disclosing information to the therapist, the therapist and patient do not agree on what to discuss during therapy, the patient does not feel valued by the therapist, the patient's motivation is low, or the patient displays chronic defenses, such as denial (Ogrodniczuk, et al., 2005).

A client's ambivalence about change can be a factor that contributes to the therapeutic alliance and to the development of alliance ruptures, and it is critical for therapists to be sensitive and to respond to ambivalence in a way that is not defensive (Urmanche et al., 2019). A patient such as Jennifer (in the next vignette) who is ambivalent, on the one hand, may wish to work through issues that are essential, and, on the other, may resist some thoughts and actions that might facilitate the resolution of these issues. Jennifer's ambivalence resulted in discomfort for her and for the therapist when she called to set up an appointment and subsequently did not show up for the session. The next section addresses terminations initiated by patients and begins with a patient's ambivalence that leads to treatment refusal prior to the first session.

Terminations Initiated by Patients

Vignette of an Example of a Termination Prior to Beginning Therapy or a Client's Ambivalence and Treatment Refusal

What if patients have a difficult time deciding what they want? Here is an example of a patient who is unsure of what she wants. This vignette focuses on patient-initiated terminations. In some cases, patients enter treatment thinking that they want help or change, but they are ambivalent. Such is the case of the patient, Jennifer, in this vignette. One part of Jennifer wishes for a different kind of life; however, another part of Jennifer fears the change or the work that may be involved to reach the desired changes. Some patients who are ambivalent may be afraid to be vulnerable, to discuss their feelings, or to trust the therapist. The scenario included in this vignette addresses a patient-initiated termination that occurs prior to the beginning of therapy. In this case, the patient, Jennifer, receives a referral, and rejects therapy prior to the first session. When clients are ambivalent about change, they may have the opportunity to engage in therapy, but refuse. They may not show up for the first session. Treatment refusal happens when a client is offered a particular treatment and then decides not to accept the intervention (Swift & Greenberg, 2015; Swift et al., 2017). Swift and colleagues (2017) report the rate of treatment refusal to be 8.2%. This vignette illustrates an example of treatment refusal, a type of patient-initiated termination.

INTRODUCTION

A client, Jennifer, age 18, who is feeling fragile, reluctantly calls a psychologist at the recommendation of a parent, and then does not show up for the first session.

DIALOGUE

Patient's statement: Uh…. Uh… Hello.

Therapist's inner thoughts: I'm hungry and tired now. I'm wondering if I should take this call.

Therapist's statement: Hello.

Patient's inner thoughts: [Long pause] I know I need to do this now. My mother said she's had it, but now that I'm on the phone with this therapist, I'm not so sure.

Patient's statement: [A long pause] Can I make an appointment, maybe?

Therapist's inner thoughts: The client seems a bit hesitant or anxious. I'm not sure what to say.

Therapist's statement: Sure. When would you like? I have a few openings next week in the afternoon.

Patient's inner thoughts: I really don't need any therapy. I don't know why I'm doing this. My mother is holding it over my head.

Patient's statement: I guess next Monday is okay.

Therapist's statement: Monday at 1 P.M. would be fine. Is that time okay with you? What is your name?

Patient's statement: Jennifer Dallio.

Patient's inner thoughts: I'm trying to get off this phone as quickly as possible.

Therapist's inner thoughts: I wonder if I should invite her to open up a bit over the phone or just wait until the appointment.

Therapist's statement: Let me give you the address of my office. It's 47 Mulberry Lane, right off the highway, Suite 240. Would you like to tell me a bit more about why you're calling prior to your appointment?

Patient's statement: OK. Got it. No. Bye.

Summary

Jennifer called the therapist to make an appointment because her mother had been requesting that she do so for several weeks. The therapist recognized that Jennifer seemed ambivalent and anxious about therapy but was not quite sure how to approach Jennifer on the phone. Jennifer did not show up for the therapy session. The therapist called Jennifer later that day, left a message, but Jennifer did not respond or return her call. This was a case of treatment refusal in a naturalistic clinical setting. A type of treatment refusal in a naturalistic clinical setting may occur when a patient fails to follow up on a referral to meet with a practitioner (Swift et al., 2017). After receiving the referral, a client may be fearful to call about the referral, may call, but not show for the first session as in the case of Jennifer, or may look into details about the referral and select not to call that particular therapist and/or any other mental health practitioner.

Do psychologists, social workers, and psychiatrists know which patients will conclude therapy in a mutually agreed way and which clients will drop out of therapy? Mental health providers often do not know which patients will terminate therapy prematurely (Maeschalck et al., 2019). Maeschalck and colleagues (2019, p. 107) point out that it is patients' ratings of the therapeutic alliance that correlate more closely with outcome than do the ratings of therapists, and that therapists are not good judges of patients' feelings about the alliance (e.g., Horvath et al., 2011). The therapeutic alliance evolves over time and depends upon the delicate balance between therapists and patients. The vignettes in this chapter include examples of some patients who may not feel supported and may test their therapists to see if they are receptive to their needs, and these patients, in particular, are attuned to the shifts over time that may take place in the alliance, from one delicate situation or minute to the next, to see if their therapists are aware of their perceptions about the durability of the bond that exists between them. Patients with a less robust therapeutic alliance are at risk for ending therapy prematurely, and it is suggested that therapists focus on decreasing premature dropout from therapy by improving the quality of the relationship (Sharf et al., 2010). The therapeutic alliance is a key component for a successful intervention (Joyce et al., 2007). Joyce and colleagues (2007, p. 144) point out that clients who drop out of therapy report that they did not have as strong a therapeutic alliance with their therapists as did clients who do not initiate a premature termination (e.g., Mohl et al., 1991; Piper et al., 1999; Tryon & Kane, 1990). da Silva and colleagues (2022, p. 183) note that there are therapist variables as well that are related to a more encouraging therapeutic outcome and the lowest incidence of premature termination, and these include factors such as a therapist's training, a therapist's professional experience, the capacity of the therapist to be flexible and to understand the patient's difficulty, and the ability of the therapist to offer psychological support (e.g., Blatt et al., 1996; Gülüm et al., 2016; Roos & Werbart, 2013).

Sometimes premature terminations are initiated by patients because of a rupture or impasse in the therapeutic alliance that may or may not be repaired. The next section includes a vignette where the patient initiates a termination that is not a result of a rupture in the therapeutic alliance.

Vignette of an Example of a Premature Termination Initiated by a Patient

INTRODUCTION

Here is an example of a patient who initiates termination. The patient, Salvadore, has been in therapy for four months. In the following vignette, Salvadore, age 33, is considering telling his therapist that he feels that he has been doing well for two weeks and believes that it is time for him to apply what he has learned on his own. Salvadore has had these thoughts during the last month, with increasing frequency during the last couple of weeks.

DIALOGUE

Patient's inner thoughts: Should I do it now? I don't want to wait because then we'll get into another topic, and we'll get to the end of the session, and I won't have spoken about ending.

Patient's statement: I have been thinking over the last few weeks that maybe it is time for me to end therapy. I think that I have made a lot of progress. I got a promotion, and I'm getting along well.

Therapist's inner thoughts: I knew he was feeling better, more self-assured, but this takes me by surprise. He is still not able to access some of his deep feelings, and I fear that this might be premature.

Therapist's statement: I have noticed that you are feeling more confident, and your promotion and the deepening of your relationship with your girlfriend are evidence that you have grown. I wonder if there is any work that is left undone that we might want to focus on before you end.

And yes, maybe things that you want to be alert to in the future. Even the ending of therapy can trigger some sadness and loss. How about we try another two months, and then see how you feel, and if you want to end then, then we end?

Patient's inner thoughts: This is perfect. I think she is right that it would be pretty hard to just stop right now. Maybe this could be helpful.

Patient's statement: Okay. This sounds like a good plan. Sounds good to me to bring up ending again after two months.

SUMMARY

In the above vignette, Salvadore is ready to end his therapy work. His external circumstances have changed, and he feels that he has accomplished what he set out as a goal in the therapy experience. He has been feeling like he wanted to end for a couple of weeks but was reluctant to share his thoughts with the therapist. Then, he lets her know. The therapist is taken by surprise. He has been a good patient. He has gained a lot from therapy. The therapist knows that he may benefit further from therapy, and she discusses the idea that he might want to look at things left undone. She does not push this but does suggest that they take some time to go through a process of ending. He is quite amenable to this idea. One of the issues that the therapist worked on with Salvadore during his four months of therapy was his need to develop a sense that he develops his own plans at his own pace without interference from family members. The therapist may continue to believe that Salvadore has deeper feelings to address; however, she accedes to his wishes in order to give him a sense that he is the captain of his own ship, a captain that feels that he develops his own wishes and plans to sail his new ship on his own. At the same time, she knows that there will be discussions during the next two months, and it is possible that Salvadore might change his mind. Either way, it is Salvadore who feels ready to end, and there's no pressing reason that he cannot end therapy if he wishes. The therapist will go along with Salvadore's plan unless he changes his mind or there is stronger indication that he needs to change his mind because he is not doing well and/or that his circumstances have changed.

Endings can evoke concern and conflict in either therapists or patients. The vignettes include examples of patients who initiate termination. The therapists in these examples seek to evaluate their work with their patients to determine that they are ready to end treatment, and determining when and how to talk about ending therapy requires reflection so that the termination process can happen in a way that reinforces the work that has occurred throughout the process. One hopes that therapists do not prolong treatment for their own personal reasons (e.g., therapists' wishes to keep a client in order not to lose income or a time slot open that might be of concern if in a group practice).

The therapist in the next vignette, in the initial therapy session, asks her patient, Tracy, that if she decides to end the therapy, she will meet for an additional session for closure. Initially, Tracy felt neutral about this request, and agreed with it. Some other patients of this therapist have been irritated by this request and have flat out disagreed with the therapist's request. Other patients have agreed in order to please this therapist. Yet, others consented at the time of the request, but reconsidered later in time. Generally, different from Tracy (next vignette), if patients do not agree that if they decide to end the therapy they will meet for an additional session for closure, therapists do not have many options, and the consequence is that there are loose ends for both. In the next vignette, although the patient, Tracy, initially agreed to an additional session for closure, she changed her mind because she was dissatisfied with therapy.

Vignette of an Example of a Rupture With a Patient Who Is Displeased With Therapy and Initiates a Unilateral Termination

INTRODUCTION

Here is an example of a client who is not satisfied with therapy and initiates a unilateral termination. The patient, Tracy, age 34, has been in therapy for seven weeks, and this is the seventh session. In this vignette, the therapist had asked Tracy, at the beginning of the first session of therapy, to agree to have a closure session prior to ending therapy. Tracy had agreed that it made sense and was committed to doing so. However, from the beginning, Tracy was dissatisfied with the therapist, and after six sessions, she became more and more dissatisfied with the course of the treatment itself. She felt that the therapist did not understand her, although she had not mentioned this source of tension in prior meetings. In what would be their last meeting, Tracy started the session saying that she wanted to evaluate where they were in the process and see if the therapy was meeting her needs.

Dialogue

Patient's inner thoughts: It's really been a drain for me. I'm not getting much out of it. But I feel so darn bad. Maybe nothing can help.

Patient's statement: [At the beginning of the seventh and last session] I don't think that this therapy has helped me much. Maybe it's time for me to stop.

Therapist's inner thoughts: I had a sense that she may not be completely satisfied but didn't realize it was this bad for her. I didn't realize the extent. I may indeed have missed some signals from her.

Therapist's statement: Can we discuss your dissatisfaction? I would like to hear more from you.

Patient's inner thoughts: I guess she is going to push me around again. She wants to know why I don't like her, but I don't feel like working for her, for having to discuss her concerns. Why do I have to tell her? She needs to be about helping me. I just want out now.

Patient's statement: Well, I haven't really felt like you were getting me. You seem to have your own view, your own agenda, and, sometimes, don't get what I was saying. I don't feel that you're out there for me.

Therapist's inner thoughts: How could I have been so blind? How do I repair this? I know that I need to be empathic and authentic.

Therapist's statement: I hear your unhappiness, and I am sorry. How can we get back? How can you continue your therapy?

Patient's inner thoughts: Again, it's all about her and her agenda. This seems all about her – how she can get me to keep continuing therapy. Why can't she just hear me, hear that it's over? Hear that I want to end, and now.

Patient's statement: I don't know. I think I want to end now.

Therapist's inner thoughts: I may have lost her. When she first began therapy, she did agree to another closure session. How can I retrieve this?

Therapist's statement: I feel sad that I missed the signals that you were not feeling that I was not getting you. We're almost at the end of our session. Can we continue this conversation so that we can understand what went wrong? When you began therapy, we agreed to have a closure session prior to ending. Will that be okay with you?

Patient's inner thoughts: I do NOT want to do that.

Patient's statement: I prefer not to. Therapy has never worked for me, and I've had it with you and therapy.

SUMMARY

In this segment, the patient, Tracy, had not engaged in the therapy process as the therapist believed was the case. The therapist did not realize the extent of Tracy's dissatisfaction with how the therapy was going. It appears that she was unaware of the signs that Tracy was not feeling understood. The therapist was blindsided. This termination is also a rupture, where the therapist has limited options in terms of repair. In these cases, the therapist may seek consultation to try to understand better why she missed the signs that Tracy was dissatisfied. In addition, there is some concern about the patient – what the potential harm may be without the opportunity for the therapist to provide any closure.

Approximately three months later, the therapist receives a call from Tracy. The therapist is stunned. The patient says that she wishes to return for one more closure session. The therapist offers the patient an appointment. The therapist is baffled, but then has some ideas.

INTRODUCTION

In the previous segment, the patient, Tracy, initiated termination without explaining, in detail, her reasons for doing so. She did not wish to honor the agreement of one last closure session to which she had agreed during the first therapy session.

DIALOGUE

Therapist's inner thoughts: Tracy seemed adamant about ending therapy. I didn't expect her to return, and I wonder what brings her back, but I will let her lead.

Patient's inner thoughts: This is somewhat embarrassing. I hope that she doesn't gloat or tell me I told you that you needed therapy. I'll walk right out if that happens. I'm so uncomfortable.

Therapist's statement: [Speaks lightly, noticing patient's discomfort] Welcome. It's nice to see you.

Patient's inner thoughts: Maybe I can tell her what's on my mind.

Patient's statement: I have a lot on my mind. Thanks for, at least, not saying I told you so and that I told you, you'd return. I'm not sure where to begin.

Therapist's statement: Wherever feels comfortable for you.

Therapist's inner thoughts: She seems weighed down.

Patient's statement: When I left, I was trying out two other therapists. Perhaps that's why it was hard for me to focus on us. I'm still not convinced at all that you're the right therapist for me, but I'm now convinced that the other two are not.

Therapist's inner thoughts: I'm going to tread lightly and see where this goes. I won't bring up the one more closure session agreement with her. I'll let her lead.

Therapist's statement: Thank you for letting me know what occurred. I'm glad that you returned. How would you like to proceed?

Summary

At times, therapists may encounter patients who attend therapy sessions with other therapists. When encountering these situations, therapists may wish to discuss the advantages and disadvantages of seeing multiple therapists at the same time. In this vignette, Tracy returned and began to explain why she dropped out of therapy the first time. The therapist decided to tread lightly and to allow the patient to discuss how she would like to proceed. The initial closure was processed upon the patient's return and in subsequent sessions.

Sometimes, a patient will return after a patient-initiated termination. In the aforementioned vignette, the patient, Tracy, returned to therapy, and the closure was processed; however, not all closures will be processed. There is a good chance that patients may not return after a patient-initiated premature termination. In the aforementioned vignette that included the patient, Tracy, the extent of the bond between therapist and patient, and thus the impact of the unprocessed closure, depend on multiple factors, including the amount of time they worked together, whether a rupture preceded the abrupt end, or whether there were unforeseen circumstances (Tracy's meeting with other therapists which was not revealed until later in time) that proceeded the closure. The inability to understand why the ending occurred, for example, in the case of Tracy who is displeased with therapy and initiates termination, can create ambiguity for both patient and therapist that is difficult to process. It is only after Tracy returns and, in subsequent sessions, that the therapist learns the reasons for the patient's initiated termination.

Unforeseen circumstances that are not a consequence of ruptures, for example, a client who changes jobs, a therapist or a client who experiences an illness, a client who lacks transportation, can result in a premature termination. These occurrences can either serve as pauses in the therapy, or they may be conclusive endings that do not afford the members of the therapeutic dyad a chance to process the therapy work, and in these situations, patient and therapist are left with unanswered questions.

After a patient-initiated termination, if the patient does not return at some later point, both the therapist and the client will have unfinished business, things left unsaid, feelings unaddressed. How do therapists and patients resolve these issues, or do they? The relationship between the therapist and the client is a meaningful one, with clients hoping to receive help and support while working on change with therapists who work to facilitate growth for clients who wish to increase their self-awareness. When therapists are faced with a lack of opportunity to process endings with clients, many therapists select to discuss the abrupt ending and their unresolved feelings about it in a supervision session scheduled to address the particular situation, for example, the situation of the newly licensed clinical psychologist in the next vignette who seeks supervision after the client, Zoey, drops out of therapy. This process is especially important for novice or intermediate therapists, but even more seasoned therapists, when stuck, can benefit from consulting with a supervisor after an abrupt termination, so that the ambiguity about the ending does not cause lasting discomfort and so that therapists can develop ways to process these occurrences in the future.

Ogrodniczuk and colleagues (2005) assert that unplanned, patient-initiated premature or unilateral terminations can be difficult for novice therapists. They explain that therapists who lose patients to premature termination may experience anger, loss, rejection, or hurt, and some therapists, particularly those therapists whose essence is connected to their capacity to help others, may experience a narcissistic injury. In the following vignette, a novice therapist is spared the fate of suffering a deeper injury because she shared her patient's initiated premature or unilateral termination with a supervisor who was sensitive to her predicament as a beginning therapist.

Vignette of an Example of a Premature Termination Initiated by a Client After a Rupture and Its Effect Upon a Therapist

INTRODUCTION

The following is an example of the impact of a client-initiated premature termination on a therapist, a newly licensed clinical psychologist. The scenario is a supervisory session between the newly licensed clinical psychologist and his former supervisor. The clinical psychologist had recently seen the client, Zoey, for five sessions, during which he recognized that Zoey was struggling with depression, marital issues, and in jeopardy of losing her job. During their last session, he thought that the relationship was building, and that Zoey was beginning to talk about her marital and job concerns more openly and to become less inclined to get depressed and give up. During that session, Zoey discussed her feelings of depression related to her marriage and her job and about her boss who chronically demanded work from her at the last minute. The therapist empathized with the client, but advised that she stay the course, no matter what, particularly since Zoey needed the money. When Zoey left, she said that she appreciated the therapist's concern, but she did not show up for her next appointment. When the therapist called, he left a message, but he received no response. The therapist was concerned about Zoey and surprised that she did not return. He called again, and Zoey said that she was fine but decided that she did not want to return to therapy. He had consulted with his former supervisor once about Zoey. Questioning himself about what he had done, he set up another appointment with his former supervisor.

DIALOGUE

Therapist's inner thoughts: I used to be his supervisee. He helped me out a lot, and I trust his opinion.

Therapist's statement: I don't know why Zoey doesn't want to return to therapy. She didn't show up, and I called twice. The first time, she didn't return my call. The second time, she picked up the phone, and said that she would not be returning to therapy. I feel bad. I don't understand what happened.

Supervisor's inner thoughts: How unfortunate that he has to experience this so soon after becoming newly licensed. He was a conscientious supervisee and therapist. This abrupt termination initiated by his client, Zoey, has created more self-doubt and insecurity for him.

Supervisor's statement: You have talked a little about Zoey, but I do not know much about her history. I think when we talked last you told me that she was quite depressed. In this case, you may be concerned because it feels to you as if Zoey is giving up, on her job, and now on her therapy.

Therapist's inner thoughts: He's trying to be supportive to me, but I know it's still my fault that Zoey dropped out.

Therapist's statement: Zoey seemed able to recognize that I'm concerned about her. She needs this job, and, given her depression, I didn't want her to give up on it too fast.

Supervisor's inner thoughts: He's a good therapist. He was concerned that her depression would get in the way of her ability to see the whole situation about her job and that Zoey might give up too soon. How to let him know that he may have overreacted by offering her advice about her job that was a bit extreme, that is, to keep at it and stay the course, no matter what.

Supervisor's statement: What do you think Zoey thought about your concerns?

Therapist's inner thoughts: My supervisor understands what happened. I overreacted, in somewhat of an extreme way by advising Zoey that she stay at her job no matter what because she needs the money. I kept giving her the message not to quit because of her depression.

Therapist's statement: Yes. I overreacted. I was so concerned that this was another situation where Zoey would be too depressed to see the whole situation and would give up quickly. Zoey doesn't like overbearing advice. I missed the mark.

Supervisor's inner thoughts: These are learning experiences. I hope that I can convey these thoughts so that his experience as a newly licensed psychologist can deepen.

Supervisor's statement: I know how difficult these unilateral terminations are. You are a conscientious therapist who wants the best for Zoey and your other clients. Zoey felt that you cared. Therapists, in general, need to focus on regulating the intensity of their responses and to attend, on a moment-to-moment basis, to clients' nonverbal and verbal responses. Being a therapist is not easy; it is human. The situation with your client, Zoey, has thrown you into a self-doubt zone, but, as you and I know, ruptures and premature terminations will occur, and some may result in dropout. I know that you recognize what occurred and can integrate it for the future.

Therapist's inner thoughts: He's right. I feel a little better. Will watch my advice-giving tendency in the future.

Therapist's statement: I know. It does not help me to ruminate, but I do feel bad. I will think about your words this week.

SUMMARY

The vignette illustrates the effect of a client-initiated premature termination on a newly licensed psychologist. The early career psychologist sought assistance in order to understand the reason that his client, Zoey, suddenly dropped out of therapy. The supervisor helped him to understand that although he was concerned about his client's tendency to give up easily, and particularly in connection to her job where she needed the money, it seemed that he overreacted as he offered advice, which Zoey had mentioned in the past that she is not seeking, and he did so in an intense way, saying to his client, "stay the course no matter what." Recognizing that this was an early career psychologist, the supervisor took care to empathize with how bad the psychologist was feeling about the dropout initiated by Zoey.

The following vignette is another example of a premature termination. It illustrates a scenario where a patient-initiated premature termination after three sessions occurred while the therapist was on vacation. In this example, the therapist did not feel that a strong therapeutic alliance had developed prior to leaving for his vacation. The patient, Miles, felt troubled and needed to speak to someone while the therapist was on vacation. Miles felt that he had hardly begun to speak when the therapist decided to go on vacation. Although the therapist offered a substitute therapist while he was on vacation, Miles felt that he needed the help of the therapist and did not feel like initiating with the temporary therapist while his therapist was away.

Vignette of an Example of an Unplanned, Premature Termination Initiated by a Patient

INTRODUCTION

A premature termination was initiated by the patient, Miles, who is 41 years old. In this scenario, the therapist has been in practice for ten years. Miles had seen the therapist for three sessions when the therapist decided to go on a two-week summer vacation. When the therapist returned, the therapist became aware that Miles left a cancellation message over the phone refusing further sessions.

DIALOGUE

Patient's inner thoughts: My therapist has decided to take a vacation right after I first met him and needed him most. What good is he? I don't believe in this whole therapy bit and don't need it. I simply won't return, but the therapist is nice, and I'm a responsible person. So, I'll let him know.

[The patient calls the therapist and leaves a message on the therapist's answering machine informing the therapist of the cancellation of the next session]

Patient's statement: [On the therapist's answering machine] I'm canceling my next session.

Therapist's inner thoughts: I wonder why Miles decided to drop out of therapy. I surely didn't see this happening. Things seemed to be going so smoothly. We seemed to be working so well together. Hmm... I wonder if this has anything to do with my vacation.

[Then, the therapist calls the patient and leaves the following message on the patient's answering machine]

Therapist's statement: I received your message and was disappointed that you decided to drop out of therapy. I realize that it might have been difficult for you to start the process and then for me to go on vacation not long after we began. I imagine that you felt that my going on vacation was poor timing and maybe even abrupt. I'm sorry if it was hurtful. I wonder if you would be willing to meet for a session so that we can discuss it.

[Miles does not respond to the call. The therapist mulls over the situation during the two weeks following the cancellation call. He reflects on what occurred to cause this premature termination]

Therapist's inner thoughts: I wonder why the patient decided to drop out of therapy altogether, not to return, wouldn't even agree to another session to discuss the matter. Maybe it had something to do with my vacation week. But I informed Miles that I would be going out of town, and I did give him a phone number of a therapist who would be covering for me while I would be away.

[The therapist decides to write the patient a nice note letting the patient know how much he has enjoyed the work with the patient and that the patient can feel free to return, if he desires]

Therapist's statement: "Dear Miles, I was disappointed that you decided to end therapy. I was encouraged by how easily we connected and by your motivation. It seemed like you were already making some changes. It is not clear to me if my going on vacation caused you to doubt me and the process. I do hope that you will consider returning to therapy. I would like that. It's been a pleasure working with you."

Patient's inner thoughts: [After receiving the letter] Wow. This therapist took time to call me and even gave a darn to treat me like a human being and write me a nice note. What a nice gesture. Somebody cares. Maybe I'll give this therapist another chance. He seems reliable and trustworthy, hard to find these days.

[Eight weeks later, Miles calls the therapist, expresses some hesitation, but sets up another appointment]

Summary

The aforementioned vignette where the therapist self-disclosed by writing a note that expressed that he enjoyed the work with the client seemed to make a difference in the client's experiential world. After receiving the therapist's letter, the client felt encouraged to continue in therapy. Sometimes situations do not turn around as in the previous vignette. They end, and they may leave the therapist and client feeling puzzled.

Farber (2010) discusses competencies in therapy from the point of view of an existential-humanistic approach. This approach underscores the therapy relationship and its reliance on the therapist's ability to be genuine, accepting, and present when engaged with the client. The therapist's genuineness and capacity to relate with congruence (Rogers, 1957) refers to a therapist's authenticity and willingness to be transparent in relating to a client (Cain, 2007, Cooper, 2007; Farber, 2010). A therapist's presence and self-disclosure in the service of promoting a client can facilitate support and security for a client (Cooper, 2007; Farber, 2010; Yalom, 1980). In the aforementioned vignette, although Miles initially dropped out of therapy, he changed his mind about prematurely terminating and felt encouraged to continue therapy after the therapist self-disclosed how he valued him as an individual.

Clients are sensitive to the behaviors and responses of their therapists to varying degrees, such as the way that the therapist reacts when greeting the client, the response to disclosures during the session, or any changes that occur in the therapy such as shifts in the calendar. As previously discussed in the chapters on ruptures in the therapeutic alliance, clients differ with respect to their vulnerability to therapists' behaviors and their reactions. Clients test therapists in many ways, such as to see if the therapist is prejudiced. Chapter 1 included a vignette of an African American client, Craig, who allowed the therapist to recover after committing a rupture that involved a microaggression with the theme of criminality. The next section explores the connection between premature terminations initiated by clients and ruptures that include racial microaggressions.

Premature Terminations and Racial Microaggressions

A previous chapter described the effect of racial microaggressions within the context of therapeutic settings. Microaggressions have been shown to be detrimental to individuals who seek mental health services (Walls et al., 2015). Imagine being in a toxic space for the entire day. This space is where patients of racial minority groups, for example, persons of color, Latinos, find themselves as they experience racial microaggressions on a daily basis. Consider how you would feel if you are an American citizen, have lived in the United States for your entire life, and heard the following interchanges directed toward you wherever you went, all day long.

> *Are you from the United States?*
> *You speak English in a sophisticated way.*
> And on and on…

These microaggressions, repeated on a daily basis, can confuse, disarm, and irritate members of racial minority groups. Psychotherapists need to try to avoid them in order to preserve the quality of the therapeutic alliance. Why is there a low use of therapy services by people of color, native Americans, Hispanic Americans, and Asians? Some attribute underutilization of therapy services by racial minority groups and premature termination, in part, to therapists' racial biases (Burkard & Knox, 2004; Kearney et al., 2005; Sue et al., 2007).

A previous chapter described a microaggression that a therapist committed at the beginning of the first therapy session. The client, Amelia, the target of the microaggression, although understandably put off at the beginning allowed the therapist to recover, perhaps, because she picked up on the therapist's caring manner. In the following vignette, a therapist commits a microaggression in the first session, and the client terminates therapy abruptly. The therapist does not get an opportunity to apologize to the patient. The vignette describes an example of a premature termination initiated by a patient; a hard, cold stop where the patient, Paul, terminates therapy prior to giving the therapist an opportunity to repair the rupture, this time because of a racial microaggression.

Vignette of an Example of a Client Who Initiated a Premature Termination After a Therapist's Racial Microaggression: A Hard Cold Stop

INTRODUCTION

Racial microaggressions come in different sizes and colors. Mental health professionals need to be aware that racial microaggressions are a constant reality for Asian Americans (Ong et al., 2013). In this therapeutic setting, an Asian American client, Paul, a junior in high school, attended his first session with a therapist in a clinic. The therapist committed a microaggression, and Paul terminated therapy. The art of repairing microaggressions is a strategy that can help therapists avoid premature terminations initiated by clients. In this vignette, Paul terminated abruptly, and the therapist did not have an opportunity to repair the rupture.

DIALOGUE

> *Patient's inner thoughts: I don't know if I'm really up to this, but the guidance counselor said I have to go, and my parents have been pushing too.*
>
> **Patient's statement:** I really don't feel like doing much of anything with the after school groups. I'm feeling kind of down and stressed lately. I dropped out of all after school activities.
>
> **Therapist's statement:** Yes. I know. Your guidance counselor at school contacted me and said that you've not been yourself lately.
>
> **Patient's statement:** Yeah. I suppose so. School requires that we join after school groups. Not really up to it now.

Therapist's thoughts: Gee. He really looks down. I want to cheer him up a bit.

Therapist's statement: [Looking at a list of activities available for students at his client's school] Well, let's see here. You can join the computer group because you folks excel at that.

Patient's inner thoughts: Oh no. Another one who has me pegged for one of those computer types. It's really not what I need now.

[Client looks down and goes silent]

Therapist's thoughts: I tried to encourage him, but it looks like I may have made a faux pas. Maybe I can recover.

Therapist's statement: It looks like I've offended you.

Client's statement: I'm sorry, but I need to go now.

[Client gets up and silently slips out the door]

Summary

The therapist, in his haste, to encourage this high school student committed a microaggression when he assumed that because his client is Asian American, he would like to join the computer group, thereby excluding a range of other opportunities for his client. Paul, accustomed to hearing this type of microaggression several times a week, did not seem to wish to engage the services of a therapist who would perpetuate this kind of slight, which he felt seemed to be daily fare for him. Furthermore, the therapist may have overstepped his bounds as he attempted to cheer up the client while he committed a microaggression. Although the therapist realized his faux pas, the client rapidly slipped out the door, and the therapist did not have the opportunity to correct his error and to begin building a therapeutic alliance.

The aforementioned example of a premature termination that can be attributed to the therapist's microaggression took place during in-person therapy. Online therapy is different from in-person therapy, and setbacks in online communication are inevitable (Weinberg et al., 2023). Chapter 1 described how a therapist was able to preserve the therapeutic alliance by repairing a rupture that ensued when a patient, Conrad, expressed his discomfort with videoconferencing during the pandemic. The next section includes a vignette that describes an example of a patient, Paisely, who initiated a premature termination during a videoconferencing session.

Vignette of an Example of a Rupture that Resulted in a Premature Termination Initiated by a Patient

Introduction

The client, Paisely, age 22, met with the therapist for her second therapy session. In the first therapy session, Paisely and the therapist experienced technical problems during the session. The therapist apologized for these problems, and the client made another appointment.

Dialogue

> *Patient's inner experience: A lot of technical hassles during the last session. Really annoying. Just when I got to several punch lines, the line went out. She didn't call me back right away. There was static. Gee. It's a pain.*
>
> **Patient's statement:** [Silence for a few minutes] It's hard getting started here. Don't know what to talk about…
>
> *Therapist's inner thoughts: I hope that the videoconferencing will hold up. I've been having trouble with the connections this week…*
>
> **Therapist's statement:** Anything that comes to your mind is fine.
>
> *Patient's inner thoughts: Maybe I'll start with my grief. My mother just died…*
>
> **Patient's statement:** My mother passed away. What? Static again? Can you hear me?
>
> *Patient's inner thoughts: Darn. The line dropped. If she cannot manage her technical stuff, how can she help me? I don't need her.*
>
> *Therapist's inner thoughts: Oh no. There's an outage. The connection dropped. I'm going to call her back right away.*
>
> [Therapist calls back twice. Phone rings, but client does not pick up. The therapist leaves a message and then sends a note but the client does not respond]

Summary

The limitation of technical problems that accompanies videoconferencing sessions rears its head during Paisley's sessions. The therapist was aware of power outages in her area that week, intermittent line breaks because of the outages, and she did what she could by calling Paisely back when the session was interrupted. It seems that Paisley's second therapy session could barely begin because of the abrupt line interruptions that resulted in an alliance rupture which the therapist was not able to repair despite her calling and writing to the client. A client-initiated premature termination ensued, and the client did not return the therapist's calls or respond to the therapist's note.

In the previous example, the client, Paisley, who initiated premature termination was 22 years old. With respect to clients and dropout from therapy, researchers have shown that clients who are younger are at a greater risk for premature termination than clients who are older (Swift & Greenberg, 2015). With respect to therapists, it was found that the rates of client dropout for therapists who were younger were not higher than the rates of client dropout for therapists who were older; however, it was shown that therapists who were in training had a greater number of clients who terminated prematurely than therapists who had concluded their training (Swift & Greenberg, 2015).

Ogrodniczuk and colleagues (2005) suggest that given that there are a myriad of factors that may be responsible for a premature termination initiated by a patient and that there is no single strategy that can be used to avoid dropout in every situation, a therapist needs to be aware of a variety of strategies that may mitigate these negative events that are obstacles to therapy and have far reaching consequences. They explain that these strategies may take place prior to therapy and during therapy, and they indicate that one of the most critical strategies for the prevention of premature termination by patients during therapy is the development of a robust therapeutic relationship. In fact, researchers assert that in order to have a strong effect on premature termination initiated by patients, it is important to develop a therapeutic alliance within the first three therapy sessions (Ogrodniczuk et al., 2005; Rainer & Campbell, 2001). Chapters 5 and 6 propose a transtheoretical model of ruptures, repair, and termination that includes ways to build a lasting therapeutic alliance and to develop strategies to decrease premature terminations.

The previous sections explored mutually agreed terminations and premature or unilateral terminations initiated by clients. Therapists with different therapeutic approaches need to be aware of the potential for abrupt or premature terminations, based on ruptures that may occur between the therapist and the patient. The following section discusses terminations initiated by therapists.

Terminations Initiated by Therapists

Terminations can be initiated by therapists as well as by clients, and often can occur as a result of a therapist's illness, a therapist's move, a change in the financial circumstances of the patient, or a therapist's retirement. Swift and colleagues (2017, p. 48) point out that when premature terminations take place, they can negatively affect clients (e.g., Björk et al., 2009; Cahill et al., 2003; Swift et al., 2009) and practitioners (e.g., Ogrodniczuk et al., 2005; Piselli et al., 2011), and that whereas it has been found that approximately 20% of patients prematurely end psychotherapy (e.g., Fernandez et al., 2015; Swift & Greenberg, 2012), 30% to 50% of patients have been shown to prematurely end pharmacotherapy (e.g., Cramer & Rosenheck, 1998; Nantz et al., 2009; Sansone & Sansone, 2012).

The ending of therapy initiated by the patient, Darci, in an earlier vignette was planned and mutually agreed by therapist and patient. The ending initiated by the patient, Paul, in an earlier vignette was abrupt and was a direct result of a rupture connected to a microaggression. Endings in therapy can be unplanned and abrupt for reasons other than a therapeutic rupture. Practical issues, such as the illness or death of the therapist, a sudden move by the therapist, or the therapist's retirement may lead to an abrupt or premature termination.

Some therapy relationships have a planned, contracted time limit. An example of a planned termination with a time limit, different from the type of planned termination in an earlier vignette with Darci and her therapist, includes therapy relationships in university counseling centers where student therapists leave at the end of the year. In these situations, the student therapist initiates the ending. Although, at university counseling centers, the members of the therapeutic dyad, from the outset of therapy, are cognizant of the therapy end date and when therapy begins to draw to an end, the therapist discusses termination and offers the patient referrals to other therapists, forced planned terminations such as these initiated by therapists may include a challenge that is different from the planned ending in the vignette with Darci.

As difficult, if not more difficult, for the patient and the therapist, is an unplanned termination initiated by the therapist, such as the one that occurs in the following vignette, an example of an unplanned, coerced, or forced termination, initiated by a therapist because of an external variable, her move to another state. Unplanned, forced terminations, such as the following one with the patient, Pat, although common, can be a particular challenge for the therapeutic dyad; however, for some patients, they may not have a large effect. The next vignette includes an example of a termination initiated by a therapist when she moved out of the state.

Vignette of an Example of a Termination Initiated by the Therapist

INTRODUCTION

In this scenario, the therapist had studied the literature on termination and was aware of the suggested steps to take. She had concern for her patients and their reactions, but she knew that she wished to live in a state which would be closer to her father so that she could help him with his illness. The therapist accepted an academic position in another state. She discussed her plan with her patients seven months prior to accepting the academic position, and the process of saying goodbye continued through the end of the seventh month. This is the story of one patient, Pat, with whom the therapist had worked for many years. During the course of therapy, Pat had suffered the loss of her mother and was fired from her job, but now felt better able to navigate several of the challenges in her personal and professional life. The following dialogue took place seven months prior to termination.

DIALOGUE

> *Therapist's inner thoughts: I am anxious about telling her about my move and accepting my new academic position out of town. Maybe I can wait until next week... No, perhaps, better to begin now.*
>
> **Therapist's statement:** I want to talk with you about our work together and let you know that I have decided to accept an academic position in another state and will no longer see patients beginning next March. We have worked well over many years. You have experienced many gains from therapy. For example, you have reached many of the goals you set when you first began therapy. I'm aware that we have worked together on many issues that run deep for you, and, from my perspective, you have developed the strength and resilience to deal with your life in a reflective manner. This will be hard for us, but we will have several months to process our feelings and develop a plan for you going forward.

Patient's inner thoughts: Oh no! I knew this day may come, but I didn't think it would be now. How am I going to manage on my own? Oh no. Oh no... How can this be happening? Oh no... This can't be happening... Not now... Not when I'm first beginning to get my footing. Why is this happening to me? Oh no... [Breathing rapidly]

Patient's statement: [Closes her eyes, then looks down. Looks up with tears in her eyes] I don't want to end therapy now. I don't know how I'll manage. Every week, I know that I can run stuff by you and get some input. You're a source of support for me. Why do these things keep happening to me? Why can't my life be smoother... I've struggled so much... I want to continue with you. Maybe you'll reconsider?

Therapist's inner thoughts: I knew this would be difficult, but I didn't think she would react strongly. She is doing well. I didn't want to upset her or stir up any past anguish...

Therapist's statement: I know this is a big surprise for you, Pat, and it will be hard, not only for you, but for me too. We have developed a bond with one another and though you don't know me in the same way that I know you, we have a connection that is strong. Lots of feelings will emerge, and I hope that we can talk about them as we proceed. In the meantime, we can continue to focus on the issues that get in the way of your managing the issues in your life.

Patient's inner thoughts: I know she wants me to hear that she's leaving, but how will I manage when she's not here anymore? Can I call her? Can I see her from time to time? Oh, trouble all the time... Although things have improved for me, I've had a lot of agony in my life. I hope she'll let me call her from time to time. I really need to stay in touch with her. I can't lose her now. This is so important for me.

Patient's statement: You would like me to hear that you're leaving, but you dropping this on me is like a bomb. Will I be able to contact you after we end, or will it just be over? Can I call you? Can I email you? Can I text you? I know you have your own life, and I've respected that in the past, but this is really hard for me... I'm not sure that I'm prepared for this... I don't want to sound unhinged, but I really need you. [Cries]

Therapist's inner thoughts: Wow, this is difficult. How do I set a firm boundary with her and be sensitive to how difficult it seems for her now? She's crying again.

Therapist's statement: I know how difficult this is for you. In the past, you have relied on me as a source of support for you. Even though we have talked about your growing strength and your progress in therapy in different parts of your life, you don't seem sure that you can manage. You are feeling a great loss.

Patient's inner thoughts: OK. But I'm still wondering about whether I could call her, whether I can even email her. Is this it, and I cannot ever contact her again? I don't know. Am I falling to pieces? What's going on with me? Oh, I'm trying to get it, but it's real hard. Really so unexpected. Breathe in slowly...

Patient's statement: But can I call you after you move in seven months? Can I email you? Can I text you? I know you're eager to move on with your life, but this is very hard for me. Please understand that I'm used to running things by you, important things. It's so hard.

Therapist's inner thoughts: This is tough. I want to set firm boundaries for when I move out of state, for me and for her, but I see how needy she is, at present.

Therapist's statement: During the next seven months, we will talk more about what happens after I leave town. We will do it together. We will come to an agreement about how to proceed.

Patient's inner thoughts: She's not really answering me now. I feel anxious.

Patient's statement: We have time yet, I know. You said you were leaving in March, right? Yeh, I suppose there will be around seven months to talk about my concerns, and I have many of them. So hard for me, but, at the same time, I can understand that you're looking forward to your new position. Must be hard seeing people like me day in and day out. Will you still be seeing patients in the new state? I want to clear all this up before you leave. It feels so bad for me.

Summary

The process of termination is delicate in many situations, whether or not it is based on external occurrences, for example, a therapist's retirement, the end of a therapist's practicum, or a move by a therapist. In this vignette, at the beginning of the termination process, the therapist initiates the termination when she decides to move and to accept an academic position in another state and to stop seeing patients. Pat and her therapist are recognizing that there will be work to do as they approach the final stages, including determining what, if any contact, there will be after the ending. Pat is feeling bereft and afraid that she will not be able to manage. The therapist is torn between wanting to be available to her client as she has been over the years of her treatment and wanting to set clear boundaries, for herself and for the client. Pat's recognition and integration of her own strength and resilience will be enhanced with a definitive closure. In addition, if the client decides to work with another therapist, having closure will enable her to form a bond unburdened by the loss of her current therapist.

Terminations occur for many reasons. They can be mutually agreed or unilateral. Some are planned, some are unplanned. Some unplanned or unilateral terminations are initiated by therapists, and some are initiated by patients. Unfortunately, the mutually agreed therapy ending and an accompanying termination letter by a therapist to a patient is not the case for every patient. The aforementioned vignette involved a premature termination initiated by the therapist. Unplanned terminations, such as premature terminations seem to be recurrent issues in psychotherapy, and they are present across patient, intervention, and therapists' approaches to psychotherapy (Swift et al., 2018). Research has shown that approximately 8% of patients refuse assigned interventions, and approximately 20% of patients select to terminate treatment prematurely (Swift et al., 2017). Premature terminations can have deleterious effects for clients and therapists (Swift et al., 2018).

Chapter Summary

Chapter 3 defined the termination process and outlined the different types of terminations. The chapter explored planned and unplanned terminations, mutually agreed terminations, and premature terminations, and it identified premature terminations that were initiated by the therapist and endings that were initiated by the patient. Although therapists strive to avoid premature terminations because of their negative effects, sometimes, as in life external to therapy, terminations from therapy may not be avoidable. This chapter highlighted the ways that therapists may think about their own thoughts related to terminations and why they may strive to avoid premature terminations.

The next chapter, "Termination Across Different Diagnoses and Theories," describes terminations that have reached their natural end and the commonalities among therapists during the termination process. It then proceeds to premature terminations. The focus of Chapter 4 is on the different types of termination that evolve for patients with different emotional and personality disorders and how therapists with different theoretical orientations navigate the termination process with their patients who have different emotional and personality disorders. Examples of the inner experiences of therapists with different theoretical orientations and of the inner thoughts of patients with different emotional difficulties during the termination process are included in the chapter.

References

Barnett, J. E. (2016, October). 6 strategies for ethical termination of psychotherapy: And for avoiding abandonment. [Web article]. Retrieved from: https://societyforpsychotherapy.org/6-strategies-for-ethical-termination-of-psychotherapy/

Bartholomew, T. T., Lockard, A. J., Folger, S. F., Low, B. E., Poet, A. D., Scofield, B. E., & Locke, B. D. (2019). Symptom reduction and termination: Client change and therapist identified reasons for saying goodbye. *Counselling Psychology Quarterly, 32*(1), 81–99. https://doi.org/10.1080/09515070.2017.1367272

Bischoff, T., Krenicki, L., & Tambling, R. (2020). Therapist reported reasons for client termination: A content analysis of termination reports. *The American Journal of Family Therapy, 48*(1), 36–52. https://doi.org/10.1080/01926187.2019.1684216

Björk, T., Björck, C., Clinton, D., Sohlberg, S., & Norring, C. (2009). What happened to the ones who dropped out? Outcome in eating disorder patients who complete or prematurely terminate treatment. *European Eating Disorders Review, 17*(2), 109–119. https://doi.org/10.1002/erv.911

Blatt, S. J., Sanislow, C. A., III Zuroff, D. C., & Pilkonis, P. A. (1996). Characteristics of effective therapists: Further analyses of data from the National Institute of Mental Health Treatment of Depression Collaborative Research Program. *Journal of Consulting and Clinical Psychology, 64*(6), 1276–1284. https://doi.org/10.1037/0022-006x.64.6.1276

Bowlby, J. (1980). *Attachment and loss: Vol. 3,* Loss: Sadness and depression. Basic Books.

Burkard, A. W., & Knox, S. (2004). Effect of therapist color-blindness on empathy and attributions in cross-cultural counseling. *Journal of Counseling Psychology, 51*(4), 387–397. https://doi.org/10.1037/0022-0167.51.4.387

Cahill, J., Barkham, M., Hardy, G., Rees, A., Shapiro, D. A., Stiles, W. B., & Macaskill, N. (2003). Outcomes of patients completing and not completing cognitive therapy for depression. *British Journal of Clinical Psychology, 42*(2), 133–143. https://doi.org/10.1348/014466503321903553

Cain, D. J. (2007). What every therapist should know, be and do: Contributions from humanistic psychotherapies. *Journal of Contemporary Psychotherapy: On the Cutting Edge of Modern Developments in Psychotherapy, 37*(1), 3–10. https://doi.org/10.1007/s10879-006-9028-7

Cooper, M. (2007). Humanizing psychotherapy. *Journal of Contemporary Psychotherapy: On the Cutting Edge of Modern Developments in Psychotherapy, 37*(1), 11–16. https://doi.org/10.1007/s10879-006-9029-6

Cramer, J. A., & Rosenheck, R. (1998). Compliance with medication regimens for mental and physical disorders. *Psychiatric Services, 49*(2), 196–201. https://doi.org/10.1176/ps.49.2.196

da Silva, A. N., Ferreira, J. F., Conceição, N., Vaz Velho, C., & Vasco, A. B. (2022). Termination in psychotherapy: Contributions of an integrative metamodel. *Journal of Psychotherapy Integration, 32*(2), 175–189. https://doi.org/10.1037/int0000235

Farber, E. W. (2010). Humanistic-existential psychotherapy competencies and the supervisory process. *Psychotherapy: Theory, Research, Practice, Training, 47*(1), 28–34. https://doi.org/10.1037/a0018847

Fernandez, E., Salem, D., Swift, J. K., & Ramtahal, N. (2015). Meta-analysis of dropout from cognitive behavioral therapy: Magnitude, timing, and moderators. *Journal of Consulting and Clinical Psychology, 83*(6), 1108–1122. https://doi.org/10.1037/ccp0000044

Fraley, R. C., & Shaver, P. R. (1999). Loss and bereavement: Attachment theory and recent controversies concerning "grief work" and the nature of detachment. In J. Cassidy & P. R. Shaver (Eds.), *Handbook of attachment: Theory, research, and clinical applications* (pp. 735–759). Guilford Press.

Gabbard, G. O. (2009). What is a "good enough" termination? *Journal of the American Psychoanalytic Association, 57*(3), 575–594. https://doi.org/10.1177/0003065109340678

Garfield, S. L. (1994). Research on client variables in psychotherapy. In A. E. Bergin & S. L. Garfield (Eds.), *Handbook of psychotherapy and behavior change* (4th ed., pp 190–228). John Wiley & Sons.

Gelman, T., McKay, A., & Marks, L. (2010). Dynamic interpersonal therapy (DIT): Providing a focus for time-limited psychodynamic work in the National Health Service. *Psychoanalytic Psychotherapy, 24*(4), 347–361. https://doi.org/10.1080/02668734.2010.513556

Goldfried, M. R. (2002). A cognitive-behavioral perspective on termination. *Journal of Psychotherapy Integration, 12*(3), 364–372. https://doi.org/10.1037/1053-0479.12.3.364

Gülüm, I. V., Soygüt, G., & Safran, J. D. (2016). A comparison of pre-dropout and temporary rupture sessions in psychotherapy. *Psychotherapy Research, 28*(5), 1–23. https://doi.org/10.1080/10503307.2016.1246765

Holmes, J. (1997). "Too early, too late": Endings in psychotherapy – An attachment perspective. *British Journal of Psychotherapy, 14*(2), 159–171. https://doi.org/10.1111/j.1752-0118.1997.tb00367.x

Holmes, J. (2009). *Exploring in security: Towards an attachment-informed psychoanalytic psychotherapy.* Routledge/Taylor & Francis.

Horvath, A. O., Del Re, A. C., Flückiger, C., & Symonds, D. (2011). Alliance in individual psychotherapy. *Psychotherapy, 48*(1), 9–16. https://doi.org/10.1037/a0022186

Joyce, A. S., Piper, W. E., Ogrodniczuk, J. S., & Klein, R. H. (2007). *Termination in psychotherapy: A psychodynamic model of processes and outcomes.* American Psychological Association.

Kealy, D., Gazzillo, F., Silberschatz, G., & Curtis, J. T. (2020). Plan-Compatible termination in psychotherapy: Perspectives from control-mastery theory. *Psychotherapy, 57*(4), 508–514. https://doi.org/10.1037/pst0000300

Kearney, L. K., Draper, M., & Barón, A. (2005). Counseling utilization by ethnic minority college students. *Cultural Diversity and Ethnic Minority Psychology, 11*(3), 272–285. https://doi.org/10.1037/1099-9809.11.3.272

Kendall, P. C., Kipnis, D., & Otto-Salaj, L. (1992). When clients don't progress: Influences on and explanations for lack of therapeutic progress. *Cognitive Therapy and Research, 16,* 269–281. https://doi.org/10.1007/BF01183281

Leibovich, L., & Zilcha-Mano, S. (2017). Integration and clinical demonstration of active ingredients of short-term psychodynamic therapy for depression. *Journal of Psychotherapy Integration, 27*(1), 93–106. https://doi.org/10.1037/int0000043

Maeschalck, C. L., Prescott, D. S., & Miller, S. D. (2019). Feedback informed treatment. In J. C. Norcross & M. R. Goldfried (Eds.), *Handbook of psychotherapy integration* (pp. 105–121). Oxford University Press.

Marmarosh, C. L. (2017). Fostering engagement during termination: Applying attachment theory and research. *Psychotherapy, 54*(1), 4–9. https://doi.org/10.1037/pst0000087

Mohl, P. C., Martinez, D., Ticknor, C., Huang, M., & Cordell, L. (1991). Early dropouts from psychotherapy. *The Journal of Nervous and Mental Disease, 179*(8), 478–481. https://doi.org/10.1097/00005053-199108000-00005

Muran, J. C., Safran, J. D., Gorman, B. S., Samstag, L. W., Eubanks-Carter, C., & Winston, A. (2009). The relationship of early alliance ruptures and their resolution to process and outcome in three time-limited psychotherapies for personality disorders. *Psychotherapy: Theory, Research, Practice, Training, 46*(2), 233–248. https://doi.org/10.1037/a0016085

Nantz, E., Liu-Seifert, H., & Skljarevski, V. (2009). Predictors of premature discontinuation of treatment in multiple disease states. *Patient Preference and Adherence, 3*, 31–43. https://doi.org/10.2147/PPA.S4633

Norcross, J. C., Zimmerman, B. E., Greenberg, R. P., & Swift, J. K. (2017). Do all therapists do that when saying goodbye? A study of commonalities in termination behaviors. *Psychotherapy, 54*(1), 66–75. https://doi.org/10.1037/pst0000097

Ogrodniczuk, J. S., Joyce, A. S., & Piper, W. E. (2005). Strategies for reducing patient-initiated premature termination of psychotherapy. *Harvard Review of Psychiatry, 13*(2), 57–70. https://doi.org/10.1080/10673220590956429

Ong, A. D., Burrow, A. L., Fuller-Rowell, T. E., Ja, N. M., & Sue, D. W. (2013). Racial microaggressions and daily well-being among Asian Americans. *Journal of Counseling Psychology, 60*(2), 188–199. https://doi.org/10.1037/a0031736

Piper, W. E., Ogrodniczuk, J. S., Joyce, A. S., McCallum, M., Rosie, J. S., O'Kelly, J. G., & Steinberg, P. I. (1999). Prediction of dropping out in time-limited, interpretive individual psychotherapy. *Psychotherapy: Theory, Research, Practice, Training, 36*(2), 114–122. https://doi.org/10.1037/h0087787

Piselli, A., Halgin, R. P., & Macewan, G. H. (2011). What went wrong? Therapists' reflections on their role in premature termination. *Psychotherapy Research, 21*(4), 400–415. https://doi.org/10.1080/10503307.2011.573819

Rainer, J. P., & Campbell, L. F. (2001). Premature termination in psychotherapy: Identification and intervention. *Journal of Psychotherapy in Independent Practice, 2*(3), 19–42.

Rogers, C. R. (1957). The necessary and sufficient conditions of therapeutic personality change. *Journal of Consulting Psychology, 21*(2), 95–103. https://doi.org/10.1037/h0045357

Roos, J., & Werbart, A. (2013) Therapist and relationship factors influencing dropout from individual psychotherapy: A literature review. *Psychotherapy Research, 23*(4), 394–418. https://doi.org/10.1080/10503307.2013.775528

Sansone, R. A., & Sansone, L. A. (2012). Antidepressant adherence: Are patients taking their medications? *Innovations in Clinical Neuroscience, 9*(5–6), 41–46.

Shahar, G., & Ziv-Beiman, S. (2020). Using termination as an intervention (UTAI): A view from an integrative, cognitive-existential psychodynamics perspective. *Psychotherapy, 57*(4), 515–520. https://doi.org/10.1037/pst0000337

Sharf, J., Primavera, L. H., & Diener, M. J. (2010). Dropout and therapeutic alliance: A meta-analysis of adult individual psychotherapy. *Psychotherapy: Theory, Research, Practice, Training, 47*(4), 637–645. https://doi.org/10.1037/a0021175

Shulman, S. R. (1999). Termination of short-term and long-term psychotherapy: Patients' and therapists' affective reactions and therapists' technical management (attachment style, therapy model). *Dissertation Abstracts International: Section B: The Sciences and Engineering, 60*(6-B), 2961.

Stroebe, M. (2002). Paving the way: From early attachment theory to contemporary bereavement research. *Mortality, 7*(2), 127–138. https://doi.org/10.1080/13576270220136267

Sue, D. W., Capodilupo, C. M., Torino, G. C., Bucceri, J. M., Holder, A. M. B., Nadal, K. L., & Esquilin, M. (2007). Racial microaggressions in everyday life: Implications for clinical practice. *American Psychologist, 62*(4), 271–286. https://doi.org/10.1037/0003-066X.62.4.271

Swift, J. K., Callahan, J., & Levine, J. C. (2009). Using clinically significant change to identify premature termination. *Psychotherapy: Theory, Research, Practice, Training, 46*(3), 328–335. https://doi.org/10.1037/a0017003

Swift, J. K., & Greenberg, R. P. (2012). Premature discontinuation in adult psychotherapy: A meta-analysis. *Journal of Consulting and Clinical Psychology, 80*(4), 547–559. https://doi.org/10.1037/a0028226

Swift, J. K., & Greenberg, R. P. (2015). Premature termination in psychotherapy: Strategies for engaging clients and improving outcomes. American Psychological Association. https://doi.org/10.1037/14469-000

Swift, J. K., Greenberg, R. P., Tompkins, K. A., & Parkin, S. R. (2017). Treatment refusal and premature termination in psychotherapy, pharmacotherapy, and their combination: A meta-analysis of head-to-head comparisons. *Psychotherapy, 54*(1), 47–57. https://doi.org/10.1037/pst0000104

Swift, J. K., Greenberg, R., Whipple, J. L., & Kominiak, N. (2012). Practice recommendations for reducing premature termination in therapy. *Professional Psychology: Research and Practice, 43*(4), 379–387. https://doi.org/10.1037/a0028291

Swift, J. K., Spencer, J., & Goode, J. (2018). Improving psychotherapy effectiveness by addressing the problem of premature termination: Introduction to a special section. *Psychotherapy Research, 28*(5), 669–671. https://doi.org/10.1080/10503307.2018.1439192

Tryon, G. S., & Kane, A. S. (1990). The helping alliance and premature termination. *Counselling Psychology Quarterly, 3*(3), 233–238. https://doi.org/10.1080/09515079008254254

Urmanche, A. A., Oliveira, J. T., Gonçalves, M. M., Eubanks, C. F., & Muran, J. C. (2019). Ambivalence, resistance, and alliance ruptures in psychotherapy: It's complicated. *Psychoanalytic Psychology, 36*(2), 139–147. https://doi.org/10.1037/pap0000237

Walls, M. L., Gonzalez, J., Gladney, T., & Onello, E. (2015). Unconscious biases: Racial microaggressions in American Indian health care. *The Journal of the American Board of Family Medicine, 28*(2), 231–239. https://doi.org/10.3122/jabfm.2015.02.140194

Wayment, H. A., & Vierthaler, J. (2002). Attachment style and bereavement reactions. *Journal of Loss and Trauma, 7*(2), 129–149. https://doi.org/10.1080/153250202753472291

Weinberg, H., Rolnick, A., & Leighton, A. (2023). Introduction. In H. Weinberg, A. Rolnick, & A. Leighton (Eds.), *Advances in online therapy: Emergence of a new paradigm* (pp. 1–17). Taylor & Francis.

Westmacott, R., & Hunsley, J. (2017). Psychologists' perspectives on therapy termination and the use of therapy engagement/retention strategies. *Clinical Psychology & Psychotherapy, 24*(3), 687–696. https://doi.org/10.1002/cpp.2037

Westmacott, R., Hunsley, J., Best, M., Rumstein-McKean, O., & Schindler, D. (2010). Client and therapist views of contextual factors related to termination from psychotherapy: A comparison between unilateral and mutual terminators. *Psychotherapy Research, 20,* 423–435. https://doi.org/10.1080/10503301003645796

Winnicott, D. W. (1953). Transitional objects and transitional phenomena: A study of the first not-me possession. *The International Journal of Psychoanalysis, 34*(2), 89–97.

Yalom, I. D. (1980). *Existential psychotherapy*. Basic Books.

Termination Across Different Diagnoses and Theories

4

Introduction

The termination phase of therapy is important for patients and their therapists. It addresses the ending of the therapeutic relationship. Termination is recognized as a major event in psychotherapy, and, in its own right, can be therapeutic (Aafjes-Van Doorn & Wooldridge, 2018; Shahar & Ziv-Beiman, 2020). Yet, there is a paucity of discussion and empirical research on therapy endings in the psychological literature (Aafjes-Van Doorn & Wooldridge, 2018; Hilsenroth, 2017). There may be less research on termination in CBT than in other therapeutic orientations given the focus of CBT on completing goals, and the fact that from the first therapy session therapists prepare clients for the end of therapy, essentially to be therapists for themselves (Beck, 1995; Okamoto et al., 2019; Vidair et al., 2017).

The previous chapter delineated Norcross and colleagues' (2017) eight core therapeutic tasks of termination that can lead to a successful course of therapy across theoretical approaches. Several models describe the common features of the process of termination, and although therapists from the majority of theoretical orientations employ many common characteristics, the manner in which the termination process is enacted may vary based on the therapist's theoretical perspective and personal elements (Norcross et al., 2017). For example, therapists with an interpersonal orientation view termination as a core part of treatment, and it is during this phase when conflicting emotions are discussed (Joyce et al., 2007). Therapists with a cognitive-behavioral orientation, on the other hand, do not consider termination as

DOI: 10.4324/9781003128489-6

a distinctive part of treatment, and the termination of the therapist-client relationship receives little focus in CBT (Goldfried, 2002; Joyce et al., 2007). These therapists emphasize the patient's development of coping skills and the patient's new capacity to apply these skills as they face new challenges with little emphasis on the ending of the patient-therapist relationship (Goldfried, 2002; Joyce et al., 2007; Nelson & Politano, 1993). Joyce and colleagues (2007, p. 82) point out that similar to therapists with an interpersonal orientation, therapists with a supportive orientation view termination as a central part of treatment; however, these therapists aim for a gradual reduction of the relationship that can stretch out over a long period of time (e.g., Werman, 1984). Therapists with an experiential orientation do not have a specific theory of termination; however, these therapists attend to the issue of separation and aim to promote discussion of new meanings that have developed for the patient during therapy (Elliott et al, 2004; Greenberg, 2002; Joyce et al., 2007).

What are the similarities among the aforementioned therapy approaches to termination? Common to the aforementioned therapy perspectives is the review of what clients have gained from therapy along with assisting them to form a feeling of empowerment at the end of therapy, the need to discuss the feelings connected to the termination of the client-therapist relationship, the study of the process of the generalization of learning to live external to the therapy setting, the minimization of what was not achieved, the paucity of discussion about dealing with new symptoms or the recurrence of old symptoms during the termination phase, and no attendance to transference resolution (Joyce et al., 2007). Joyce and colleagues (2007) found that, in general, there are distinctions with respect to the amount of focus that the process of ending therapy receives, and these particularities depend upon the different therapy approaches. They explain that the more that a therapist attends to the client's relationships during therapy, whether internal to the therapy setting or external to it, the more the therapist attends to the process of ending therapy. Endings are composed of a realistic recognition of treatment and the therapeutic relationship; however, there are no perfect endings (Joyce et al., 2007).

Termination, similar to therapy itself, is not the same for every client. The process of ending differs depending upon the client and the context, and therapists need to tailor the process to the needs of the client. Chapter 4, "Termination Across Different Diagnoses and Theories," illustrates the process of termination across different diagnoses and theoretical orientations, for example, humanistic, psychodynamic, integrated, or cognitive-behavioral. It underscores how termination occurs for therapists from different theoretical orientations who navigate the termination process with patients with different emotional disorders. Examples of the inner thoughts of therapists from different theoretical orientations and patients with differing diagnoses are interspersed throughout this chapter.

The chapter begins by describing therapists' activities and the common-alities among therapists during the termination process. The differences among therapists during the termination process are explored as well. First, the chapter looks at terminations that have reached their natural end, and a vignette of a full-term termination is explored. Then, the chapter proceeds to premature terminations and addresses the differences by theory based on multiple factors related to patient characteristics including diagnosis.

Termination as a Central Event

Unpacking the termination process begins with a recognition that termin-ation is a primary event in the course of therapy and in the continuity beyond therapy. According to Norcross and colleagues (2017), there are specific ther-apist activities that are common across different models of termination. The following are a few examples of the common therapist activities during termination:

Confirming Gains Garnered by Patients During Therapy Sessions (Norcross et al., 2017)

In addition to discussing with the client the content of the meaningful moments during therapy, the therapist might discuss the pace of the gains. Sometimes these gains may go slowly or may not be noticed. At the end of therapy, here is what one client, Will, reported as his gains:

> *I felt that you didn't take me for granted. You recognized me for who I was. You accepted me. I felt included in a larger sense. More than what I gained during the therapy sessions themselves, were the times when I sensed that you were with me when I was not in session. I appreciated that you were there for me even then. For example, sometimes, when I panicked, you listened to me over the phone for ten minutes, and it was then that I knew that you cared that I got back on track, even though it wasn't during the therapy session itself. What helped me progress during the therapy sessions themselves was the fact that*

I knew that I could count on you when something urgent occurred and that you would get back to me. The sense of care that I felt when you were my therapist is what was important for me. For the most part, I felt safe during and in between sessions.

Discussing the Favored Times That Took Place During Therapy Sessions (Norcross et al., 2017)

During the termination process, a therapist asked a client, Alice, to list her favorite times during therapy sessions. The client said:

My best times during therapy were the humorous moments that we shared. There were times that you laughed with me when I joked. You weren't rigid. Prior to seeing you, I went to another therapist. I left him after the fourth session. He had no sense of humor, and he said that I was using humor as a defense, that I was resistant. With you, it was different. You genuinely appreciated my sense of humor. And you also were able to cry with me when I cried. That told me that you didn't dismiss or disregard me. It said to me that you heard me, that you cared. That you were HUMAN. Thank you.

Following an Ethical Approach for the Termination Process (Norcross et al., 2017)

An ethical approach suggests that therapists take care to avoid abandoning clients (Norcross et al., 2017; Vasquez et al., 2008). Here is an example of how a therapist who needed to retire his practice suddenly because of a terminal illness made plans to avoid abandoning his clients. During the therapy process with Kirk, the therapist became sick with a life-threatening illness. Kirk had difficulty parting with the therapist. In order to avoid abandoning Kirk, here is how he prepared his client:

As we discussed last week, the timing of termination has been coerced for you and for me because of my illness. As you know, I will need to retire my practice as soon as possible. During our work together, you've let me know how attached you feel toward me, and you have told me that you are sad that you'll no longer be able to see me. I have set up a temporary therapist for my clients to see until they seek out the referrals that I have provided. This therapist will see you until you are able to find a new therapist, and if you wish to see her as a therapist in the future, she is pleased to accommodate. I can be reached for administrative questions from 2 P.M. to 4 P.M. on Mondays and Wednesdays for the next month. Please feel free to call me with your questions, and the therapist who is replacing me will work with me and with you to help connect you with a new therapist. If you need paperwork processed, the therapist who is replacing me will be pleased to help you with these issues. Again, I am sorry that I need to retire my practice, we have worked well together, and I aim to assist you with your difficult transition.

In their article, "Using Termination as an Intervention (UTAI): A View From an Integrative, Cognitive-Existential Psychodynamics Perspective," Shahar and Ziv-Beiman (2020) propose a version of ending in therapy, and this version relies on Howard and colleagues' (1986) phase framework of therapy outcome that suggests that benefits in therapy emerge along the following phases: Remoralization, remediation, and rehabilitation. They recommend that termination or ending in therapy be viewed as a primary intervention that leads to the patient's remoralization (e.g., Howard et al., 1986). Remoralization takes place when individuals who feel demoralized by their difficulties and stuck to the point that they cannot mobilize their own coping capacity begin to believe that therapy will help them incorporate long-term changes (Howard et al., 1986; Shahar & Ziv-Beiman, 2020).

For some individuals, determining a preset date for termination in psychotherapy helps to facilitate a perception of agency and can serve to extend the recognition of one's schemas (Shahar & Ziv-Beiman, 2020). In cases that are not prematurely or unilaterally terminated, a predetermined end date is set, and the patient and therapist work toward that end (Norcross et al., 2017).

Although there are common therapist activities during termination, there are variations related to termination as well. The next portion focuses on the differences in the termination process based on a therapist's theoretical orientation.

Are There Differences in the Termination Process Based on a Therapist's Theoretical Approach?

There are varying degrees of subtlety in how therapists with different theoretical orientations engage in the termination process. In his article, "What is a 'Good Enough Termination?',", Gabbard (2009) explains that a key consideration when reflecting on ending therapy is whether a pathway has been set out to facilitate the potential for ongoing self-analysis. He does not view termination as an end, but as a beginning for analysands to continue the process of working through their separation from the analyst in other relationships. Bartholomew and colleagues (2019) point out that whereas there are some psychoanalysts who consider that an ending to therapy occurs with the resolving of patients' infantile issues and resistance, others do not view endings in therapy as readily discernible and view termination as tailored to the individual needs of patients (e.g., Pedder, 1988). They note that whereas psychotherapy approaches such as interpersonal process therapy or tailored approaches focus on the effect of ending a meaningful relationship with a therapist (e.g., Teyber & Teyber, 2017), cognitive-behavioral frameworks specify that termination takes place when symptoms are decreased (for a minimum of two months) and when patients can apply their new skills to their daily lives and hold onto their progress that they made in therapy (e.g., Jakobsons et al., 2007).

Chapter 3 described therapist behaviors during termination that, for the most part, are common to therapists with different approaches. Although Norcross and colleagues (2017) agree that there are common therapist behaviors that need to take place during termination, they recognize that there are occasional differences depending upon a therapist's theoretical orientation (e.g., psychodynamic, experiential, cognitive-behavioral). For example, they point out that with respect to a cognitive-behavioral approach, it is suggested that during termination, the therapist does not emphasize feelings of separation or underscore the relationship between the patient and the therapist (e.g., Goldfried, 2002). Rather, during the termination process, the cognitive-behavioral therapist assists the client to hold onto the gains of the intervention per se, decreases the number of sessions during termination, and discusses the new skills that the client has learned while encouraging the client to apply these skills to work on their own problems, with minimal therapist intervention (Goldfried, 2002; Norcross et al., 2017). Wachtel (2002) points out that unlike proponents of an experiential (e.g., Greenberg, 2002) and a cognitive-behavioral approach (e.g., Goldfried, 2002), who view the tapering of therapy sessions as a critical part of ending therapy, proponents of a psychoanalytic approach are reluctant to taper because of their view that tapering can contribute toward the patient's denial of the reality of terminating therapy.

Mutually Agreed Terminations

Different types of termination, full-term or mutually agreed and premature, may interact with the therapist's approach. See Table 4.1.

The next section explores the themes of full-term terminations of cognitive-behavioral, psychodynamic, and humanistic therapists along with the dialogue and the inner thoughts of the client and the therapist. The following vignette offers an example of termination with a cognitive-behavioral therapist.

Vignette of an Example of a Mutually Agreed Termination With a Cognitive-Behavioral Therapist

INTRODUCTION

Dolores is a 51-year-old client with a three-year history of dysthymia or persistent depression. Dolores has been diagnosed with dysthymia or persistent depression, a type of depression that stays with an individual for a period of several years. Dolores' depression was relentless. It stuck with her. She felt sad, hopeless, and pessimistic most of the time for many years. Recently, she saw a cognitive-behavioral therapist when she began thinking about suicide in a more serious way. After the death of her adolescent, she had trouble functioning during the day, she slept only about three hours a night, although she rarely got out of bed at all.

Table 4.1 Vignettes: Types of Termination From Therapy and Theoretical Approach

Theoretical Approach of Therapist	Mutually Agreed Termination	Premature Termination
Cognitive-Behavioral	Dolores	
Psychodynamic	Melissa	
Cognitive-Behavioral	Miguel	
Integrated	Colette	
Cognitive		Dana
Humanistic		Darren

Dialogue

> *Therapist's inner thoughts: Dolores seems deeply depressed. I want to gently inquire if Dolores wishes to harm herself.*
>
> **Therapist's statement:** Are you able to tell me how you're feeling today?
>
> *Patient's inner thoughts: I don't really care if I live or die now. What the heck if I walk into the street and get hit by a car? I have nothing left to live for. The stars have never been in my favor, and things are not getting better now.*
>
> **Patient's statement:** [Patient's head is down] I've not ever attempted suicide, but lately, I've been feeling that dying might be an option for me.
>
> [During the course of therapy, the cognitive-behavioral therapist conducted a thorough assessment and employed a specific cognitive-behavioral program for depression, Cognitive Behavior Analysis System of Psychotherapy (CBASP) (McCullough, 2000), a model that integrates cognitive-behavioral and interpersonal methods.]
>
> [After approximately a year and a half of CBASP sessions twice a week, Dolores and the therapist began to explore the process of a full-term, planned, mutually agreed upon termination.]

Dialogue (cont)

> *Therapist's inner thoughts: It's been almost two years since Dolores first contacted me. It seems that she is feeling better. I'd like to check where she is.*
>
> **Therapist's statement:** How are you feeling today?
>
> *Patient's inner thoughts: These days I'm feeling less fatigued and less like I'm dragging myself through the day.*
>
> **Patient's statement:** I feel somewhat better. I've resumed my interests. I joined a gardening class, and I'm meeting new people. I think that I'm ready to think about ending therapy now. Do you think that's okay?
>
> **Therapist's thoughts:** *Dolores seems to have made progress in therapy, and she seems to be less distressed, and although I know that her self-esteem is better, that she feels less helpless, and that she may be ready to end therapy, I have gnawing concerns about whether she can maintain the gains. I better put in place some precautions if Dolores relapses.*

Therapist's statement: I know that you rarely think about dying these days, that you have accomplished many of the goals that we defined together, and that you're coping better despite your deep loss and the hard, cold winter. Let's try to taper your sessions. I would suggest that you decrease the number of sessions per month, perhaps to two sessions a month and then to one a month as a trial for termination to see if you can maintain your gains. Then, at approximately month eight, if you still feel like ending, we can end. During the next session, let's discuss the plan further. How does that sound to you?

Patient's inner thoughts: I'm okay with this plan because it can give me an opportunity to see if I slide.

Patient's statement: Hmm… This sounds okay to me. Gives me a chance to practice how I do on my own without therapy.

Summary

Dolores and her cognitive-behavioral therapist agreed that she could end therapy in eight months provided that she could maintain her gains over the next year. The planned, mutually agreed termination process was put into place.

Norcross and colleagues (2017) note that practitioners and researchers with different theoretical perspectives may approach termination from various points of view. They explain, for example, that from a psychodynamic perspective, recommendations may be as specific as those of Curtis (2002) who suggests the following particular therapist termination activities:

Facilitate the patient's determination of the termination.
Decrease the number of sessions as termination approaches.
Facilitate a conversation about the patient's past and present ways of dealing with stress and discuss gains and plans for the future.
Discuss therapy activities that have felt beneficial and activities that have not assisted.
Inquire if the patient is terminating because of not being satisfied.
Strive for an equality in the therapeutic relationship.
Invite the patient to call with later updates.

The next example is one of a fully planned, mutually agreed termination process with a psychodynamic therapist. The therapist facilitates a conversation about how the patient dealt with stress in the past and how she deals with it in the present, and the therapist asks the patient about the portions of therapy that she found helpful and the activities that she did not find useful.

Vignette of an Example of a Planned, Mutually Agreed Termination With a Psychodynamic Therapist

INTRODUCTION

Melissa is a 41-year-old client with a two-year history of anxiety. She has been seeing a psychodynamic therapist when her worrying increased after her third child. After her third child was born, Melissa said that she barely had time for herself, felt that her self-esteem was faltering, had too many demands placed upon her, had little support from her husband, and was fatigued from taking care of her mother who was ill. Her thoughts prior to her first session revolved around feelings of being overwhelmed by life: "My anxiety is out of control. I don't get enough sleep. I have little confidence in myself anymore. My husband expects me to take care of everything, and berates me if I don't, and I'm falling apart." During the third therapy session, Melissa shared with the therapist that she feels like she is going crazy. The psychodynamic therapist decided to help Melissa experience a better sense of self.

After approximately three years of twice a week psychodynamic therapy, Melissa mentioned the possibility of ending therapy in a few months. She said that she felt more confident in her ability to attend to her own needs rather than to comply with the demands of members of her family.

DIALOGUE

Therapist's inner thoughts: I'm pleased to see that Melissa has learned to consider herself more.

Therapist's statement: You seem more confident about your ability to speak up to family members and others about your own needs.

Patient's inner thoughts: Thanks to this therapist and my good relationship with her, I'm functioning better.

Patient's statement: In the past, I used to put everyone's demands before my own needs. I no longer do this. Now I feel more comfortable with myself, and my husband no longer berates me. I'm assertive about what I will and won't do, and today, I feel that I'm a different person than when I began therapy. In general, I worry less. I think that I'm ready to end therapy, but I'll miss you.

Therapist's inner thoughts: Melissa has shown progress in therapy, she seems to be less worried, her self-esteem is better, and she is more likely to express her own needs. Today, I have a sense that Melissa displays more self-cohesion than she did when she first began therapy. She may be ready to end therapy, and I'll begin by inquiring whether Melissa wishes to discuss closing issues within a period of a few months.

Therapist's statement: I agree with you that we can discuss the termination process that you mentioned last week. During this process, you can let me know what you have gained, and, if you wish, we can discuss our relationship. Do you have an idea about which therapy activities you felt were beneficial and which haven't felt like they were helpful?

Patient's inner thoughts: In the past, I would be afraid to tell the therapist my thoughts for fear that she would disagree with me, but now I feel somewhat comfortable doing so. I'll be assertive.

Patient's statement: Although I appreciated your interpretations and thought they were, for the most part, correct, I sometimes needed more support because of the difficulties that I was experiencing with my husband and my mother.

Therapist's inner thoughts: I'm glad that Melissa is able to express her needs. I want to confirm the importance of being assertive for her.

Therapist's statement: We have worked a lot on you recognizing that your needs are as worthy, if not more important, than the needs of others, and we worked on your ability to be assertive about your needs. I encourage you to continue to do so. Please let me know in the future what you need from me. If I'm offering an interpretation that is not helpful and/or if the timing is not helpful, please let me know that it's not suitable for me to do so. Ending therapy is on the horizon in a few months, depending upon your needs and wishes. Next time, we can discuss what you wish to talk about until we end.

Summary

This example is one of a fully planned, mutually agreed termination process with a psychodynamic therapist. When Melissa inquired about ending therapy, she showed positive signs that she was able to tell the therapist about the therapist's mistakes, and the therapist saw Melissa's newly learned assertiveness skills as a sign that she was able to express her own needs to others, for example, her husband and her mother, rather than placing her needs on hold and the requests of her husband and mother ahead of her own. The therapist agreed that they could begin the collaborative termination process and that Melissa could end therapy in a few months.

The goal is a termination that is mutual, an ending phase with which both client and therapist feel comfortable, and although proponents of different psychotherapy approaches disagree about the manner of termination, they agree that the termination process needs to be shared between patient and therapist (DeBerry & Baskin, 1989). Whereas therapists with an interpersonal or short-term approach aim for a specific agreed upon number of therapy sessions, therapists with a psychoanalytic orientation aim for an open-ended approach with a mutually agreed upon process of termination (DeBerry & Baskin, 1989).

Norcross and colleagues (2017) note that from an experiential perspective, recommendations may be as specific as those of Greenberg (2002) who suggests the following therapist termination activities:

Strive for clients to decide on termination.
Accept that clients will make changes post therapy.
Assist clients to work on issues linked to loss.
Inform clients that change can be credited to their endeavors.
Discuss new understandings of the therapy work and its relationship to
    clients' views about themselves and others.
Recognize that there could be relapses in the future.
Decrease the number of sessions prior to the last session.
Inform the client that there is opportunity if the client wishes future sessions.

Norcross and colleagues (2017) highlight that the similarities in therapist behaviors during the termination process are of greater importance than the differences in therapist termination activities based on various theoretical orientations. They explain that during terminations with successful outcomes, the therapist and patient collaborate by determining an end date, and they plan together to work through material toward that end. The crux of the matter related to termination is that the similarities at termination override the differences. The therapists described in this chapter aim for effective terminations that include most of the common characteristics, but the termination may be described differently depending upon the language and underpinnings of the particular theory.

There are full-term, collaborative endings and premature or unilateral terminations. As discussed in Chapter 3, these endings can be initiated either by the therapist or the patient, and there are many variables that may be considered for each ending and for each member of the therapeutic dyad. According to Vidair and colleagues (2017), the last CBT session needs to focus on a plan for the prevention of a relapse. In the next vignette of an example of a fully planned, mutually agreed termination between a client and a therapist with a cognitive-behavioral orientation, the focus is on the completion of the client's goals, the emphasis is on the prevention of relapse, and the inner thoughts of the client and the cognitive-behavioral therapist are illustrated throughout the vignette.

Vignette of an Example of a Mutually Agreed or a Full-Term Termination: A Therapist With a Cognitive-Behavioral Orientation

INTRODUCTION

In this vignette, a 26-year-old client, Miguel, has been in CBT for a period of 11 months. The scenario includes a concluding therapy session where the therapist and the client have agreed that he has accomplished his goals to be less dependent on others and that he can complete therapy. In a previous session, Miguel brought up ending therapy, and the therapist discussed a plan with Miguel. See Figure 4.1.

DIALOGUE

Therapist's statement: This is our last session. We have discussed the goals of your therapy throughout the time that we have worked together, and we have changed some goals and added others. Today, maybe we can summarize the progress that you have made.

Patient's inner thoughts: [Assertive] *This is good that she is asking me that. I learned a lot, especially that I can make my own decisions, and I don't need to rely on others. I don't have to ask everyone else what to do, or wake up thinking whom I'm going to call the next day to help me.*

Patient's statement: It feels good to be making my own decisions, and I learned to have confidence in myself, but I know that sometimes my confidence plummets quickly. If I start calling a lot of people for advice during the day, I'll focus on the program that I learned during therapy, the manual that you gave me, and the notes that I have recorded in my notebook. These things really help me. They are concrete, and I can sink my teeth into them if the going gets rough.

Therapist's inner thoughts: He seems to have a good indication of how's he faring. Let's turn to the prevention of relapse.

Therapist's statement: Yes. You seem to have a good handle on your thoughts now. Do you remember what you can say to yourself when you start feeling the need to rely excessively on others?

Patient's inner thoughts: She's challenging me. Maybe she wants to make sure that I know what to do when I slip. I do know what to do. Breathe deeply. Stop being the clingy, dependent person that I used to be. I don't like that person who's so needy.

Patient's statement: I know how to catch myself now. When I make a mistake, I need to tell myself that I can take my time. I can collect my thoughts first. I have to breathe and go off to a private place if I need to. I don't need to call people or to ask them to help me because I can rely on myself until I get home. I can look at my strategy book and review how to take charge rather than fall back and be that clingy, dependent person I used to be.

Therapist's inner thoughts: He seems to have integrated the strategy that he worked on in therapy.

Therapist's statement: It's been a pleasure working with you. I am confident that you are able to make more informed decisions for yourself, that your judgment is as good as, if not better than, others. I wish you well. It has been rewarding for me to work with you as you developed this confidence and the capacity to make your own decisions. I trust that you will be able to manage going forward.

Patient's inner thoughts: I feel grateful that I was able to work this through to my satisfaction.

Patient's statement: Thanks for helping me. I'm off to meet my friends now. Bye.

SUMMARY

In this vignette, Miguel and his therapist agreed on a planned termination. The last CBT session focused on the plan for the prevention of a relapse. The therapist encouraged Miguel to express confidence in his ability to move forward on his own. Miguel seemed pleased that he had met his goals.

The next portion turns, once again, to a vignette of an example of a fully planned or mutually agreed upon termination; however, this time the scenario is between a client, Colette, and a therapist with a humanistic orientation. The focus during this course of therapy is on the patient's death anxiety and meaning in life. The patient, Colette, reported that since she learned that her best friend has been admitted to the hospital with cancer, she has been experiencing panic attacks, and she feels as if she cannot breathe.

Whereas the previous vignette illustrated a termination with a focus on relapse with a cognitive-behavioral therapist, this scenario highlights the work of a therapist with an integrated psychotherapy approach of humanistic theory and psychodynamic theory. The theme for the termination process of the therapist with an integrative psychotherapy approach is the consolidation of the client's new perspective in light of the client's initial difficulty with death anxiety. The inner thoughts of the client and the therapist are illustrated in the vignette.

Vignette of an Example of a Mutually Agreed Full-Term Termination With a Therapist That has an Integrated Humanistic and Psychodynamic Psychotherapy Approach

INTRODUCTION

Existential issues are related to many of the emotional disorders that involve anxiety. Death is a common existential problem that most people share.

According to Yalom (2017), in order to reassure patients with death anxiety, rather than ignore talking about death, therapists need to discuss the patient's anxiety about death in a direct and matter-of-fact way. At the beginning of therapy, Colette, a 29-year-old client, reported that her best friend had colon cancer and had been admitted to the hospital. Since her friend's hospital admission, Colette began having panic attacks, and she feared that she could not breathe. Colette expressed a fear that her best friend would die and that she, herself, would die early as her own mother did. During the course of therapy, the therapist calmly inquired of Colette about the specifics of her fear about death, which was connected to her concern that her best friend would die. Colette has been in humanistic therapy for more than two years. Initially, she presented with her feeling that she could not get enough air into her lungs. The therapist referred her to a physician, and the physician provided a clean bill of health. The following scenario includes the communication between the therapist and Colette during the next to last therapy session.

Several weeks ago, Colette hinted that she might be ready to end therapy. The therapist offered positive indication that it would be okay to end soon, proposed a plan for an ending, and the client agreed with the therapist's plan to end within five months. In the next to last session, the therapist and the client continue their collaborative discussions during the termination process. Here the client, Colette, lets the therapist know that she understands some of the issues that comprise her new perspective, one where she has become aware that her concerns about death with accompanying anxiety and panic have been related to her sense of the early loss of her mother when she was eight years old.

DIALOGUE

Therapist's statement: Throughout our time when we have explored your anxiety about death, you have informed me that you often felt that you cannot get enough breath in, and then you start to panic further. During these times, you said that you feel like you're going to die.

Patient's inner thoughts: [Takes a deep breath through her nose, a pause, sits upright, and stops to think] This is good that she is reviewing the way I have felt. Turns out that I now understand that some of the fears that I have that I'm going to die are related to having observed my mother falling ill when I was younger. My mother had a heart attack and died when I was eight years

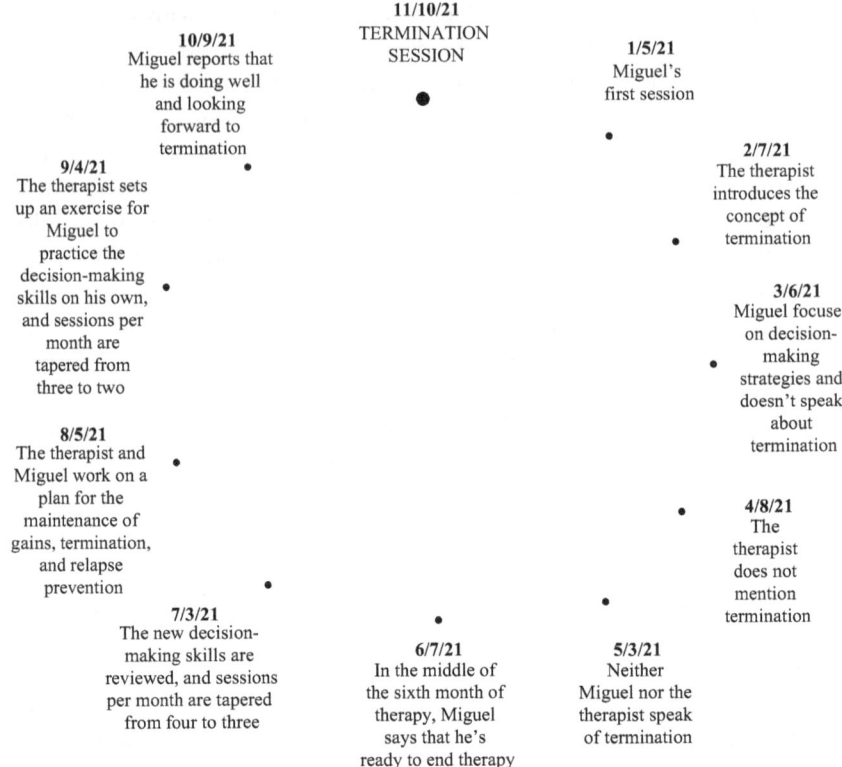

Figure 4.1 Circle of Time for Miguel: A Full Termination with a Cognitive-Behavioral Therapist

Note. This figure illustrates a monthly timeline of the discussion of Miguel's full termination from beginning to end.

old. I felt like I was going to fall down when I saw my mother pass out. I called 911 but didn't know what else to do. All my life, I felt guilty like I could hardly breathe when I thought about it.

Patient's statement: I appreciate you being there for me when I panic. I think I have a fair sense now of what happens when I start to feel that I cannot get enough air in, and then I tend to escalate and make matters worse.

Therapist's inner thoughts: She seems to have a handle on the situation at this time, and she recognizes the vicious cycle of hyperventilation that repeats itself each time she quickly draws in deeper and deeper breaths of air. In the sessions that are left, I'd like to discuss with her how her perspective fits in with her new endeavors.

Therapist's statement: Yes. You seem to be more aware now that your breathing is connected to an image that you remember when you were young when you saw your mother collapse, and you felt helpless. And you now know that none of this is your doing. The tragic passing of your mother happened when you were with her, by yourself, at eight years of age, and you acted heroically by calling 911.

Patient's inner thoughts: She's mentioning the death of my mother again, but I no longer feel panicked.

Patient's statement: I know now that everyone is occasionally concerned about death, that we all think about it, but it no longer overwhelms me, and if I get a panic attack, it's mild, and I pull out of it quickly by not taking in a lot of air at once, realizing that I have people to call on if I need help, and understanding a particular episode's connection to the loss of my mother when I was young.

Therapist's inner thoughts: She seems to have developed a deeper understanding of what has transpired. I'd like to talk with her about other meaningful parts of her current life.

Therapist's statement: I think that you and I agree that you are ready to end therapy. It's been a pleasure working with you. In the sessions that are left, I'm wondering if we can talk some more about your ideas that have been percolating about your future.

Patient's inner thoughts: I feel grateful that I had someone to call when I needed. Just knowing that she was here for me helped me to rely on myself better and to be able to focus on my future plans. I have friends outside of therapy who said they would be there for me now that I revealed this problem to them.

Patient's statement: Thanks for helping me. I have been accepted at a graduate school in an architecture program. And now that I have revealed my problem to others, I can count on my three close friends if need be. Before therapy, I hadn't confided in them because I was ashamed about the breathing and panic problem. Just knowing that they now know and having their reassurance that I can call on them helps me to rely on myself. I decided to take the part-time job working in the center for the deaf, and that gives me satisfaction that I can share with others.

Therapist's statement: Seems like you're headed in a way you wish. Let's meet for one last session, as planned. If you feel that you need assistance in the future, and I'm not suggesting that you will, there's a counseling center at your new university.

SUMMARY

In this vignette, Colette and her therapist collaborated on termination. The last few sessions focused on an integrative approach of humanistic themes such as consolidating her perspective that death is part of life and psychodynamic themes, such as her new understanding that her sense of panic and death anxiety seem connected to the feeling of the loss of her mother at an early age. During therapy, Colette and her therapist with an integrated humanistic and psychodynamic approach discussed overarching themes such as alienation, loneliness, and death while the therapist helped Colette understand the connection between her past history that included the death of her mother and her symptoms today. Colette and the therapist agreed to a fully planned, mutually agreed termination, and the above session was an excerpt from the next to last therapy session.

This section with its illustrated examples of fully planned, mutually agreed terminations by therapists with different theoretical orientations, e.g., cognitive-behavioral, psychodynamic, humanistic, integrated, concludes the discussion of full-term terminations. The next portion underscores the inner thoughts of therapists as they think about premature or unilateral, rather than fully planned terminations, and it delves into the interactions between premature termination and therapist variables, including the therapist's theoretical orientation.

Premature Terminations

Premature Termination and Therapist Variables

Previous sections described the association between full-term terminations and the different theoretical approaches of therapists. This section addresses the relationship of premature termination, discontinuation, or dropout from therapy and therapists' variables.

One may wonder when, during the course of therapy, premature endings take place. Do they generally take place at the beginning, at the midpoint, or at the end of a course of therapy? Muran and colleagues (2009) note that most dropouts from therapy have been shown to take place within the first few therapy sessions, and the median treatment length is approximately six sessions (e.g., Garfield, 1994). Furthermore, how do different therapists' theoretical orientations fare with respect to premature endings? Constantino and colleagues (2008) point out that the dropout rate for cognitive therapy was found to be 20.4% (e.g., De Maat et al., 2006) and that there were fewer premature terminations in BRT (20%) than there were in brief psychodynamic therapy (46%) and CBT (37%) (e.g., Muran et al., 2005). They suggest the use of strategies of rupture repair to promote the completion of treatment.

Dropout from therapy has been linked to different therapist variables, and it is suggested that the different ways that therapists navigate the process of therapy and their relationship with a patient during a session can impact whether a client stays the course of therapy. For example, Philips and colleagues (2018) point out therapist factors that are associated with premature termination, and they note that studies that include trainees as therapists have higher rates of premature termination than studies that include therapists who are experienced (e.g., Swift & Greenberg, 2012). They explain that therapists' overestimation of patients' symptoms and the time that patients need to be in therapy can result in ruptures and client dropouts from therapy (e.g., Berghofer et al., 2002; Roos & Werbart, 2013) and that therapists' negative behaviors, for example, hostility or rejection, can lead to higher premature termination rates (e.g., Mahon et al., 2001; Ogrodniczuk et al., 2005).

There are different reasons for premature termination or discontinuation from therapy, for example, ruptures or disagreements between a patient and a therapist. A rupture is the impetus for the premature termination or patient dropout in the next example of an early career therapist with a cognitive approach who, in general, has concerns about the unilateral termination of his clients during the first or second session of therapy. In this case, the rupture can be attributed to the therapist's variables. For many of his patients, this early career therapist, generally, tends to rely on pharmacotherapy, to overestimate the symptoms of his patients, and his patients tend to initiate premature terminations early in therapy. The following is a vignette that illustrates an example of a segment of the second session with an early career therapist with a cognitive approach who is self-focused, self-conscious, and who tends to overestimate the symptoms of the patient, Dana, who drops out of therapy prematurely during the second session.

Vignette of an Example of an Early Career Cognitive Therapist Whose Patients Tend to Prematurely Terminate or to End Therapy After One or Two Sessions

INTRODUCTION

The patient, Dana, is a 51-year-old dermatologist who reported a few altercations with her husband about the upcoming wedding of the youngest of her two sons. This excerpt is from the second therapy session. The couple has been married for 25 years. Both spouses had been previously married and widowed. During the first session Dana said that she has been working a lot and feels like she is going to have a nervous breakdown.

DIALOGUE

Therapist's inner thoughts: What a load she has. Today, in my abnormal psychology class, I just learned about the diagnosis of borderline personality disorder. I wonder if she's displaying signs of borderline personality disorder. After all, she's saying that she feels like she's going to have a nervous break-down and fights with him a lot. It's hard for me to deal with her stuff. She reminds me of my mother who divorced my father. I wonder if she can use a bit of medication so that she doesn't drive me nuts. Her thinking processes may be way off. I am also concerned about how my supervisor is going to evaluate my progress with this case. Dana is much older than I am. Gee, I hope this doesn't end soon like my last client. Lately, I've been losing a lot of clients.

Therapist's statement: Last time, you mentioned that you felt like you were going crazy. I wonder if a little medication could help you calm down and get you thinking straight. I wouldn't want you to start fighting with me like you fight with your husband. You may need to be in therapy for quite some time.

Patient's inner thoughts: Oh my gosh! He's making me feel worse. I don't need any medication. That's the last thing I need. He's a bit young, and somewhat obtuse, and self-focused.

Patient's statement: WHAT! I don't need medication.

Therapist's inner thoughts: I thought she'd calm down a bit. Instead, she seems angry. I wonder why. I was only trying to help. I don't want her spewing her messed-up stuff on me. That's all I need now. She may need both medication and a lot of therapy in the future. Oh no. What is my supervisor going to say about this…

Therapist's statement: I did not mean to anger you, but I thought a little medication can help you calm down and clear your thought processes, and I can refer you to a psychiatrist at the clinic.

Patient's inner thoughts: He doesn't understand my concerns at all. I think I'll end it here.

Patient's statement: I think that I need to end here. This is not helping me. Here's what I owe you for today and the last time. Goodbye.

Summary

This early career therapist seems surprised and confused about why the patient left. The way that this cognitive therapist approached Dana is not a correct approach. With many of his patients, rather than delving into the issues of his client, he tends to prefer to make inappropriate pharmacotherapy referrals. The novice therapist learns about disorders in school, tries to apply them to his patient, but does so incorrectly. The therapist in this example tends to focus on himself, and he overestimates the patient's symptoms, for example, his assigning a diagnosis of borderline personality to her when she mentions that she feels like she is going to have a nervous breakdown. The therapist prefers to latch on to a newly learned diagnosis, borderline personality disorder, and does not sufficiently consider Dana's current stressors. He is afraid to face his supervisor because he is clueless about what he has done wrong. The beginning therapist in this vignette is new to the profession, self-focused, and is concerned about his own adequacy. He may not be feeling comfortable in his own skin. He would rather use medication than explore his patient's concerns. He would rather latch onto diagnoses that he learns about in school, but does not fully understand, than to speak to Dana about the current concerns in her life. The therapist is self-conscious and becomes concerned about how he will discuss this case with his supervisor. He may benefit from supervision and/or from his own therapy that focuses on exploring his concerns about his entering the profession and seeing clients with a vast array of life experiences whose concerns are different from his own experiences.

This section illustrated that therapist variables such as a therapist's tendency to overestimate the symptoms of patients and the negative behaviors of the therapist that include self-focused behaviors can impact the therapy process. Ruptures were the impetus for the client's premature termination in this segment. The takeaway is that regardless of the theoretical orientations of therapists, there are relational strategies that therapists can employ to reduce ruptures and avoid premature terminations. Had this cognitive therapist initiated a relational rupture-repair strategy during this session, the premature termination may not have occurred. Whereas the focus of this section was on discontinuation from therapy and therapist variables, the next section focuses on the association between premature termination, discontinuation, or dropout from therapy and patient variables.

Premature Termination and Patient Variables

A vignette in a previous chapter explored the case of the client, Pat, where the therapist initiated a forced termination because of a move to another state. A premature termination can occur because of a client-initiated termination as well, a premature termination that happens because a client moves to another state. Such was the case with the patient, Darren, in the next vignette where a therapist uses positive relational skills to help the client, Darren, sort out his problems and make a decision that is satisfying to him. Although the client is satisfied with the humanistic therapist who uses relational strategies, and there are no ruptures, Darren initiates a premature termination. After much back and forth about his job versus school conflict, he decides to drop out of therapy in order to move to another state. The client's move to another state is the impetus for the premature termination in the next vignette.

Vignette of an Example of a Premature or Forced Termination Initiated by a Client Who Decides to Move to Another State

INTRODUCTION

In this vignette, the client, Darren, reports a job-school conflict to the therapist, and he requests that the therapist listen to him about his job and school choices without offering him explicit advice. This is Darren's eleventh session with the therapist. Throughout the course of therapy, the therapist listens attentively, reflects the here and now for Darren, and uses relational strategies to build a solid relationship with the client. However, during the eleventh session, Darren expresses satisfaction to the therapist, and then initiates a premature termination when he informs her that he will be moving because he was accepted in the English department of a graduate school at a major university in a different state.

DIALOGUE

Therapist's inner thoughts: He seems somewhat tense today.

Therapist's statement: You look like you have something on your mind.

Patient's inner thoughts: I appreciate that she listens to me, takes me seriously, and doesn't give me advice. The members of my family don't seem to be hearing my needs. They want me to take the job that I was offered after I graduate from college, but yesterday, I found out that I was accepted in the graduate program of my choice in a different state. And I have been wanting to live in this new state for a long time because I like the environs better than the one I'm in now, and I have several friends there too. This therapist seems like she cares, and I feel sorry to leave this therapist because I don't know if I'll be able to find another one who understands me as well.

Patient's statement: [Hesitantly] I think that I've made up my mind. My father is against my decision, my mother is neutral, and my brother can't make up his mind. Last time, I told you that I may be close to having the opportunity to go to graduate school full time and to quit my job, but then I don't know how I'll be able to pay my bills. I'm able to get a loan, but my father is against it. You and I know that he has the wherewithal to help me out, but he wants me to stay in town… Also, I received a part-time scholarship to study in the English department in the graduate school of my choice, and a work-study position, but it may not cover all costs. I do have some savings.

Therapist's inner thoughts: I'm hoping that this can be a positive experience for him despite the lack of support that he's receiving at home.

Therapist's statement: Congratulations, Darren! I'm excited for you. The new graduate school program in the English department seems like a good opportunity for you, and you've been planning it and mulling it over, back and forth, for so long.

Patient's inner thoughts: At last. Some support for my decision and hard work.

Patient's statement: Thank you. I still feel a bit unsure, but I know that it's the right choice for me. I really would like to live in the new state permanently because of what it offers, because my friends are there, and now I have the chance to go to the graduate program of my choice, receive a scholarship, and a work-study position. I think that if the members of my family were with me more in spirit, I would feel better. Also, if I accept, I will be moving in six weeks after graduation from college. My problem now is that I feel that I still need therapy but realize that I may not be able to continue with you if I make a permanent move and establish residency in the new state.

Therapist's inner thoughts: Darren seems to wish to continue in therapy, but he has decided to move out of state permanently. There's a short period of time to talk about termination issues such as separation and loss and exploring different means of financial support. At the same time, it's important for me to empower his decision to move because he's been wanting to move to this new state for several years, and now he's received an acceptance at a graduate program in this state along with a scholarship and work-study position.

Therapist's statement: I'm proud that you've made a positive decision for yourself. I know it was hard for you. At the same time, we need to prepare for termination in therapy. How many sessions will we have given your upcoming move?

Patient's inner thoughts: I will really miss this therapist. She gets it.

Patient's statement: I have a lot to discuss with you before I leave such as financial stuff, and I'll miss this therapy. I'm hoping for four or five more sessions.

Therapist's inner thoughts: I need to help him establish a relationship with another therapist in the state where he will have permanent residence.

Therapist's statement: During our last few sessions, let's continue to discuss a plan for termination, to talk over issues related to separation, and to explore financial options for you. I will be helping you to make the transition to a new therapist. I have two colleagues in that state, and I wish to consult with them prior to offering you a few referrals.

Summary

During his therapy sessions, Darren was able to explore and to make an important decision in his life. At the same time, although Darren expressed satisfaction with the therapist, Darren initiated a premature termination because of his decision to move to another state and establish permanent residency in the new state, a path that he had explored for several years. The tasks of termination for this dyad included discussion of separation, empowering the client's independent decision, discussions of the reality of finances, and finding a new therapist. Whereas ruptures were the impetus for premature termination in the vignette with Dana, the impetus for premature termination from therapy with Darren was his move to another state.

In summary, premature terminations, initiated by patients, can occur because of ruptures, a patient's loss of insurance, a move by a client, a client's illness, or other patient-initiated unilateral terminations. In the previous vignette, a client initiated a forced termination because of a move to another state. Premature terminations initiated by clients, at times, may occur because of clients' particular issues, for example, a client's style of attachment and/or for reasons unknown to the therapist or to the client. The next segment explores premature terminations initiated by clients that are related to the client's diagnosis.

Premature Termination and Patient Diagnosis

The previous vignette highlighted the experience of a client, Darren, who was satisfied with his therapist. The impetus for his initiated premature termination was his decision to permanently move out of state rather than a rupture during therapy or his diagnosis. Are there particular kinds of individuals who tend to drop out of therapy, for example, individuals with specific characterological problems? There are several patient variables that can predict premature termination. Patient variables that predict premature termination include a patient's substance abuse, and more severe emotional disorders such as personality disorders (Cluster B) and psychosis (Philips et al., 2018). This section focuses on the relationship between a patient's diagnosis and a premature termination initiated by a patient.

Dropout rates for patients who are diagnosed with different emotional disorders can vary (Swift & Greenberg, 2015). Swift and Greenberg (2015) found that patients with personality disorders and patients with eating disorders have the highest dropout rate, and patients with personality disorders were found to have a higher dropout rate than patients with eating disorders. They explain that it is no surprise that patients with personality and eating disorders would have the highest rates of premature discontinuation as these disorders are distinguished by rigidity, and the development of the treatment process can be slow. Philips and colleagues (2018, p. 208) point out that a median rate of therapy dropout of 37% was found for patients with personality disorders (e.g., McMurran et al., 2010) and that dropout among these patients is related to a lower level of education and occupation, a younger age, having a mother and father who divorced prior to the patient reaching age 10, and a past filled with neglect during childhood (e.g., McMurran et al., 2010).

With respect to eating disorders, Jordan and colleagues (2017, p. 979) note that premature termination for patients with anorexia nervosa is common, and it has been shown that 30–40% of adult clients with anorexia nervosa do not complete therapy in outpatient settings (e.g., DeJong et al., 2012). They found that treatment credibility, the patient's report of whether the intervention is logical, applicable, and helpful, was a variable that predicted dropouts from therapy for patients with anorexia nervosa. Swift and colleagues (2017, p. 48) point out that for patients with anorexia, it was found that the termination rate for medication was higher than for psychotherapy or a combination of psychotherapy and medication (e.g., DeJong et al., 2012), and for GAD, no difference was found in the rates of termination whether psychotherapy or medication was used (e.g., Gonçalves & Byrne, 2012). They note that for social anxiety, patients were almost two times more likely to refuse medication over therapy; for depression, patients were a bit over two times more likely to refuse medication over therapy; for panic disorder, almost three times more likely to refuse medication over therapy; however, for PTSD, mixed anxiety disorders, obsessive-compulsive disorder, GAD, and eating disorders, no differences in rates of treatment refusal were found between medication and therapy. Furthermore, it has been shown that patients with depression, social anxiety disorder, and panic disorder will be more likely to commence treatment if they are offered the choice of receiving psychotherapy (Swift et al., 2017).

According to Gamache and colleagues (2018), early termination has been associated with deleterious results for clients, such as poorer outcomes for clients with narcissistic (Ronningstam et al., 1995), borderline (e.g., Gunderson et al., 1989; Yeomans et al., 1994), and anti-social personality (e.g., Cacciola et al., 1995; Woody et al., 1985) disorders. The following vignette illustrates an example of a client, Scott, with a substance use disorder who quits therapy suddenly.

Vignette of an Example of a Client with a Substance Use Disorder Who Initiates Termination Prematurely: A Hard Cold Stop

INTRODUCTION

It has been shown that therapy for individuals with personality disorders is characterized by a high proportion of premature termination (Gamache et al., 2018). Philips and colleagues (2018, p. 208) point out that the likelihood of premature termination is greater for patients with a diagnosis of a personality disorder and with substance use disorder (e.g., Bohart & Wade, 2013).

In the following example, the patient, Scott, is 42 years old, and it is his first encounter with therapy. In a previous session, he informed the therapist that he wants to be the number one salesman in his company. During the middle of his second session, he quits, stomps out of the room, and does not return.

DIALOGUE

Patient's inner thoughts: I'm not sure that I feel right being here. This is very different than I've ever experienced. I'm not sure that this is for me. I usually do things on my own. I don't need to consult anybody in therapy because I know most things. I don't know how my friends would react if they knew I were going to therapy. I'll tell her a few things.

Therapist's inner thoughts: Scott looks uncomfortable and angry. I wonder if now would be a good time to bring it up with him. But I don't know him well enough. I think I'll tread lightly.

Patient's statement: Last night, the guys and I had a few beers. They've been watching me work on my house. I've been working on my house for some time. It needs fixing, and I don't really have a hand from anyone. People need to do what I want. It's ridiculous the way things have been going. I told the guy in the hardware store that I need the tools [Shouts] NOW, not yesterday.

Therapist's statement: Tell me more about the house and the work. Have you been working on it alone up until now?

Patient's statement: [Cracks open his second beer] Hal said he'd be out to help on the roof. But he didn't show up last week. I called him last week, and I'm really angry about it. [Scott's phone is ringing, and he answers his phone. Scott shouts at Hal over the phone in the therapist's office for about five minutes] That was Hal. He said that he can't be out to help me in the next month because he has some other business. I really was counting on him. [Scott's phone rings again, and he answers. Scott speaks to Sarina for about five minutes] Oh. That was Sarina. I told her that I would be by her house when I'm ready! [Scott lights up a second cigarette. Takes a gulp of his beer]

Therapist's inner thoughts: I wonder if he saw the building sign downstairs that said no smoking. My office is a small room, and it's filling with smoke.

Therapist's statement: I'm interested in hearing more about your arrangement with Hal, but I'm wondering if I can ask you to put out the cigarette. This building has a no smoking policy.

Patient's statement: What! Goodbye. [Slams the door] I don't need anyone else telling me what to do.

Summary

In this vignette, the patient, Scott, a patient with a personality disorder and a substance use disorder initiates a premature termination when the therapist informs him about the no smoking sign in the building. It is questionable whether the patient began to engage in therapy at all. Scott does not respond to the note that the therapist sends him in the mail a week later, and he does not call or return to therapy.

The next scenario describes a premature termination initiated by a patient with a personality disorder who thinks that individuals are in love with him. In this vignette, the patient, Randy, makes explicit advances on an early career therapist who consults with her supervisor about her discomfort with this patient.

Vignette of an Example of a Premature Termination Initiated by a Patient With a Narcissistic Personality Disorder

Introduction

The following is an example of a patient, Randy, who is obsessed with the thought that people are in love with him. Randy terminated therapy prematurely after the third appointment. Prior to the third session, the therapist, a novice clinician who works in a clinic discusses her discomfort about this patient with her supervisor. The therapist knows that she is not looking forward to the advances of this patient and decides to discuss her thoughts with the patient. The therapist's supervisor supports her intention to maintain a firm approach with Randy and advises her to have the clinic secretary stay in the reception room during the patient's next session. Prior to the session, the therapist is thinking: *This patient continues to make explicit and nuanced advances throughout the session as he has done during previous sessions, and he thinks that I want to go out on a date with him. I know that I have done nothing to give him this impression. Yet he continues his advances, and I have told my supervisor that I am uncomfortable with his advances. My supervisor and I have discussed his narcissistic personality disorder and his tendency toward erotomania.*

Dialogue

Patient's statement: [Dramatically] Ooo… Don't you look precious today. [Patient smiles broadly] You remind me of that girl in my biology class who I'm 100% certain wants me to date her. In fact, I went up to her after the first class and I told her that we could go out after class.

Therapist's inner thoughts: There he goes again, making the same advances as he did before. I'm so uncomfortable. How can he believe I want to go out on a date with him? I didn't do anything to bring this on. Or did I? And my supervisor agrees that I have to stay firm.

Therapist's statement: [Firmly] Some of the comments that you have been directing toward me and other individuals are unacceptable, and they need to stop now!

Patient's inner thoughts: [Ignores the therapist's statement] I'll tell the therapist about the new place I'm thinking about, and how I can pick her up after her last patient to take her there for a good time. I know from the last session that she's looking forward to going out with me. Maybe, I'll pick some flowers outside. She's sure to want to go with me then.

Patient's statement: Well, that girl in my biology class was busy, but I found a cool place that I wanted to take her. You'd like the place. Maybe we can go after your last patient? I'm sure you'll have a great time.

Therapist's inner thoughts: How am I going to get through this session? He jumps to the conclusion that I, similar to the girl in his biology class, want to go out with him. I am so angry. I need to speak to him firmly.

Therapist's statement: [Speaks clearly and firmly] I understand that sometimes you have intense feelings that people are in love with you; however ...

Patient's statement: [Misreads and cuts off therapist] I knew it. You'll go on a date with me! I can pick you up after your last patient. I think that's at 6 P.M. I watched your office last week, and I see that's when you usually leave. I've been watching for a few weeks so that I can know when you leave and have flowers ready for you when I pick you up. We'll have a grand time, and I love to eat at this place with my favorite person. A romantic evening for me and you. Just what I need.

Therapist's inner thoughts: Oh no. He's stalking me too. I need to be even firmer. Okay. Here goes.

Therapist's statement: I was saying that will not be possible because...

Patient's statement: [Irate and shouting] What do you mean won't be possible? What are you talking about? I know that you love me more than your other patients. You even wore my favorite colors last session. You remind me of that girl in my biology class who was also a tease. After the first class, I knew she loved me, but then she ended up ditching me. [Patient continues to rant angrily] All women are teases. You're like the rest of them. No different. A tease is a tease is a tease is a tease. [Patient is ranting] I'm sick and tired of this business. Here, I do my best to please you, talk about flowers, and a nice time. I do not need you. I have others waiting who think that I am charming and want to go on a date with me tonight. [Patient is shouting, slams door, and leaves]

SUMMARY

The patient in this vignette has a narcissistic personality disorder, a grandiose belief of one's importance accompanied by little or no empathy for others, with a tendency toward erotomania, an individual's irrational belief that another is in love with the individual. Despite the therapist's repeated efforts to curtail his advances, he continued with the enduring thought that people are attracted to him, think him charming, and fall in love with him when, in reality, they barely know him. The therapist's supervisor supported her decision to maintain a firm approach toward this patient in the face of his unreasonable and persistent demands, which presented the therapist with an uncomfortable challenge.

This section highlighted the relationship between the client's makeup, for example, a personality disorder, and premature termination. The therapist needs to take into consideration the client's diagnosis, for example, narcissistic personality disorder, borderline personality disorder, and each client's capacity for attachment given the diagnosis of a personality disorder.

Previous sections have explored the connection between a therapist's theoretical orientation, for example, psychodynamic, cognitive-behavioral, humanistic, and premature termination separately from the connection between the patient's diagnosis and dropout from therapy. The next part explores the way in which these variables, premature termination, therapist theoretical orientation, and patient diagnosis, interact with each other.

Premature Termination, Therapists' Theoretical Orientation, and Patients' Diagnosis

Is there an interaction between patient-initiated premature termination, therapist theoretical orientation, and patient diagnosis? According to Swift and Greenberg (2015), the rate of dropout does not vary considerably depending upon a therapist's theoretical orientation unless crossed with particular diagnoses. For example, it was found that for depression and PTSD (where significant variation among different theoretical approaches was found), integrative therapy approaches (approaches to psychotherapy that draw from many therapy models and are developed into a comprehensive framework that transcends the limitations of a single model) were shown to have the lowest rates of dropout (Swift & Greenberg, 2015). Rates of dropout were shown not to differ considerably between treatment orientations for nine emotional disorders studied by Swift and Greenberg (2015), for example, GAD, panic disorder, obsessive-compulsive disorder, social phobia, and others; however, these researchers found significant differences for rates of dropout for PTSD, eating disorders, and depression. Swift and Greenberg (2015) point out that with respect to PTSD, the highest average rate of premature discontinuation was shown for CBT, and the lowest average rate of premature termination was shown for an integrative orientation. It is suggested that practitioners who use a theoretical orientation with a high rate of dropout such as CBT for PTSD recognize the high risk for premature termination and use other strategies to decrease dropout (Swift & Greenberg, 2015).

The following vignette illustrates an example of the interaction between the variables, premature termination, theoretical orientation, and patient diagnosis. In this scenario, the therapist needed to consider the likelihood that the patient, Hank, would drop out when, during a rupture, he persisted in using a manualized cognitive-behavioral approach to treat Hank. Hank has PTSD. Had the therapist switched to a relational or integrative approach when he became aware that Hank was experiencing anxiety and trauma rather than rigidly adhering to his theoretical orientation, the therapist would have had a greater chance of retaining the patient.

Vignette of an Example of a Patient With Post-Traumatic Stress Disorder Who Prematurely Terminates Therapy and a Cognitive-Behavioral Therapist

INTRODUCTION

This vignette illustrates an example of the interaction of a patient with a diagnosis of PTSD and a cognitive-behavioral therapist. In this scenario, Hank, a 32-year-old patient, has been discharged from the service because he was found wondering in a field, off course from the rest of his unit. For the last half of a year, he has been having recurring nightmares about his own death. This is the third session with the cognitive-behavioral therapist.

DIALOGUE

Patient's inner thoughts: Maybe I can get a job as a sniper somewhere else because I know I messed up in the service, and they don't want me back. I might be okay as a sniper if I could concentrate again and focus on the right stuff. But now I'm so messed up. I don't know what's wrong with me. I didn't used to be like this. Really hard for me. Why when I first arrived in Afghanistan, I was being showered with compliments from the sergeant.

Therapist's inner thoughts: He's army. I don't know why he's not progressing with the exposures. I'm doing the exposure therapy the way I learned it and applied it for the last 15 years.

Patient's statement: I still can't sleep at night. I keep having bad dreams. My wife says I'm not the same since I returned. The exercises aren't helping me.

Therapist's statement: You need to stick with the homework. It will eventually help. It usually does.

Patient's inner thoughts: To heck with this. I'm elsewhere.

Therapist's inner thoughts: He looks out of it, but I want to stick with my protocol. [Silence. Patient approaches the window]

Therapist's statement: Where are you going?

[Patient looks dazed, out of it. Sitting on ledge of the windowsill without speaking]

Therapist's statement: You need to be practicing your exercises now.

Patient' statement: I'm not sure that I want to live anymore, let alone do your crummy exercises.

Therapist's statement: It's really important for you to give these exercises a fair shake. We need to end for the day. Same time next week?

Patient's statement: I don't think so. I knew I shouldn't have ever told my wife that I'd try therapy. I did it only because she wanted it, but I'm sorry for it now. Never again!

Summary

The way that this cognitive-behavioral therapist approached the client with PTSD is not a correct approach. Although individuals with PTSD can present challenges to therapists, the therapist's behavior is inexcusable. The therapist in this vignette wished to preserve his theoretical approach, CBT, and sacrificed a relationship with Hank who suffered from PTSD. He clearly did not have the patient's interests at the top of his agenda. The therapist missed crucial cues, for example, Hank's suicidal ideation. His issues, similar to those of other therapists in the vignettes who do not have a cognitive-behavioral approach, interfered with his work with Hank. Rather than relying on a manualized, one-size-fits-all approach for individuals with PTSD, an adequate therapeutic response, at least, needs to be attuned to the unique issues of the patient. Integrative strategies may help patients with PTSD (Swift & Greenberg, 2015); however, in this case, the therapist rigidly adhered to one theoretical approach, CBT, despite the patient's refusal.

Chapter Summary

Research has demonstrated that rates of refusal for medication have been shown to be approximately two times more than refusal rates for therapy, particularly for patients with depression, panic, and social anxiety disorders (Swift et al., 2017). Chapter 4, "Termination Across Different Diagnoses and Theories," described the relationship between ending in therapy and therapist variables and between termination from therapy and patient variables. It focused on the different types of termination, fully planned and premature, that evolve for patients with different emotional and personality disorders, how therapists with different theoretical orientations navigate the termination process, and the interaction between therapist theoretical orientation and patient diagnosis and its impact on the termination process. Examples of the inner experiences of the therapist and patient during the process of full-term terminations and premature or unilateral terminations were included throughout the chapter. See Table 4.2

Chapter 5, "The I_{rt} – CARE Transtheoretical, Psycholinguistic Model of Ruptures and Repairs," presents a transtheoretical model that encourages the patient to consolidate the work of the therapeutic process across various theories. This model, with its emphasis on the covert or inner experiences of therapists, emphasizes the dynamic between a therapist and a patient and describes the critical phases in the therapy process so that these difficult transitions can be navigated with skill and compassion. It emphasizes the notion that disagreements, in therapy and beyond, happen, and it is the move toward repair or resolution that is the crux of the matter rather than the therapy rupture itself. The integrative model embraced in Chapter 5 recognizes the ruptures and repairs that take place in the therapeutic alliance and explores an educative view of strategies for avoiding and repairing ruptures across theoretical orientations.

Table 4.2 Vignettes: Premature Termination, Patient Diagnosis, and Therapist Approach

Diagnosis			
Theoretical Approach of Therapist	Personality Disorder With Substance Use Disorder	Narcissistic Personality Disorder	Posttraumatic Stress Disorder
	Scott	Randy	
Cognitive-Behavioral			Hank

References

Aafjes-Van Doorn, K., & Wooldridge, T. (2018). The complexity of loss during a forced termination: A case illustration. *British Journal of Psychotherapy, 34*(2), 285–299. https://doi.org/10.1111/bjp.12362

Bartholomew, T. T., Lockard, A. J., Folger, S. F., Low, B. E., Poet, A. D., Scofield, B. E., & Locke, B. D. (2019). Symptom reduction and termination: Client change and therapist identified reasons for saying goodbye. *Counselling Psychology Quarterly, 32*(1), 81–99. https://doi.org/10.1080/09515070.2017.1367272

Beck, J. S. (1995). *Cognitive therapy: Basics and beyond.* Guilford Press.

Berghofer, G., Schmidl, F., Rudas, S., Steiner, E., & Schmitz, M. (2002). Predictors of treatment discontinuity in outpatient mental health care. *Social Psychiatry and Psychiatric Epidemiology, 37,* 276–282. https://doi.org/10.1007/s001270200020

Bohart, A. C., & Wade, A. G. (2013). The client in psychotherapy. In M. J. Lambert (Ed.), *Bergin and Garfield's handbook of psychotherapy and behavior change,* (6th ed., pp. 219–257). Wiley.

Cacciola, J. S., Alterman, A. I., Rutherford, M. J., Snider, E. C. (1995). Treatment response of antisocial abusers. *The Journal of Nervous and Mental Disease, 183*(3), 166–171. https://doi.org/10.1097/00005053-199503000-00007

Constantino, M. J., Marnell, M. E., Haile, A. J., Kanther-Sista, S. N., Wolman, K., Zappert, L., & Arnow, B. A. (2008). Integrative cognitive therapy for depression: A randomized pilot comparison. *Psychotherapy: Theory, Research, Practice, Training, 45*(2), 122–134. https://doi.org/10.1037/0033-3204.45.2.122

Curtis, R. (2002). Termination from a psychoanalytic perspective. *Journal of Psychotherapy Integration, 12*(3), 350–357. https://doi.org/10.1037/1053-0479.12.3.350

DeBerry, S., & Baskin, D. (1989). Termination criteria in psychotherapy: A comparison of private and public practice. *The American Journal of Psychotherapy, 43*(1), 43–53. https://doi.org/10.1176/appi.psychotherapy.1989.43.1.43

DeJong, H., Broadbent, H., & Schmidt, U. (2012). A systematic review of dropout from treatment in outpatients with anorexia nervosa. *International Journal of Eating Disorders, 45*(5), 635–647. https://doi.org/10.1002/eat.20956

De Maat, S., Dekker, J., Schoevers, R., & De Jonghe, F. (2006). Relative efficacy of psychotherapy and pharmacotherapy in the treatment of depression: A meta-analysis. *Psychotherapy Research, 16*(5), 566–578. https://doi.org/10.1080/10503300600756402

Elliott, R., Watson, J. C., Goldman, R. N., & Greenberg, L. S. (2004). *Learning emotion-focused therapy: The process-experiential approach to change.* American Psychological Association.

Gabbard, G. O. (2009). What is a "good enough" termination? *Journal of the American Psychoanalytic Association, 57*(3), 575–594. https://doi.org/10.1177/0003065109340678

Gamache, D., Savard, C., Lemelin, S., Côté, A., & Villeneuve, E. (2018). Premature psychotherapy termination in an outpatient treatment program for personality disorders: a survival analysis. *Comprehensive Psychiatry, 80,* 14–23. https://doi.org/10.1016/j.comppsych.2017.08.001

Garfield, S. L. (1994). Research on client variables in psychotherapy. In A. E. Bergin & S. L. Garfield (Eds.), *Handbook of psychotherapy and behavior change* (4th ed., pp. 190–228). John Wiley & Sons.

Goldfried, M. R. (2002). A cognitive-behavioral perspective on termination. *Journal of Psychotherapy Integration, 12*(3), 364–372. https://doi.org/10.1037/1053-0479.12.3.364

Gonçalves, D. C., & Byrne, G. J. (2012). Interventions for generalized anxiety disorder in older adults: Systematic review and meta-analysis. *Journal of Anxiety Disorders, 26*(1), 1–11. https://doi.org/10.1016/j.janxdis.2011.08.010

Greenberg, L. S. (2002). Termination of experiential therapy. *Journal of Psychotherapy Integration, 12*(3), 358–363. https://doi.org/10.1037/1053-0479.12.3.358

Gunderson, J. G., Frank, A. F., Ronningstam, E. F., Wachter, S., Lynch, V. J., & Wolf, P. J. (1989). Early discontinuance of borderline patients from psychotherapy. *The Journal of Nervous and Mental Disease, 177*(1), 38–42. https://doi.org/10.1097/00005053-198901000-00006

Hilsenroth, M. J. (2017). An introduction to the special issue on psychotherapy termination. *Psychotherapy, 54*(1), 1–3. https://doi.org/10.1037/pst0000106

Howard, K. I., Kopta, S. M., Krause, M. S., & Orlinsky, D. E. (1986). The dose-effect relationship in psychotherapy. *American Psychologist, 41*(2), 159–164. https://doi.org/10.1037/0003-066X.41.2.159

Jakobsons, L. J., Brown, J. S., Gordon, K. H., & Joiner, T. E. (2007). When are clients ready to terminate? *Cognitive and Behavioral Practice, 14*(2), 218–230. https://doi.org/10.1016/j.cbpra.2006.09.005

Jordan, J., McIntosh, V. V., Carter, F. A., Joyce, P. R., Frampton, C. M., Luty, S. E., & Bulik, C. M. (2017). Predictors of premature termination from psychotherapy for anorexia nervosa: Low treatment credibility, early therapy alliance, and self-transcendence. *International Journal of Eating Disorders, 50*(8), 979–983. https://doi.org/10.1002/eat.22726

Joyce, A. S., Piper, W. E., Ogrodniczuk, J. S., & Klein, R. H. (2007). *Termination in psychotherapy: A psychodynamic model of processes and outcomes*. American Psychological Association.

Mahon, J., Bradley, S. N., Harvey, P. K., Winston, A. P., & Palmer, R. L. (2001). Childhood trauma has dose–effect relationship with dropping out from psychotherapeutic treatment for bulimia nervosa: A replication. *International Journal of Eating Disorders, 30*(2), 138–148. https://doi.org/10.1002/eat.1066

McCullough, J. P., Jr. (2000). *Treatment for chronic depression: Cognitive behavioral analysis system of psychotherapy (CBASP)*. Guilford Press.

McMurran, M., Huband, N., & Overton, E. (2010). Non-completion of personality disorder treatments: A systematic review of correlates, consequences, and interventions. *Clinical Psychology Review, 30*(3), 277–287. https://doi.org/10.1016/j.cpr.2009.12.002

Muran, J. C., Safran, J. D., Gorman, B. S., Samstag, L. W., Eubanks-Carter, C., & Winston, A. (2009). The relationship of early alliance ruptures and their resolution to process and outcome in three time-limited psychotherapies for personality disorders. *Psychotherapy: Theory, Research, Practice, Training, 46*(2), 233–248. https://doi.org/10.1037/a0016085

Muran, J. C., Safran, J. D., Samstag, L. W., & Winston, A. (2005). Evaluating an alliance-focused treatment for personality disorders. *Psychotherapy: Theory, Research, Practice, Training, 42*(4), 532–545. https://doi.org/10.1037/0033-3204.42.4.532

Nelson, W. M., & Politano, P. M. (1993). The goal is to say "goodbye" and have the treatment effects generalize and maintain: A cognitive-behavioral view of termination. *Journal of Cognitive Psychotherapy, 7*(4), 251–264. https://doi.org/10.1891/0889-8391.7.4.251

Norcross, J. C., Zimmerman, B. E., Greenberg, R. P., & Swift, J. K. (2017). Do all therapists do that when saying goodbye? A study of commonalities in termination behaviors. *Psychotherapy, 54*(1), 66–75. https://doi.org/10.1037/pst0000097

Ogrodniczuk, J. S., Joyce, A. S., & Piper, W. E. (2005). Strategies for reducing patient-initiated premature termination of psychotherapy. *Harvard Review of Psychiatry, 13*(2), 57–70. https://doi.org/10.1080/10673220590956429

Okamoto, A., Dattilio, F. M., Dobson, K. S., & Kazantzis, N. (2019). The therapeutic relationship in cognitive–behavioral therapy: Essential features and common challenges. *Practice Innovations, 4*(2), 112–123. https://doi.org/10.1037/pri0000088

Pedder, J. R. (1988). Termination reconsidered. *International Journal of Psycho-Analysis, 69*(4), 495–505.

Philips, B., Karlsson, R., Nygren, R., Rother-Schirren, A., & Werbart, A. (2018). Early therapeutic process related to dropout in mentalization-based treatment with dual diagnosis patients. *Psychoanalytic Psychology, 35*(2), 205–216. https://doi.org/10.1037/pap0000170

Ronningstam, E., Gunderson, J., & Lyons, M. (1995). Changes in pathological narcissism. *The American Journal of Psychiatry, 152*(2), 253–257. https://doi.org/10.1176/ajp.152.2.253

Roos, J., & Werbart, A. (2013). Therapist and relationship factors influencing dropout from individual psychotherapy: A literature review. *Psychotherapy Research, 23*(4), 394–418. https://doi.org/10.1080/10503307.2013.775528

Shahar, G., & Ziv-Beiman, S. (2020). Using termination as an intervention (UTAI): A view from an integrative, cognitive-existential psychodynamics perspective. *Psychotherapy, 57*(4), 515–520. https://doi.org/10.1037/pst0000337

Swift, J. K., & Greenberg, R. P. (2012). Premature discontinuation in adult psychotherapy: A meta-analysis. *Journal of Consulting and Clinical Psychology, 80*(4), 547–559. https://doi.org/10.1037/a0028226

Swift, J. K., & Greenberg, R. P. (2015). Premature termination in psychotherapy: Strategies for engaging clients and improving outcomes. American Psychological Association. https://doi.org/10.1037/14469-000

Swift, J. K., Greenberg, R. P., Tompkins, K. A., & Parkin, S. R. (2017). Treatment refusal and premature termination in psychotherapy, pharmacotherapy, and their combination: A meta-analysis of head-to-head comparisons. *Psychotherapy, 54*(1), 47–57. https://doi.org/10.1037/pst0000104

Teyber, E., & Teyber, F. H. (2017). *Interpersonal process in therapy: An integrative model* (7th ed.). Cengage Learning.

Vasquez, M. J., Bingham, R. P., & Barnett, J. E. (2008). Psychotherapy termination: Clinical and ethical responsibilities. *Journal of Clinical Psychology, 64*(5), 653–665. https://doi.org/10.1002/jclp.20478

Vidair, H. B., Feyijinmi, G. O., & Feindler, E. L. (2017). Termination in cognitive-behavioral therapy with children, adolescents, and parents. *Psychotherapy, 54*(1), 15–21. https://doi.org/10.1037/pst0000086

Wachtel, P. L. (2002). Termination of therapy: An effort at integration. *Journal of Psychotherapy Integration, 12*(3), 373–383. https://doi.org/10.1037/1053-0479.12.3.373

Werman, D. S. (1984). *The practice of supportive psychotherapy.* Brunner/Mazel.

Woody, G. E., McLellan, A. T., Luborsky, L., & O'Brien, C. P. (1985). Sociopathy and psychotherapy outcome. *Archives of General Psychiatry, 42*(11), 1081–1086. https://doi.org/10.1001/archpsyc.1985.01790340059009

Yalom, I. D. (2017). *The gift of therapy: An open letter to a new generation of therapists and their patients.* Harper Perennial.

Yeomans, F. E., Gutfreund, J., Selzer, M. A., Clarkin, J. F., Hull, J. W., & Smith, T. E. (1994). Factors related to drop-outs by borderline patients: Treatment contract and therapeutic alliance. *The Journal of Psychotherapy Practice and Research, 3*(1), 16–24.

Part III

A Transtheoretical Model

Introduction

The following is a brief excerpt of a dialogue from the fifth session of a 41-year old female client, Candace, who is a graduate student in the engineering department. Candace contacted the university's counseling center because she is dissatisfied with her graduate program, and she is having difficulty keeping up with her work. The therapist is a client-centered therapist, and the members of the therapeutic dyad are about to hit a rocky patch.

Dialogue

Patient's inner thoughts: The therapist is a nice person, and we seem to be getting on well, but I'm nowhere with my goals. I'm at the same place that I started when I had my first session. I need some concrete stuff.

Patient's statement: I keep talking to you, but I'm not getting anywhere. Can't you give me some advice about how to proceed here?

Therapist's inner thoughts: I've been using a humanistic, client-centered approach, with active listening, throughout the sessions; however, the client does not seem to be satisfied. I've practiced Rogerian therapy for three years.

Therapist's statement: You seem to be asking me for homework ideas about your course of study in the engineering department. Can you tell me more?

DOI: 10.4324/9781003128489-7

Patient's inner thoughts: Oh, no! Not another session where I do all the talking.

Patient's statement: I don't like my graduate school program. I don't know what to do...

Summary

In the aforementioned brief segment, the patient, Candace, is frustrated with the therapist and with what she is getting from the therapy. The therapist is using a client-centered approach; however, Candace is requesting feedback, advice, and guidance from the therapist. A confrontation rupture occurs, and Candace lets the therapist know that she feels unhappy with her studies, needs a response from the therapist, and is, generally, dissatisfied because her needs are not being met.

Part III, "A Transtheoretical Model," develops an overarching two-part model that addresses the connection between ruptures and termination, a model that relies on concepts from psycholinguistics in order to assist therapists who wish to avoid ruptures. When ruptures occur, the model can help therapists understand why they occur and how to repair them. Part III consists of Chapter 5, "The I_{rt} – CARE Transtheoretical, Psycholinguistic Model of Ruptures and Repairs," and Chapter 6, "The I_{rt} – CARE Transtheoretical, Psycholinguistic Model of Termination: The Termination or the Ending Process of Therapy."

Chapter 5, "The I_{rt} – CARE Transtheoretical, Psycholinguistic Model of Ruptures and Repairs," includes a transtheoretical framework of the rupture and repair process in the therapeutic alliance that relies on psycholinguistic components. The model underscores how therapists think and speak about their work and highlights their understanding of the inner experiences of their own and of their patients, provides a blueprint that emphasizes the verbal, paralinguistic, and nonverbal dynamic between a therapist and a patient, and describes the therapy process so that the difficult moment-to-moment transitions during a rupture can be navigated with skill and compassion. The I_{rt} – CARE model relies on the verbal and nonverbal nuances of language as well as on paralinguistic elements to inform therapists about how to avoid ruptures and how to repair them. It encourages therapists to focus on the details of the dyadic dialogue so that the members of the dyad become less stuck during a rupture, so that the rupture does not become irreparable.

Each of the letters of the psycholinguistic I_{rt} – CARE model represents different aspects or concepts of ruptures, repairs, and termination, and the concepts may intersect. This transtheoretical model relies on psycholinguistic elements. The letter "I" stands for inner or immediacy, the letter "r" (subscript) of I_{rt} for rupture, the letter "t" (subscript) of I_{rt} for termination, the letter "C" for covert, curiosity, compassion, the letter "A" stands for awareness, alliance, attunement, or authenticity, the letter "R" for repair or resolution, and the letter "E" for empathy or ending. The model includes a psycholinguistic framework that can inform therapists about the verbal and nonverbal nuances of language as well as paralinguistic features necessary to understand what is happening in the therapeutic alliance.

Chapter 6, "The I_{rt} – CARE Transtheoretical, Psycholinguistic Model of Termination: The Termination or the Ending Process of Therapy," develops a transtheoretical model that can help therapists to navigate termination in the context of differing theoretical orientations. Similar, but somewhat different from the representations of the letters of the model that were described in Chapter 5, in the portion of the model described in Chapter 6, the I_{rt} – CARE Transtheoretical, Psycholinguistic Model of Termination: The Termination or the Ending Process of Therapy, the letter "I" stands for inner (covert), the letter "r" (subscript) of I_{rt} for rupture, the letter "t" (subscript) of I_{rt} for termination, the letter "C" for covert or consolidation, the letter "A" stands for awareness or alliance, the letter "R" for repair or resolution, and the letter "E", for ending or empathy. The psycholinguistic model in Chapter 6 can inform therapists about the verbal and nonverbal nuances of language as well as paralinguistic features necessary to understand what is happening during the termination process and entails a compass that can guide therapists and patients as they navigate difficult transitions during the end phase of therapy.

The I$_{rt}$ – CARE Transtheoretical, Psycholinguistic Model of Ruptures and Repairs

5

Introduction

The contribution of the therapeutic alliance to the progress of clients is underscored throughout the book, *Navigating Ruptures, Repairs, and Termination Within the Therapeutic Process*. Previous chapters have suggested that ruptures or breaks in communication during therapy and beyond are not infrequent, that they are humbling experiences for therapists and clients, and that repairing these tensions or deteriorations in the therapeutic alliance is a challenge to therapists, regardless of their theoretical orientation, for example, cognitive-behavioral, psychodynamic, humanistic (e.g., Eubanks et al., 2023; Muran et al., 2023). Luo and colleagues (2022, p. 642) point out that the term "rupture" and the negative process between clients and therapists that it connotes is transtheoretical, and it is used to convey the tensions or disruptions that occur across different therapeutic perspectives (e.g., Safran et al., 2011a; Safran & Muran, 2006). Difficulties in the alliance are present across theoretical orientations, and no matter the therapeutic orientation, tensions will ensue, ruptures will vary by type, for example, confrontation or withdrawal, and many tensions will be repaired (Macdonald et al., 2023). Previous chapters have described the feelings of discomfort and vulnerability that therapists and patients experience during ruptures and their difficulty in knowing how to proceed.

Regardless of their theoretical orientation, it is important for therapists to attend to ruptures during therapy sessions (Safran & Kraus, 2014; Safran et al.,

DOI: 10.4324/9781003128489-8

2011a). There is a relationship between rupture resolution and a decrease in a client's tendency to prematurely drop out of therapy, and given the often subtle or nuanced nature of ruptures, a therapist's responsiveness is vital in the repair process (Eubanks, Muran, et al., 2019; Eubanks, Sergi, et al., 2021). The therapist as well as the patient are involved in the creation of a rupture, and the therapist and the patient need to be involved in its repair (Muran et al., 2023). It is critical for therapists to be aware of subtle movements so that they can respond to them (Eubanks, Sergi, et al., 2021). There are several ways that therapists can repair ruptures. It is suggested that therapists take initiative to help to repair a rupture by encouraging patients to express their negative thoughts about therapy and what they would want changed, by taking responsibility for contributing to the rupture, and by interpreting ruptures according to what transpires for patients external to the therapy session (Kline et al., 2019; Safran et al., 2001; Safran et al., 2011b).

Ruptures can be viewed from different perspectives. Chapter 5 views ruptures from a psycholinguistic perspective and relies on the verbal, paralinguistic, and nonverbal elements of a psycholinguistic framework. The chapter includes a transtheoretical or overarching psycholinguistic model of the rupture and repair process in the therapeutic alliance. The transtheoretical framework, the I_{rt} – CARE Transtheoretical, Psycholinguistic Model of Ruptures and Repairs, incorporates a view of the linguistic styles of therapists and patients and encourages therapists to integrate elements from various theories that address the particularities of the patient, treatment, personal history, and personality style. The I_{rt} – CARE Transtheoretical, Psycholinguistic Model of Ruptures and Repairs underscores how therapists think and speak about their work as well as their understanding of the inner experiences of their own and of their patients, provides a blueprint that emphasizes the verbal, paralinguistic, and nonverbal dynamic between a therapist and a patient, and describes the therapy process so that the difficult moment-to-moment transitions during a rupture can be navigated with skill and compassion. The model emphasizes the delicate moment-to-moment interactions between clients and therapists, and the psycholinguistic framework can help therapists focus on and study the details of the dyadic dialogue so that they become less stuck during a rupture and so that the rupture does not become irreparable. On a minute-to-minute basis, therapists need to be aware of their responses to clients, regulate their expressions, and strive to find out how clients think about their inner world (Gelso & Perez-Rojas, 2017; Wolf et al., 2013). The extent to which therapists' interpretations are effective may depend on how they think and feel about themselves and clients during a particular minute and at other times (Gelso & Perez-Rojas, 2017).

The model included in this chapter, the I$_{rt}$ – CARE Transtheoretical, Psycholinguistic Model of Ruptures and Repairs, is transtheoretical in that it can be useful across theories and treatments. Each of the letters of the psycholinguistic I$_{rt}$ – CARE model represents different aspects or concepts of ruptures and repairs, and the concepts may intersect. This transtheoretical model includes a psycholinguistic framework that can inform therapists about the verbal and nonverbal nuances of language as well as paralinguistic features necessary to understand what is happening in the therapeutic alliance. The letter "I" of the I$_{rt}$ – CARE Transtheoretical, Psycholinguistic Model of Ruptures and Repairs stands for inner or immediacy, the letter "r" (subscript) of I$_{rt}$ for rupture, the letter "t" (subscript) of I$_{rt}$ for termination, the letter "C" for covert, curiosity, or compassion, the letter "A" for awareness, alliance, attunement, or authenticity, the letter "R" for repair or resolution, and the letter "E" for empathy or ending. See Figure 5.1.

The I$_{rt}$ – CARE Transtheoretical, Psycholinguistic Model of Ruptures and Repairs is transtheoretical because it emphasizes the use of conceptualizations, cognitions, affective nuances, and language from different therapy approaches. It is suggested that therapists use therapeutic concepts and methods from various therapy orientations during rupture sessions; however, when therapists are challenged by alliance ruptures, it is recommended that they use a moderate level, rather than a high or low level, of therapeutic method diversity, and the implementation of a moderate approach to a range of therapeutic methods will result in an improvement in clients' functioning

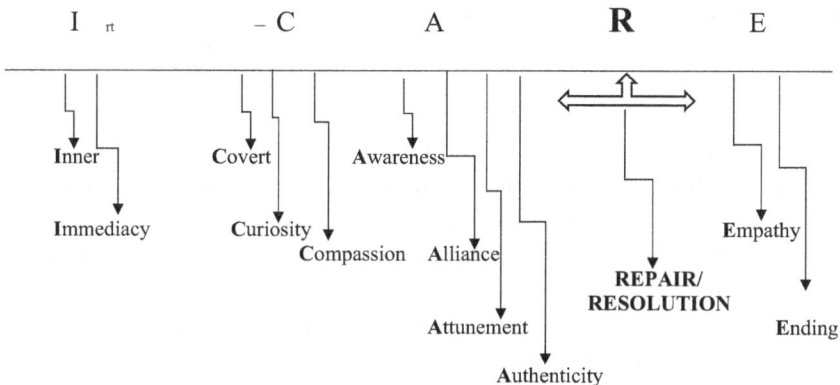

Figure 5.1   I$_{rt}$ – CARE Model of Ruptures and Repairs

Note. This figure illustrates the components of the transtheoretical model, the I$_{rt}$ – CARE Transtheoretical, Psycholinguistic Model of Ruptures and Repairs.

during rupture sessions (Chen et al., 2020). Chen and colleagues (2020) found that when therapists use a narrow (low) or a wide (high) range of different therapeutic methods, client functioning was reduced in the therapy sessions post ruptures. They explain that during ruptures, when therapists integrate an abundance of different therapeutic methods, their patients may feel overwhelmed; however, therapists who integrate few methods may not address their patients' needs. They assert that their results are consistent with research that finds the moderate use of different methods to be the most effective (e.g., Barber et al., 2006; McCarthy et al., 2016).

Tensions, impasses, or ruptures during therapy involve a dyad that is comprised of the client and the therapist. Chapter 2 explained the difficulty that clients and therapists face during ruptures in communication or impasses in the therapeutic relationship. Luo and colleagues (2022, p. 643) note that disruptions or breaks (ruptures) that go unresolved can challenge the therapeutic alliance and result in the unilateral termination of clients (e.g., Eubanks, Muran, et al., 2018; Sharf et al., 2010), and termination is discussed further in Chapter 6. Previous chapters have illustrated the importance of identifying a rupture and how lost and/or defeated patients can feel during a break in the therapeutic alliance. During a rupture, patients may view their therapists as individuals with whom they are not satisfied. It is suggested that the investigation of within-person changes is a way to delineate fluctuations in the therapeutic alliance from one minute to the next during a therapy session (Falkenström & Larsson, 2017; Luo et al., 2022). If patients are feeling that the therapist is against them during a rupture, therapists may invite patients to collaborate in order to understand the shared dilemma that presents itself as a rupture in the moment (Muran & Eubanks, 2020). Previous chapters have illustrated that this process may not work in some situations, at some times, and with some individuals.

The vignettes included in this book show that, sometimes, it is difficult for patients and therapists to discuss ruptures and terminations or endings, that it takes effort to realize that ruptures can, at times, occur more often than either therapists or patients would like to imagine. Given that ruptures are part of the therapy process itself, and of life beyond therapy, looking at them from the perspective of the inner experiences of the therapeutic dyad may help therapists and patients to embrace opportunities for repair. The opportunity for repair can pose a challenge for both patients and therapists, and it is this challenge that the transtheoretical psycholinguistic model seeks to address.

The importance of the therapeutic alliance for therapists and clients cannot be underestimated. Muran and Eubanks (2020) highlight the critical nature of a robust supervisory alliance as well. They explain that supervisors need to be attuned to the supervisory alliance in a similar way that therapists need to pay attention to the working alliance, and therapists and supervisors need to be attuned to how, when, and why therapeutic ruptures takes place.

The I_rt – CARE Transtheoretical, Psycholinguistic Model of Ruptures and Repairs

Previous chapters discussed the importance of therapists' responsiveness to changes in the therapeutic alliance in order to repair ruptures. Therapists need to facilitate the therapeutic alliance by internally monitoring what occurs in the relationship between client and therapist from one moment to the next and by focusing on the core skill of resolving ruptures in the therapeutic alliance (Negri et al., 2019; Safran & Kraus, 2014). The I_rt – CARE Transtheoretical, Psycholinguistic Model of Ruptures and Repairs relies on core concepts from different theoretical orientations. It suggests that therapists meet patients in the moment in order to provide an intervention that has the potential to offer an opportunity for change. In order to reflect on the processes that underlie changes in therapy, it is helpful to examine the therapeutic setting within the context of fields such as psycholinguistics and cognitive psychology (Bucci, 2013). Members of the therapeutic dyad, therapists and patients, use verbal and nonverbal language, for example, eye contact (e.g., Yildirim et al., 2014), to communicate their thoughts. The client signals the therapist with verbal and nonverbal language. The I_rt – CARE Transtheoretical, Psycholinguistic Model of Ruptures and Repairs encompasses the verbal, the nonverbal, and the paralinguistic. For example, Berger and Packard (2022) suggest that the use of language can signal an impending rupture or breakup in the relationship (e.g., Seraj et al., 2021). Interpersonal negotiation is needed if misattunements during therapy are to be repaired so that patients can benefit (Muran, 2019; Zlotnick et al., 2020).

What are some of the components of the psycholinguistic I_rt – CARE model of ruptures? The model is composed of a psycholinguistic framework that relies on the verbal and nonverbal nuances of language as well as on paralinguistic elements to understand what is happening in the therapeutic alliance and to inform therapists about how to avoid ruptures and how to repair them. Language can provide insight about how an individual is feeling (Berger & Packard, 2022; Schwartz et al., 2014). Language and its complexity may be realized from different angles, such as psychology, neuroscience, linguistics, literature, and sociology (Wampold & Flückiger, 2023).

The I_{rt} – CARE Transtheoretical, Psycholinguistic Model of Ruptures and Repairs included in this chapter can help therapists to become aware of the verbal and nonverbal language of the therapy session, to understand the linguistic and psychological styles of patients and therapists during confrontation, withdrawal, and mixed ruptures, to study the rupture repair and termination processes that emerge during therapy sessions, and the model includes a paralinguistic thread as well. How therapists process the language of their patients and how patients process the language of their therapists and the interaction between these processes are of concern to therapists who study the cycles of ruptures and repairs. The model can inform therapists about the content of the language during a therapy session, about what patients say, as well as about what patients do not say, and about how patients say it or do not say it. It is important for therapists to understand the linguistic and paralinguistic components of the psycholinguistic I_{rt} – CARE model, so that they can attend to the nuances of the rupture-repair process as well as to the termination or ending phase of therapy (discussed in Chapter 6). Chapter 5 discusses the portion of the model, the I_{rt} – CARE Transtheoretical, Psycholinguistic Model of Ruptures and Repairs, that focuses specifically on ruptures. Chapter 6 discusses the portion of the model, the I_{rt} – CARE Transtheoretical, Psycholinguistic Model of Termination: The Termination or the Ending Process of Therapy, that focuses specifically on termination or ending in therapy.

I for Inner or Immediacy

Inner (or Covert)

The letter "I" of the I_{rt} – CARE Transtheoretical, Psycholinguistic Model of Ruptures and Repairs stands for inner or immediacy. Inner refers to the inner experiences of therapists as well as to the inner cognitions of the client. The "I" for inner in the model embraces the notion of how the inner thoughts of the therapist resonate with the inner thoughts of the patient. Ruptures are frequently composed of inner or covert processes (e.g., Watson & Greenberg, 2000). The I_{rt} – CARE Transtheoretical, Psycholinguistic Model of Ruptures and Repairs focuses on discerning when and how ruptures occur. The model underscores the need for therapists to consider their inner thoughts. According to Safran and Segal (1996), the inner thoughts of therapists hold important indications about patients' styles of thought and interpersonal patterns. Therapists can help clients to benefit by recognizing their own inner experiences and by managing their countertransference (Gelso & Perez-Rojas, 2017). Therapists need to be willing to commit to attend to their own inner thoughts as well as to the inner experiences of their clients (Eubanks, Sergi, et al., 2021). An essential consideration of the vignettes in Chapters 1 through 4 was on the inner experiences of clients and therapists. The I$_{rt}$ – CARE Transtheoretical, Psycholinguistic Model of Ruptures and Repairs included in this chapter can help therapists to recognize their own inner experiences and to intuit the inner experiences of their clients.

Immediacy

The letter "I" of the I$_{rt}$ – CARE Transtheoretical, Psycholinguistic Model of Ruptures and Repairs stands for immediacy as well. Kasper and colleagues (2008) note that the immediacy of the interpersonal therapist refers to disclosures during therapy about the therapist's feelings about the patient or about the relationship between the therapist and the patient (e.g., Hill, 2004), and that Kiesler (1988) uses the term, "metacommunication," to refer to immediacy. They distinguish between the intervention of immediacy and transference interpretations by explaining that whereas therapists who use immediacy encourage the client's awareness in the moment of difficult interpersonal repetitions, therapists who use transference interpretations encourage awareness of the source of displaced repetitions of interaction by offering a reason for the patient's actions. Navigating ruptures can facilitate a corrective experience for how to explore relational disruptions and can promote learning that is interpersonal (Luo et al., 2022).

Chapter 2 described a supervision program that offers AFT (e.g., Eubanks-Carter et al., 2015; Muran et al., 2010). This program focuses on metacommunication, a skill that is used to address ruptures in the alliance (Muran & Eubanks, 2020; Safran & Muran, 2000). Muran and colleagues (2023, p. 10) point out that metacommunication, the process of communicating about communication or what is being played out in the relationship, has been suggested as a guide for therapists who wish to repair ruptures (e.g., Kiesler, 1996; Safran & Muran, 2000). For example, let's say a patient, Melanie, and her therapist have been communicating for a few minutes when suddenly Melanie stops speaking, and falls silent for some period of time. The therapist might say, "I'm wondering what you may be thinking." Or the therapist may say, "Melanie, I notice that you were engaged in telling me about your experience at your parents' house the other day, and then you paused for a few moments. I'm curious about your thoughts." The aforementioned statements are examples of immediacy or metacommunication, which has been described as a type of "mindfulness-in-interaction" (Muran, 2019; Muran et al., 2023). The concept of mindfulness has been used in religion to guide one's self-awareness to the present moment (Safran & Reading, 2008). Mindfulness is used in secular settings as well. For example, in a secular setting such as a therapy session, therapists use metacommunication that is therapeutic, a type of mindfulness in action (e.g., Safran & Muran, 2000), where the therapist invites the patient to collaborate in order to explore patterns that emerge in the therapeutic relationship (Safran & Reading, 2008). When therapists meta-communicate, they reflect on their inner thoughts and feelings, and they explore dialogues with their clients in the present (Muran, 2019). In the aforementioned scenario with Melanie, the therapist used immediacy or metacommunication to make Melanie's inherent message more explicit in order to explore it. Therapists use metacommunication to help clients express inner thoughts and covert needs, and through the process of immediacy, clients may become more able to approach their interpersonal problems in their relationships beyond therapy (Cashdan, 1988; Hill & Knox, 2009; Safran & Muran, 2000). Metacommunication can generate the latent material of a dialogue in its reference to relational aspects or content (Tannen, 1986; Winther & Dindler, 2018). When using metacommunication, therapists join their clients to work on the interchange between them in the moment, thereby fostering awareness of each other's experience in the present, which facilitates the repair of ruptures (Eubanks, Warren, et al., 2021). For example, Chapter 2 included the vignette with the example of Curtis (with a dismissive attachment style) where the therapist used an exploratory type of metacommunication to invite Curtis to express his experience.

It has been shown that therapists' moment-to-moment responses that are interpersonal are critical in the formation of ruptures (Luo et al., 2022). The I_{rt} – CARE Transtheoretical, Psycholinguistic Model of Ruptures and Repairs recognizes the importance of the therapist's use of immediacy or metacommunication to repair alliance ruptures and for therapists to be cognizant of their own countertransference responses when they use immediacy.

C for Covert, Curiosity, Compassion

Covert

The letter "C" of the I_{rt} – CARE Transtheoretical, Psycholinguistic Model of Ruptures and Repairs stands for covert (inner), curiosity, or compassion.

The words, covert and inner, are used interchangeably. See the section, "I" for inner, above. (The letter "C" that stands for consolidation is used to describe the ending of therapy and is discussed in Chapter 6, which embraces a psycholinguistic model for the termination phase of therapy.)

Curiosity

Curiosity is a key concept for researchers who discuss the therapeutic alliance (Eubanks et al., 2023; Muran et al., 2023). Curiosity is an important attitude that therapists need to cultivate when they think about the rupture-repair process (Muran & Eubanks, 2020; Muran et al., 2023). How inquisitive is the therapist about the patient? Is the patient curious about the therapy process? What is happening in the therapeutic relationship? Muran and colleagues (2023, p. 11) point out that when therapists ask questions that are good during a session, the answers may surprise clients and therapists (e.g., Stern, 1997). Curiosity can help therapists to recognize the subjectivity of their clients and to stay engaged with clients who display aggressive behaviors (Eubanks et al., 2023). In short, individuals who are curious about others make efforts to elicit and care about the viewpoints of others. They want to know what others are thinking, how they are thinking, and the reasons that they are thinking in specific ways. They take time to find out what is on the mind of others, what matters to others, while attending to the perspective of others. Individuals who are curious wish to know how the thoughts of others are different from their own ideas. The AFT program (Eubanks-Carter et al., 2015; Muran et al., 2010), a program that focuses on metacommunication which is a skill that is used to address ruptures in the alliance (Muran & Eubanks, 2020; Safran & Muran, 2000), encourages supervisees who are training to be therapists to cultivate an open and accepting attitude of curiosity about themselves and their patients (Muran & Eubanks, 2020).

Compassion

The letter "C" of the I$_{rt}$ – CARE term of the model stands for compassion. Eubanks, Sergi, et al. (2021) suggest that compassion is an important attitude that therapists need to cultivate particularly during the time that ruptures occur. They explain that therapists need to understand that if they address ruptures with irritation, the patient may feel criticized. At the same time, therapists need to cultivate self-compassion, and with this attitude they will better be able to recognize their own errors during ruptures, learn to explore them, and recognize them as possibilities for progress (Eubanks, Sergi, et al., 2021).

A for Awareness, Alliance, Attunement, or Authenticity

Awareness

The letter "A" of the I_{rt} – CARE term of the model stands for awareness, alliance, attunement, or authenticity, and the portion of the model included in this section emphasizes the importance of the nature of the therapist's self-awareness, the need for therapists to have self-insight, considered to be critical regardless of theoretical orientation (e.g., Gelso & Perez-Rojas, 2017; Reik, 1948; Rogers, 1957). How aware are therapists of their own inner thoughts and experiences? McConnaughy (1987) points out that by accepting their own inner cognitions that lead therapists to a deeper recognition of the self, therapists can more easily encourage the self-awareness of their patients (e.g., Reik, 1948; Rogers, 1957). Attuning to one's inner thoughts can help therapists to unpack the inner thoughts of patients and to uncover the inward matter, to hear, in depth, the patients' inner voice, the true voice of the self that may be drowned out by rational cognition (McConnaughy, 1987; Reik, 1948), and by managing their inner experiences, therapists can further benefit patients without affecting patients in negative ways (Gelso & Perez-Rojas, 2017).

It is important for therapists to be self-aware, to accept themselves, and to develop an inner truthfulness (McConnaughy, 1987; Reik, 1948). By understanding their own inner feelings, therapists can become more self-aware, thus encouraging the self-awareness of their patients (McConnaughy, 1987; Reik, 1948). Humanistic theories highlight the critical nature of the therapist as a human being in the therapy endeavor (McConnaughy, 1987). McConnaughy (1987, p. 306) points out that the understanding of oneself is a prerequisite for a therapist who can succeed (e.g., Rogers, 1939). In their clinical practices, behavioral therapists would agree that the qualities of a psychotherapist are essential; however, generally, they have not emphasized therapists' personal features (McConnaughy, 1987). It is suggested that therapists, whether novice, mid-career, or seasoned, be open to personal therapy, individual supervision or consultation, and continuing education experiences that can assist to cultivate awareness of self and others while building interpersonal skills and deepening knowledge about self and others (McConnaughy, 1987).

It may not be easy for therapists or patients to recognize that a rupture is occurring. A goal of AFT is to heighten the capacity of therapists to recognize ruptures in the therapeutic alliance by elevating their self-awareness (Eubanks-Carter et al., 2015). When therapists meta-communicate about ruptures, it is important for them to draw on their self-awareness so that they realize that a rupture is occurring (Eubanks-Carter et al., 2015). Eubanks-Carter and colleagues (2015, p. 169) point out that AFT is a resolution strategy that involves the resolution of ruptures or the communication about therapist-client dialogues (e.g., Kiesler, 1996). They suggest that therapists meta-communicate in the present, aim to increase awareness of their clients' and their own immediate experiences, recognize that the exploration of ruptures may result in further ruptures, that the process of rupture repair is ongoing, and that therapists need to be flexible during the course of shifts in the interpersonal dialogue.

Alliance, Attunement, and Language Style Matching (LSM; Borelli et al., 2019; Gonzales et al., 2010; Niederhoffer & Pennebaker, 2002)

Previous chapters delved into the importance of the therapeutic alliance. The I$_{rt}$ – CARE Transtheoretical, Psycholinguistic Model of Ruptures and Repairs set forth in this chapter focuses on the need of therapists to deepen their understanding of the therapeutic alliance and change processes during therapy by concerning themselves with language, verbal and nonverbal, with what clients say, how they speak, and the way that patients signal their therapists. Negri and colleagues (2019) explain that a strong therapeutic alliance during the intake session encourages clients to begin engaging with their inner world. They note that individuals who are rated as more affectively engaged as they talk about their experiences, and as they reflect on these experiences in the middle of a therapy session, have elevated scores in the therapeutic alliance at the end of the therapy session. The connection between heightened engagement and the therapeutic alliance, not necessarily linked to patients' emotional disorders, suggests that the interpersonal variables that encourage the elaboration of a client's inner experience are associated with the unfolding of an early alliance (Negri et al., 2019).

It is critical to monitor what is unfolding relationally for the members of the therapeutic dyad throughout the course of therapy in order to reflect on the ebb and flow of the therapeutic alliance (Negri et al., 2019). Negri and colleagues (2019) assert that a way to study the development of the therapeutic relationship is to analyze the verbal contents or words and the linguistic style, both of which reveal what is taking place interpersonally between the patient and the therapist with respect to affective participation and reflection, which are key change processes. Their conceptual model and methods, drawn from Bucci's Multiple Code Theory (1997), focuses on the association between the alliance and the mental processes of the therapeutic dyad, as represented by linguistic markers.

How do individuals communicate? "Language is everywhere." (Berger & Packard, 2022, p. 525). Therapists and patients use language to communicate, and moment-to-moment language signals during a therapy session may be at the verbal or nonverbal level. Berger and Packard (2021, p. 526) point out that it is possible to think of language as an individual's or group's fingerprint or signature (e.g., Pennebaker, 2011) given that individuals make use of terms differently, and people who produce language reveal their own specific attentional focus (e.g., Boyd & Schwartz, 2021). For example, Pennebaker and colleagues (2003) emphasize the need to study particles, e.g., prepositions, pronouns, that hold the verbs and nouns together and signify social identity, affective state, and styles of thinking. Berger and Packard (2022, pp. 533–534) note that although an individual may feel depressed and not express depression explicitly, an analysis of the language may signal that the individual is depressed (e.g., Eichstaedt et al., 2018). A psycholinguistic model can help practitioners to recognize and track subtle verbal and nonverbal shifts and to respond to them.

The I_{rt} – CARE Transtheoretical, Psycholinguistic Model of Ruptures and Repairs suggests that therapists consider the dimension of linguistic elements that relate to the verbal organization of the members of the therapy dyad, the LSM (Borelli et al., 2019) between the therapist and the patient. LSM refers to the extent to which rates of function or grammatical words, for example, prepositions, pronouns, are similar in dyadic communications and is concerned with how individuals who share a conversation naturally coordinate their styles of language to realize a common purpose (Aafjes-van Doorn et al., 2020). This section points out the connection between the linguistic notion of language style matching (LSM) and the letter "A" for alliance or attunement of the I_{rt} – CARE Transtheoretical, Psycholinguistic Model of Ruptures and Repairs. Borelli and colleagues (2019) describe the path of patient-therapist LSM across therapy sessions. They explain that LSM refers to the extent to which unconscious elements of one individual's language mimic that of the other individual during an interaction, and it offers insight into the therapeutic alliance. LSM (Gonzales et al., 2010) measures how often different kinds of function or grammatical words, for example, prepositions, pronouns, are used by the interactional individuals of a dyad, assesses the interaction quality between patient and therapist, and offers a deeper understanding of the patient-therapist bond (Borelli et al., 2019). Borelli and colleagues (2019, p. 10) point out that function or grammatical words, for example, conjunctions, prepositions, and pronouns (different from content words, for example, adjectives and nouns), occur in the absence of conscious awareness and are generated at elevated frequencies during interactive speech (e.g., Gonzales et al., 2010; Ireland & Pennebaker, 2010; Pennebaker & King, 1999). They explain that these aspects of language reflect how individuals speak rather than the substance of the speech, and thus the degree of matching is considered to be independent of the topic of the material that is discussed (e.g., Ireland & Pennebaker, 2010). The I$_{rt}$ – CARE Transtheoretical, Psycholinguistic Model of Ruptures and Repairs aims to promote the "A" or attunement between the client and the therapist both on a conscious and an unconscious level.

What is the potential for and/or the actualization of a good match between the members of a therapeutic dyad? How do clients and therapists who are matched feel when or if they are on the same wavelength? What level of satisfaction during therapy sessions do members of a therapeutic dyad feel from the relational level of their interactions? A higher degree of LSM reflects an elevated degree of attunement in conversation to another individual, rather than agreement on the content of the conversation (Borelli et al., 2019; Pennebaker, 2011). According to Borelli and colleagues (2019), LSM that is higher early on in the therapy reflects a high-quality bond between patient and therapist, a better therapist-patient fit, which can lead to the patient feeling more in tune with the therapist. The matching of the unconscious characteristics of the therapeutic alliance may be as or more beneficial for a client's growth as the matching of the explicit or conscious features of the alliance (McWilliams, 2011). Borelli and colleagues (2019) view LSM as an index of the value of interactions between patients and therapists. The LSM evaluates synchrony in speech characteristics that are generated on a level that is not conscious, and variations in this matching metric may suggest a lack of attunement between members of a dyad that is not accessible on a conscious level (Borelli et al., 2019). The I$_{rt}$ – CARE Transtheoretical, Psycholinguistic Model of Ruptures and Repairs emphasizes the letter "A" of the word CARE in order to underscore the critical need for therapists to be aware of the need for attunement between patients and therapists. Practitioners who are interested in the therapy process, therapists who care about the potential to deepen the therapy alliance, may wish to study linguistic features that relate to the verbal organization of the members of the therapy dyad, for example, LSM. This concludes the section on the association between LSM and the alliance or attunement components of the I_{rt} – CARE Transtheoretical, Psycholinguistic Model of Ruptures and Repairs.

Authenticity

The letter "A" of the I_{rt} – CARE model stands for authenticity as well. This portion turns to the importance of authenticity in the therapeutic alliance. Humanistic therapists hold that authenticity involves notions about the self that reflect the tendency of individuals to actualize their capacity (Polkinghorne, 2015). According to the client-centered approach (Erekson & Lambert, 2015; Rogers, 1951), a humanistic perspective, therapists are responsible for the therapeutic alliance and need to relate to the client in an authentic way (Koole & Tschacher, 2016). The effectiveness of therapy, regardless of theoretical approach, depends on therapists' establishing an authentic relationship with clients (Rogers, 1957). The humanistic concept of congruence (e.g., Rogers, 1961) is used to portray the notion of authenticity, and to be authentic is to recognize one's feelings, to be one with them, and to share them with others when suitable (Sutton, 2020). The takeaway is that in their communications with clients, therapists need to aim toward being themselves, being genuine and sincere, without pseudo-sophisticated or feigned facades aimed at impressing their clients with their knowledge or skills. To repair ruptures, therapists need to allow themselves to be open and fearless about their imperfections, to be and to live their authentic selves. The process of repairing ruptures creates a space for members of the therapeutic dyad to free themselves from communications that are not authentic.

R for Repair or Resolution

The letters "I", "C", "A", and "E", of the I_{rt} – CARE term of the I_{rt} – CARE Transtheoretical, Psycholinguistic Model of Ruptures and Repairs surround the letter "R" that stands for repair or resolution and buttress the notion that the elements or conditions represented by the surrounding letters can be used to navigate the rupture in order to repair and/or resolve the ruptures or impasses in the therapeutic alliance. For example, the following section considers how the last letter "E" of the I_{rt} – CARE Transtheoretical,

Psycholinguistic Model of Ruptures and Repairs that stands for empathy can help therapists to navigate during a rupture or difficult moments of a therapy session.

E for Empathy or Ending

Empathy

The letter "E" in the I$_{rt}$ – CARE Transtheoretical, Psycholinguistic Model of Ruptures and Repairs stands for empathy (discussed in this chapter) or ending or termination from therapy (discussed in Chapter 6). Empathy refers to the extent to which therapists can identify with the inner perspective of patients (e.g., Gelso & Perez-Rojas, 2017). How empathetic are therapists with different theoretical perspectives, for example, client-centered, psychodynamic, or behavioral, to the experiences of their patients? Empathy within the context of a client-centered framework and countertransference from a psychodynamic perspective are utilized to talk about the therapists' inner experiences (Omylinska-Thurston & James, 2011). Gelso and Perez-Rojas (2017) point out that empathy has been noted as a condition of change in therapy or as a facilitative condition (e.g., Rogers, 1957), and that therapists feel empathic recognition of their clients' internal experiences, take part in their clients' inner worlds, and communicate empathy to their clients. Although behavioral therapists do not underscore the role of the personal features of the therapist as much, Lazarus (1985) emphasized that empathy is critical in behavior therapy (McConnaughy, 1987). Nof and colleagues (2021) point out that conductance of the skin suggests perceived empathy on the part of the therapist (e.g., Marci et al., 2007).

Earlier chapters have illustrated (with brief vignettes of the statements and inner thoughts of patients and therapists) how ruptures or tensions during the therapy session can emerge to undermine the therapeutic alliance and how important it is for therapists to pay attention to markers of the therapeutic alliance ruptures and to try to resolve ruptures. Much support has been garnered for the association between rupture repair and positive outcome in therapy (Safran & Kraus, 2014; Safran et al., 2011a). When resolving ruptures, it is important to elicit clients' experiences of the rupture and to empathize with clients' negative concerns about therapy or the therapist (Eubanks, Muran, et al., 2018; Negri et al., 2019). According to Borelli and colleagues (2019), LSM can predict outcomes in relationships as demonstrated in dyads composed of patients and therapists where an association exists between a higher language style matching and a greater degree of therapist empathy (e.g., Lord et al., 2015) and as shown in dyads composed of children and parents where an association exists between a higher LSM and children's greater degree of attachment security and reduced reactivity (e.g., Borelli et al., 2017; Rasmussen et al., 2017).

The I$_{rt}$ – CARE Transtheoretical, Psycholinguistic Model of Ruptures and Repairs: The Linguistic and the Paralinguistic

The I$_{rt}$ – CARE Transtheoretical, Psycholinguistic Model of Ruptures and Repairs encourages psychotherapists to avail themselves of linguistic and paralinguistic concepts to study the communication of their patients in order to understand the rupture and repair process. With respect to the linguistic, for example, the model proposes that therapists become familiar with psychotherapy discourse and conversation analysis, in order to understand ruptures and their repairs. Conversation analysis involves the examination of the unfolding of sequences of patients' and therapists' interactions and can be applied to study change in therapy (Voutilainen et al., 2011).

The Linguistic

An Introduction to Psychotherapy Discourse, Conversation Analysis, and Situations: Common Ground and the Therapeutic Alliance

The I$_{rt}$ – CARE Transtheoretical, Psycholinguistic Model of Ruptures and Repairs is informed by conversation analysis and suggests that therapists draw on an understanding of psychotherapy discourse in order to help them understand the reason for ruptures or conversations that deteriorate. This scenario calls for an emphasis on the situation and on the repair process rather than on the rupture itself. Buchholz (2016, p. 135) suggests the use of conversation analysis to study situations that take place between therapists and patients, and he points out that negative events or errors in therapy conversations or interactions are less important than their repair (e.g., Barnett, 1980; Castonguay & Hill, 2012). He suggests studying these errors in a micro-analytic way by using conversation analysis and that the occurrence of problems during psychotherapy interactions may be unavoidable; however, it is the lack of repair that matters most rather than the occurrence of the error during conversation. In his analysis of psychotherapy discourse, he stresses the importance of the notion of "Common Ground" (e.g., Enfield, 2006; Stalnaker, 2002), an activity with a linguistic dimension. In order to know that other people understand their words, individuals create Common Ground by guiding attention to a common object in a shared environment (Buchholz, 2016). For example, a patient might say, "I like the rug in your office." The therapist may respond with "Yes, it's been with me since the beginning..." Buchholz (2016) would consider the therapist's "yes" to be a perceptual object that is transitioned into a conversational object, which then becomes connected to other experiences. He proposes a situationist view with a focus on micro-analytic observation of small segments of conversations between therapists and patients, delicate moments that can either decrease the quality of a good relationship or instill a flat relationship with deeper affect. Buchholz (2016) explains that Common Ground, with its linguistic side, adjusts the speed difference between fast thoughts or cognition and slow conversation. He proposes that Common Ground activities are complex and therapist-client interaction can fail if the Common Ground is at risk of deterioration or is not established. According to Buchholz (2016), the notion of Common Ground is related to the therapeutic alliance (e.g., Safran & Muran, 2000), which assumes a lot of Common Ground activity, and the focus on how a conversation begins is an integral part of conversation analysis. He suggests that in order to help therapists to recognize what takes place during a conversation and how to attend to important moments with their patients, the focus of study needs to include the situation rather than only the therapist, only the therapy method, or only the matching of therapist and client.

Linguistic Style and the Therapeutic Alliance

How is linguistic style connected to the alliance? It is possible in the first therapy session to distinguish strong and weak therapeutic alliances by examining the linguistic style of the members of the dyad (Negri et al., 2019). For example, Negri and colleagues (2019) found that in the beginning of the initial therapy session there was a positive association between a robust therapeutic alliance and fewer references to bodily activities. They indicated that in the middle of an intake session, a stronger alliance was linked to the ability of clients to take time to talk about themselves. In the last part of an intake session, a stronger therapeutic alliance was related to clients' speech that included fewer words that signify neutral emotion or defensiveness (Negri et al., 2019). The I_{rt} – CARE Transtheoretical, Psycholinguistic Model of Ruptures and Repairs encourages therapists and patients to reflect on the verbal style of the intake and other therapy sessions with attention to both rupture and non-rupture sessions. A model that inspires therapists to pay attention to the linguistic style of their patients can offer therapists a peek into the complexities of patients' inner thoughts during ruptures. For example, it was found that in sessions where ruptures do not occur, the speech of therapists and clients was more disfluent, clients utilized fewer words that contained emotion, and therapists used a greater number of words that were related to communication (Negri et al., 2019). Furthermore, Negri and colleagues (2019) showed that by studying the linguistic style of the members of the therapeutic dyad, it was possible to predict the quality of the therapeutic alliance at intake.

The I_{rt} – CARE Transtheoretical, Psycholinguistic Model of Ruptures and Repairs suggests that therapists incorporate both linguistic and paralinguistic dimensions when considering the therapeutic alliance and ruptures during therapy sessions. This section described the association between linguistic style and the therapeutic alliance and underscored the content of therapy sessions. The next part discusses the relationship between verbal and non-verbal synchrony and alliance ruptures.

Synchrony and the Therapeutic Alliance

Verbal Synchrony: The Linguistic

What is synchrony and how does it relate to the therapeutic relationship and the communication that ensues between patients and their therapists? Language is a primary feature of interpersonal synchrony, and the way in which language contributes to psychotherapy encourages curiosity about linguistic synchrony in the collaboration between patients and therapists (Tay & Qiu, 2022). Linguistic synchrony (LS) refers to an association between more than one individual's linguistic behavior, a relationship between individuals' language dynamics (indicated by constant words spoken) that have a pattern in form and timing (Shapira et al., 2022). Shapira and colleagues (2022, p. 159) point out that synchrony, taking place over time, is an essential change mechanism that has an impact on the therapy bond, and, if the synchrony or alignment between the therapist and the patient is satisfactory, synchrony can lead to a better treatment outcome (e.g., Koole & Tschacher, 2016; Paulick et al., 2018).

The I$_{rt}$ – CARE Transtheoretical, Psycholinguistic Model of Ruptures and Repairs suggests that therapists pay attention to the LS of patients and therapists because the language used by patients and therapists reflects their inner thoughts and how they feel about their relationship. The study of language during the therapy session embraces the notion of LS or alignment in the therapeutic dyad (Tay & Qui, 2022). Tay and Qui (2022) study LS or alignment in therapeutic dyads within the context of different theoretical orientations, for example, humanistic, cognitive-behavioral, and psychoanalytic. They view LS as a similar style of linguistic selections of patients and therapists that represent the dyad's socio-psychological perspectives, and they suggest that therapists apply their method to their sessions with clients and study how their alignment styles change with different patients and at different times.

What does LS have to do with the therapeutic alliance, and why is it important in therapy? Shapira and colleagues (2022) found that the LS of therapists and patients holds clues about whether the members of a therapeutic dyad can work well together and can adjust their language to each other's style, which may result in a better treatment outcome. They found that there is a relationship between a more elevated linguistic similarity and a higher alliance. Tay and Qiu (2022, p. 2) note that an example of a distributional measure of synchrony is LSM (Niederhoffer & Pennebaker, 2002) (discussed in the section under "A" for attunement) with its focus on the similarity, or lack thereof, of independent units.

The Paralinguistic

The Paralanguage of Patients and Therapists

The previous section highlighted the centrality of LS to the therapeutic alliance. The I$_{rt}$ – CARE Transtheoretical, Psycholinguistic Model of Ruptures and Repairs suggests that therapists pay attention to the paralinguistic synchrony of patients and therapists as well. De Pasquale and colleagues (2019) assert that a relationship exists between elevated levels of synchrony or coordination during therapy and the building of rapport. They explain that prosodic accommodation is an example of a coordinative behavior in speech that contributes to successful conversations and that speakers who are conversing tend to adapt their levels of voice intensity, their pitch, and speech rate (e.g., De Looze & Rauzy, 2011; Edlund et al., 2009).

This chapter included a previous section on attunement and the alliance that described the relationship between the therapeutic alliance and LSM. The I_{rt} – CARE Transtheoretical, Psycholinguistic Model of Ruptures and Repairs suggests to therapists that the paralinguistic dimension may be as important as the linguistic component in the work of developing the therapeutic relationship. What is the paralinguistic dimension of communication, and what is its relationship to the therapeutic alliance? Paralinguistic, paraverbal, or proto-language refers to the vocal and the extra-verbal components of communication, for example, rate, volume, level of voice, complements the verbal and nonverbal levels, and can help therapists to explore hidden affect (Sikorski, 2012). Beebe and colleagues (2000, p. 100) point out that paralinguistic elements such as rhythm and timing serve as core unifying principles of interpersonal interactions, with rhythm underlying behavior (e.g., Lenneberg, 1967). When individuals consider relatedness to others, they attend to fluctuations such as the nuanced changes in timing, for example, hesitations or long pauses between the turn of one individual and another, and this timing is accompanied by gaze or facial expression (Beebe et al., 2000). Variations in tempo, pitch, and intensity as well as pauses and stutters are included in the study of paralanguage (Duncan et al., 1968; Trager, 1958). For example, whereas talking slowly, in a long way, and with a low and falling voice along with pauses is a paralanguage that characterizes depression, speaking quickly and with a breathy and anxious voice tone characterizes fearfulness of situations or others (Sikorski, 2012). Sikorski (2012, p. 51) points out that characteristics of the voice, for example, can influence the building of the therapeutic relationship (e.g., Ellgring & Scherer, 1996; Heaton & Bartosik, 2003; Ostwald, 1961).

If you are a therapist, have you ever jumped in to speak after what seemed like too long a period of time of silence from a patient? Paralinguistic features include the silences during the therapy session. For example, Sikorski (2012) notes that silence on the part of patients may communicate a lot and may have different meanings. It can mean that the patient may not find the correct words to express something, that the patient may not want to talk about an issue, that the patient is concerned that someone else may overhear what is being said, and many other possibilities. Many novice practitioners are concerned about silence to the point that they may talk prior to understanding the reason that the patient is silent (Sikorski, 2012).

De Pasquale and colleagues (2019, p. 3043) note that the way in which therapists speak to their patients is as important as what they say, and there has been much discussion on gestures, posture, and nonverbal mannerisms (e.g., Weiste & Peräkylä, 2014). It has been found that therapists' paralinguistic behaviors can differentiate valued therapy time from poor therapy time, and whereas therapists' paralinguistic activities during a valued therapy hour showed that the therapist seemed relaxed and warm, therapists' paralanguage during a poor therapy time showed that the voice of the therapist sounded flat, dull, and lacked involvement (Duncan et al., 1968).

The Paralinguistic Dimension: The Relationship Between Changes in the Therapeutic Alliance and Acoustic Markers

The I$_{rt}$ – CARE Transtheoretical, Psycholinguistic Model of Ruptures and Repairs emphasizes a focus on paralinguistic elements such as acoustic data, which can assist therapists to discern ruptures or breaks in the therapeutic alliance. For example, consider the paralinguistic feature of pitch. Dolev-Amit and colleagues (2022) point out that elevated levels of corresponding measures of pitch between clients and psychotherapists are associated with a lower quality therapeutic alliance (e.g., Reich et al., 2014). Researchers have suggested that acoustic data can signal markers for ruptures, that acoustic markers include speech and vocal parameters that measure the physical characteristics of speech production, and that examples include fundamental frequency (F0) (pitch of the sound), articulation rate, shimmer, and pause proportion (e.g., De Cheveigné & Kawahara, 2002; Dolev-Amit et al., 2022; Rochman & Amir, 2013). The F0-span gauges the voice alterations during an utterance and refers to the degree of speech that is monotonic as compared to lively, or when one considers intonation that is restricted or monotonic versus varied or playful, one is referring to the F0-span (Dolev-Amit et al., 2022; Knowles & Little, 2016). Articulation rate means the pace of the generation of speech segments, shimmer refers to a shaky quality of voice, and pause proportion to the silences during conversation (Dolev-Amit et al., 2022). What do the aforementioned paralinguistic features have to do with ruptures in the therapeutic alliance? Dolev-Amit and colleagues (2022) show that confrontation ruptures are related to a higher pause proportion and F0-span than regular speech and that withdrawal ruptures are associated with a higher pause proportion, F0-span, and shimmer, but a lower articulation rate than regular speech. They suggest that therapists receive training relevant to how to use their ears to increase their skill in discerning ruptures or tensions in communication during the therapy session. For example, Dolev-Amit and colleagues (2022) explain that a therapist who detects an acoustic alteration such as a client's rapid speech rate might say to the client, "You seem to be speaking quicker now. Your voice may be offering us a clue about what is going on now. Can you share your thoughts and feelings at this point?" They suggest that the training of therapists to utilize their ears to detect acoustic changes can enhance their capacity to detect impasses or tensions during therapy.

This section underscored the relationship between verbal synchrony, the linguistic and the paralinguistic, the therapeutic alliance, and ruptures. The next portion is devoted to the association between nonverbal synchrony and ruptures in the therapeutic alliance.

The Relationship Between Nonverbal Synchrony and Alliance Ruptures

The previous section suggested the need to consider the verbal synchrony of the therapeutic dyad regardless of the therapist's theoretical orientation. Aafjes-van Doorn and colleagues (2020, p. 510) point out that what may be most central to psychotherapy is the way or manner in which content is shared rather than the verbal content itself (Hölzer et al., 1996; Reyes et al., 2008). The I_{rt} – CARE Transtheoretical, Psycholinguistic Model of Ruptures and Repairs proposes that rather than considering only linguistic and para-linguistic verbal synchrony, therapists become attuned to the nonverbal syn-chrony between patients and therapists, how nonverbal synchrony impacts the alliance, and its effect upon ruptures or misattunements in the thera-peutic alliance. What is nonverbal synchrony, and what is its relationship to the therapeutic alliance and to ruptures or impasses during therapy sessions? Nonverbal synchrony refers to the coordination of movement between individuals who interact, regardless of their gestures or postures (Condon & Ogston, 1966; Deres-Cohen et al., 2021; Ramseyer & Tschacher, 2011). Schoenherr and colleagues (2019, p. 504) note that nonverbal synchrony can be thought of as the amount of contact between individuals, and the con-cept of synchrony offers the perception of an interrelationship between the behaviors of the persons who are interacting (e.g., Altmann, 2013; Bernieri & Rosenthal, 1991). In therapy, synchrony can refer to the nonverbal com-ponent of engaging fully with a client (Deres-Cohen et al., 2021). Generally, there is an association between dyadic nonverbal synchrony and a better relationship when the therapeutic relationship is rated by patients (Paulick et al., 2018).

Ramseyer and Tschacher (2011, p. 284) note that nonverbal or movement synchrony is a common, nonconscious aspect of the interaction of the client-therapist dyad, and the nonverbal behavior of a therapist affects the therapeutic alliance (e.g., Philippot et al., 2003). Higher synchrony was observed in CBT than in psychodynamic therapy, and synchrony that took place early in therapy was associated with a stronger alliance later in therapy and decreased interpersonal difficulties at termination (Altmann et al., 2020; Ramseyer, 2020). Ramseyer and Tschacher (2011) assert that individuals with more elevated nonverbal synchrony have more secure attachment, lower interpersonal distress, display fewer symptoms, and report elevated self-efficacy.

What has synchrony to do with ruptures or tensions in the therapeutic alliance, the concern of this chapter? Nonverbal or movement synchrony can serve as a marker of the therapeutic alliance, and, specifically, has been shown to be strongly related to confrontational rather than withdrawal ruptures (Deres-Cohen et al., 2021). When therapists are challenged by difficulties with the therapeutic relationship during a therapy session, they tend to seek a higher degree of nonverbal synchrony with clients in order to strengthen the therapeutic alliance (Deres-Cohen et al., 2021). Deres-Cohen and colleagues (2021) recommend that clients and therapists be provided with suggestions about their nonverbal markers of ruptures because this process can assist therapists to become aware of confrontation ruptures and address them, and therapists will be able to know if the methods that they are using during a session help to decrease a rupture's intensity. In short, the takeaway is that nonverbal synchrony suggests important components of the therapy process (Ramseyer & Tschacher, 2011).

Chapter Summary

The repair of ruptures is a challenge for therapists, no matter what their theoretical approach. How can therapists proceed if there are ruptures during the therapy session? Eubanks, Burckell, and colleagues (2018, p. 61) point out that if, during a rupture, therapists continue by using their usual treatment methods, the therapeutic alliance may deteriorate further (e.g., Castonguay et al., 1996; Piper et al., 1999). In the face of a rupture, rather than continuing with their usual interventions, therapists need to shift the focus of their efforts to the rupture itself (Eubanks, Burckell, et al., 2018). The I$_{rt}$ – CARE Transtheoretical, Psycholinguistic Model of Ruptures and Repairs alerts therapists to attend to the interspace created by ruptures and suggests ways to address impasses and tensions so that ruptures may be resolved. The transtheoretical model included in this chapter emphasizes how therapists can become aware of the rupture in order to employ strategies for its repair. Addressing the rupture and validating the patient during the impasse comprise key steps in the process of rupture resolution (Eubanks, Burckell, et al., 2018; Safran & Muran, 2000). The overarching linguistic, paralinguistic, and nonverbal constructs of the transtheoretical model described in this chapter can assist therapists to chart their course toward rupture resolution. See Figure 5.2.

The book, *Navigating Ruptures, Repairs, and Termination Within the Therapeutic Process*, accentuates the notion that ruptures happen more often than therapists would like to admit, and this chapter embraces a transtheoretical model that addresses these ruptures. Luo and colleagues (2022, p. 643) note that therapeutic alliance ruptures take place in 30%–50% of therapy sessions

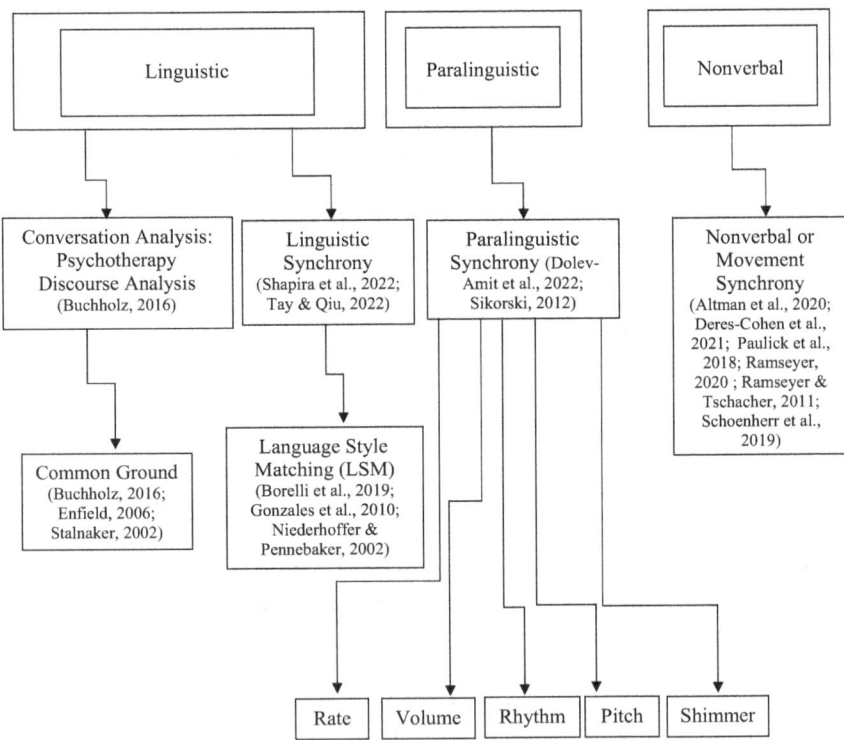

Figure 5.2 I_{rt} – CARE Transtheoretical, Psycholinguistic Model of Ruptures and Repairs

Note. This figure illustrates the different components of the psycholinguistic model.

according to clients' or therapists' reports; in 80%–100% of sessions, according to observer ratings (e.g., Eubanks, Muran, et al., 2018). This chapter embraces a transtheoretical model, the I$_{rt}$ – CARE Transtheoretical, Psycholinguistic Model of Ruptures and Repairs, a psycholinguistic framework that can inform the therapeutic alliance and the rupture-repair process. It is transtheoretical in that it relies on concepts from different theoretical orientations to inform the alliance, the rupture-repair process, and the termination stage of therapy. Relying on psycholinguistic concepts, the model can inform therapists about the various verbal and nonverbal components of language that can be used to understand what is taking place on a moment-to-moment basis between the therapist and the patient. It highlights the need for therapists to be attuned to their own as well as their patients' inner thoughts, to the use of language that may suggest a rupture, and it suggests that therapists pay attention to what patients say, how they say it, and what patients do not say.

The next chapter discusses how the I$_{rt}$ – CARE Transtheoretical, Psycholinguistic Model of Termination: The Termination or the Ending Process of Therapy can contribute toward an understanding of the termination process in therapy, describes how the transtheoretical model furthers the connection between ruptures, their repairs, and termination or ending in therapy, and how the psycholinguistic framework of the model can help therapists to be aware of the therapeutic space in order to avoid the premature termination of their clients.

References

Aafjes-van Doorn, K., Porcerelli, J., & Müller-Frommeyer, L. C. (2020). Language style matching in psychotherapy: An implicit aspect of alliance. *Journal of Counseling Psychology*, 67(4), 509–522. https://doi.org/10.1037/cou0000433

Altmann, U. (2013). *Synchronisation nonverbalen Verhaltens: Weiterentwicklung und Anwendung zeitreihenanalytischer Identifikationsverfahren* [*Synchronization of nonverbal behavior: Development and Application of time series analysis methods*]. Springer-Verlag. https://doi.org/10.1007/978-3-531-19815-6

Altmann, U., Schoenherr, D., Paulick, J., Deisenhofer, A.-K., Schwartz, B., Rubel, J. A., Stangier, U., Lutz, W., & Strauss, B. (2020). Associations between movement synchrony and outcome in patients with social anxiety disorder: Evidence for treatment specific effects. *Psychotherapy Research*, 30(5), 574–590. https://doi.org/10.1080/10503307.2019.1630779

Barber, J. P., Gallop, R., Crits-Christoph, P., Frank, A., Thase, M. E., Weiss, R. D., & Connolly Gibbons, M. B. (2006). The role of therapist adherence, therapist competence, and the alliance in predicting outcome of individual drug counseling: Results from the National Institute Drug Abuse Collaborative Cocaine Treatment Study. *Psychotherapy Research*, 16(2), 229–240. https://doi.org/10.1080/10503300500288951

Barnett, J. (1980). Cognitive repair in the treatment of the neuroses. *Journal of the American Academy of Psychoanalysis, 8, 39–55*.

Beebe, B., Jaffe, J., Lachmann, F., Feldstein, S., Crown, C., & Jasnow, M. (2000). System models in development and psychoanalysis: The case of vocal rhythm coordination and attachment. *Infant Mental Health Journal, 21*(1–2), 99–122.

Berger, J., & Packard, G. (2022). Using natural language processing to understand people and culture. *American Psychologist, 77*(4), 525–537. https://doi.org/10.1037/amp 0000882

Bernieri, F. J., & Rosenthal, R. (1991). Interpersonal coordination: Behavior matching and interactional synchrony. In R. S. Feldman & B. Rimé (Eds.), *Fundamentals of nonverbal behavior* (pp. 401–432). Editions de la Maison des Sciences de l'Homme; Cambridge University Press.

Borelli, J. L., Ramsook, K. A., Smiley, P., Bond, D. K., West, J. L., & Buttitta, K. H. (2017). Language matching among mother–child dyads: Associations with child attachment and emotion reactivity. *Social Development, 26*(3), 610–629. https://doi.org/10.1111/sode.12200

Borelli, J. L., Sohn, L., Wang, B. A., Hong, K., DeCoste, C., & Suchman, N. E. (2019). Therapist–client language matching: Initial promise as a measure of therapist–client relationship quality. *Psychoanalytic Psychology, 36*(1), 9–18. https://doi.org/10.1037/pap 0000177

Boyd, R. L., & Schwartz, H. A. (2021). Natural language analysis and the psychology of verbal behavior: The past, present, and future states of the field. *Journal of Language and Social Psychology, 40*(1), 21–41. https://doi.org/10.1177/0261927X20967028

Bucci, W. (2013). The referential process as a common factor across treatment modalities. *Research in Psychotherapy: Psychopathology, Process and Outcome, 16*(1), 16–23. https://doi.org/10.4081/ripppo.2013.86

Buchholz, M. B. (2016). Conversational errors and common ground activities in psychotherapy – Insights from conversation analysis. *International Journal of Psychological Studies, 8*(3), 134–153. https://doi.org/10.5539/ijps.v8n3p134

Cashdan, S. (1988). *Object relations therapy: Using the relationship*. W. W. Norton & Co.

Castonguay, L. G., Goldfried, M. R., Wiser, S., Raue, P. J., & Hayes, A. M. (1996). Predicting the effect of cognitive therapy for depression: A study of unique and common factors. *Journal of Consulting and Clinical Psychology, 64*(3), 497–504. https://doi.org/10.1037/0022-006X.64.3.497

Castonguay, L. G., & Hill, C. E. (Eds.) (2012). *Transformation in psychotherapy: Corrective experiences across cognitive behavioral, humanistic, and psychodynamic approaches*. American Psychological Association. https://doi.org/10.1037/13747-000

Chen, R., Rafaeli, E., Ziv-Beiman, S., Bar-Kalifa, E., Solomonov, N., Barber, J. P., Peri, T., & Atzil-Slonim, D. (2020). Therapeutic technique diversity is linked to quality of working alliance and client functioning following alliance ruptures. *Journal of Consulting and Clinical Psychology, 88*(9), 844–858. https://doi.org/10.1037/ccp0000490

Condon, W. S., & Ogston, W. D. (1966). Sound film analysis of normal and pathological behavior patterns. *The Journal of Nervous and Mental Disease,143*(4), 338–347. https://doi.org/10.1097/00005053-196610000-00005

De Cheveigné, A., & Kawahara, H. (2002). YIN, a fundamental frequency estimator for speech and music. *The Journal of the Acoustical Society of America, 111*(4), 1917–1930. https://doi.org/10.1121/1.1458024

De Looze, C., & Rauzy, S. (2011, August 27–31). Measuring speakers' similarity in speech by means of prosodic cues: Methods and potential. *Proceedings of the Annual Conference of the International Speech Communication Association, INTERSPEECH,* Florence, Italy, 1393–1396. https://doi.org/10.21437/interspeech.2011-457

De Pasquale, C., Cullen, C., & Vaughan, B. (2019, September 15–19). An investigation of therapeutic rapport through prosody in brief psychodynamic psychotherapy. *Proceedings of INTERSPEECH,* Graz, Austria, 3043–3047. https://doi.org/10.21437/Interspeech.2019-2551

Deres-Cohen, K., Dolev-Amit, T., Peysachov, G., Ramseyer, F. T., & Zilcha-Mano, S. (2021). Nonverbal synchrony as a marker of alliance ruptures. *Psychotherapy, 58*(4), 499–509. https://doi.org/10.1037/pst0000384

Dolev-Amit, T., Nof, A., Asaad, A., Tchizick, A., & Zilcha-Mano, S. (2022). The melody of ruptures: Identifying ruptures through acoustic markers. *Counselling Psychology Quarterly, 35*(4), 724–743. https://doi.org/10.1080/09515070.2020.1860906

Duncan, S., Jr., Rice, L. N., & Butler, J. M. (1968). Therapists' paralanguage in peak and poor psychotherapy hours. *Journal of Abnormal Psychology, 73*(6), 566–570. https://doi.org/10.1037/h0026597

Edlund, J., Heldner, M., & Hirschberg, J. (2009, September 6–10). Pause and gap length in face-to-face interaction. Proceedings of the Annual Conference of the International Speech Communication Association, INTERSPEECH, Brighton, UK, 2779–2782.

Eichstaedt, J. C., Smith, R. J., Merchant, R. M., Ungar, L. H., Crutchley, P., Preoţiuc-Pietro, D., Asch, D. A., & Schwartz, H. A. (2018). Facebook language predicts depression in medical records. Proceedings of the National Academy of Sciences of the United States of America, *115*(44), 11203–11208. https://doi.org/10.1073/pnas.1802331115

Ellgring, H., & Scherer, K. R. (1996). Vocal indicators of mood change in depression. *Journal of Nonverbal Behavior, 20*(2), 83–110. https://doi.org/10.1007/BF02253071

Enfield, N. J. (2006). Social consequences of common ground. In S. C. Levenson & N. J. Enfield (Eds.), *Roots of human sociality. Culture, cognition and interaction* (pp. 399–430). Berg.

Erekson, D. M., & Lambert, M. J. (2015). Client-centered therapy. In R. L. Cautin & S. O. Lilienfeld (Eds.), *The encyclopedia of clinical psychology* (pp. 1–5). Wiley. https://doi.org/10.1002/9781118625392.wbecp073

Eubanks, C. F., Burckell, L. A., & Goldfried, M. R. (2018). Clinical consensus strategies to repair ruptures in the therapeutic alliance. *Journal of Psychotherapy Integration, 28*(1), 60–76. https://doi.org/10.1037/int0000097

Eubanks, C. F., Muran, J. C., & Safran, J. D. (2018). Alliance rupture repair: A meta-analysis. *Psychotherapy, 55*(4), 508–519. https://doi.org/10.1037/pst0000185

Eubanks, C. F., Muran, J. C., & Safran, J. D. (2019). Repairing alliance ruptures. In J. C. Norcross & M. J. Lambert (Eds.), *Psychotherapy relationships that work: Evidence-based therapist contributions* (3rd ed., pp. 549–579). Oxford University Press. https://doi.org/10.1093/med-psych/9780190843953.003.0016

Eubanks, C. F., Samstag, L. W., & Muran, J. C. (2023). Conclusion: Don't be afraid to get messy – Points of convergence in rupture and repair. In C. F. Eubanks, L. W. Samstag, & J. C. Muran (Eds.), *Rupture and repair in psychotherapy: A critical process for change* (pp. 305–317). American Psychological Association.

Eubanks, C. F., Sergi, J., & Muran, J. C. (2021). Responsiveness to ruptures and repairs in psychotherapy. In J. C. Watson & H. Wiseman (Eds.), The responsive psychotherapist: Attuning to clients in the moment (pp. 83–103). American Psychological Association. https://doi.org/10.1037/0000240-005

Eubanks, C. F., Warren, J. T., & Muran, J. C. (2021). Identifying ruptures and repairs in alliance-focused training group supervision. *International Journal of Group Psychotherapy*, *71*(2), 275–309. https://doi.org/10.1080/00207284.2020.1805618

Eubanks-Carter, C., Muran, J. C., & Safran, J. D. (2015). Alliance-focused training. *Psychotherapy*, *52*(2), 169–173. https://doi.org/10.1037/a0037596

Falkenström, F., & Larsson, M. H. (2017). The working alliance: From global outcome prediction to micro-analyses of within-session fluctuations. *Psychoanalytic Inquiry, 37*(3), 167–178. https://doi.org/10.1080/07351690.2017.1285186

Gelso, C. J., & Perez-Rojas, A. E. (2017). Inner experience and the good therapist. In L. G. Castonguay & C. E. Hill (Eds.), *How and why are some therapists better than others?: Understanding therapist effects* (pp. 101–115). American Psychological Association. https://doi.org/10.1037/0000034-007

Gonzales, A. L., Hancock, J. T., & Pennebaker, J. W. (2010). Language style matching as a predictor of social dynamics in small groups. *Communication Research, 37*(1), 3–19. https://doi.org/10.1177/0093650209351468

Heaton J. A., & Bartosik, J. (2003). *Podstawy umiejętności terapeutycznych*. GWP.

Hill, C. E. (2004). *Helping skills: Facilitating, exploration, insight, and action* (2nd ed.). American Psychological Association.

Hill, C. E., & Knox, S. (2009). Processing the therapeutic relationship. *Psychotherapy Research*, *19*(1), 13–29. https://doi.org/10.1080/10503300802621206

Hölzer, M., Mergenthaler, E., Pokorny, D., Kächele, H., & Luborsky, L. (1996). Vocabulary measures for the evaluation of therapy outcome: Re-studying transcripts from the Penn Psychotherapy Project. *Psychotherapy Research, 6*(2), 95–108. https://doi.org/10.1080/10503309612331331618

Ireland, M. E., & Pennebaker, J. W. (2010). Language style matching in writing: Synchrony in essays, correspondence, and poetry. *Journal of Personality and Social Psychology, 99*(3), 549–571. https://doi.org/10.1037/a0020386

Kasper, L. B., Hill, C. E., & Kivlighan, D. M., Jr. (2008). Therapist immediacy in brief psychotherapy: Case study I. *Psychotherapy: Theory, Research, Practice, Training, 45*(3), 281–297. https://doi.org/10.1037/a0013305

Kiesler, D. J. (1988). *Therapeutic metacommunication: Therapist impact disclosure as feedback in psychotherapy*. Consulting Psychologist Press.

Kiesler, D. J. (1996). *Contemporary interpersonal theory and research: Personality, psychopathology, and psychotherapy*. John Wiley & Sons.

Kline, K. V., Hill, C. E., Morris, T., O'Connor, S., Sappington, R., Vernay, C., Arrazola, G., Dagne, M., & Okuno, H. (2019). Ruptures in psychotherapy: Experiences of therapist trainees. *Psychotherapy Research*, *29*(8), 1086–1098. https://doi.org/10.1080/10503307.2018.1492164

Knowles, K. K., & Little, A. C. (2016). Vocal fundamental and formant frequencies affect perceptions of speaker cooperativeness. *Quarterly Journal of Experimental Psychology, 69*(9), 1657–1675. https://doi.org/10.1177/03010066221135472

Koole, S. L., & Tschacher, W. (2016). Synchrony in psychotherapy: A review and an integrative framework for the therapeutic alliance. *Frontiers in Psychology, 7*, Article 862.

Lazarus, A. (1985). Setting the record straight. *American Psychologist, 40*(12), 1418–1419. https://doi.org/10.1037/0003-066X.40.12.1418.b

Lenneberg, E. H. (1967). *Biological foundations of language.* Wiley.

Lord, S. P., Sheng, E., Imel, Z. E., Baer, J., & Atkins, D. C. (2015). More than reflections: Empathy in motivational interviewing includes language style synchrony between therapist and client. *Behavior Therapy, 46*(3), 296–303. https://doi.org/10.1016/j.beth.2014.11.002

Luo, X., Liu, S., Levendosky, A. A., Good, E. W., Turchan, J. E., & Hopwood, C. J. (2022). Idiographic and nomothetic relationships between momentary interpersonal behaviors, interpersonal complementarity, and alliance ruptures in psychotherapy. *Journal of Counseling Psychology, 69*(5), 642–655. https://doi.org/10.1037/cou0000619

Macdonald, J., Elliott, R., & Couto, A. B. (2023). Relational dialogue in emotion-focused therapy: Process analysis and comparison with the alliance-focused training model. In C. F. Eubanks, L. W. Samstag, & J. C. Muran (Eds.), *Rupture and repair in psychotherapy: A critical process for change* (pp. 187–220). American Psychological Association. https://doi.org/10.1037/0000306-009

Marci, C. D., Ham, J., Moran, E., & Orr, S. P. (2007). Physiologic correlates of perceived therapist empathy and social-emotional process during psychotherapy. *The Journal of Nervous and Mental Disease, 195*(2), 103–111. https://doi.org/10.1097/01.nmd.0000253731.71025.fc

McCarthy, K. S., Keefe, J. R., & Barber, J. P. (2016). Goldilocks on the couch: Moderate levels of psychodynamic and process-experiential technique predict outcome in psychodynamic therapy. *Psychotherapy Research, 26*(3), 307–317. https://doi.org/10.1080/10503307.2014.973921

McConnaughy, E. A. (1987). The person of the therapist in psychotherapeutic practice. *Psychotherapy: Theory, Research, Practice, Training, 24*(3), 303–314. https://doi.org/10.1037/h0085720

McWilliams, N. (2011). *Psychoanalytic diagnosis: Understanding personality structure in the clinical process* (2nd ed.). Guilford Press.

Muran, J. C. (2019). Confessions of a New York rupture researcher: An insider's guide and critique. *Psychotherapy Research, 29*(1), 1–14. https://doi.org/10.1080/10503307.2017.1413261

Muran, J. C., & Eubanks, C. F. (2020). Therapist performance under pressure: Negotiating emotion, difference, and rupture. American Psychological Association. https://doi.org/10.1037/0000182-000

Muran, J. C., Eubanks, C. F., & Samstag, L. W. (2023). Introduction: Rupture in a wicked and wonderful world. In C. F. Eubanks, L. W. Samstag, & J. C. Muran (Eds.), *Rupture and repair in psychotherapy: A critical process for change* (pp. 3–20). American Psychological Association. https://doi.org/10.1037/0000306-001

Muran, J. C., Safran, J. D., & Eubanks-Carter, C. (2010). Developing therapist abilities to negotiate alliance ruptures. In J. C. Muran & J. P. Barber (Eds.), *The therapeutic alliance: An evidence-based guide to practice* (pp. 320–340). The Guilford Press.

Negri, A., Christian, C., Mariani, R., Belotti, L., Andreoli, G., & Danskin, K. (2019). Linguistic features of the therapeutic alliance in the first session: A psychotherapy process study. *Research in Psychotherapy: Psychopathology, Process and Outcome, 22*(1), 71–82. https://doi.org/10.4081/ripppo.2019.374

Niederhoffer, K. G., and Pennebaker, J. W. (2002). Linguistic style matching in social interaction. *Journal of Language and Social Psychology, 21*(4), 337–360. https://doi.org/10.1177/026192702237953

Nof, A., Amir, O., Goldstein, P., & Zilcha-Mano, S. (2021). What do these sounds tell us about the therapeutic alliance: Acoustic markers as predictors of alliance. *Clinical Psychology & Psychotherapy, 28*(4), 807–817. https://doi.org/10.1002/cpp.2534

Omylinska-Thurston, J., & James, P. E. (2011). The therapist's use of self: A closer look at the processes within congruence. *Counselling Psychology Review, 26*(3), 20–33. https://doi.org10.53841/bpscpr.2011.26.3.20

Ostwald, P. F. (1961). The sounds of emotional disturbance. *Archives of General Psychiatry, 5*(6), 587–592. https://doi.org/10.1001/archpsyc.1961.01710180071008

Paulick, J., Deisenhofer, A.-K., Ramseyer, F., Tschacher, W., Boyle, K., Rubel, J., & Lutz, W. (2018). Nonverbal synchrony: A new approach to better understand psychotherapeutic processes and drop-out. *Journal of Psychotherapy Integration, 28*(3), 367–384. https://doi.org/10.1037/int0000099

Pennebaker, J. W. (2011). The secret life of pronouns. *New Scientist, 211*(2828), 42–45. https://doi.org/10.1016/S0262-4079(11)62167-2

Pennebaker, J. W., & King, L. A. (1999). Linguistic styles: Language use as an individual difference. *Journal of Personality and Social Psychology, 77*(6), 1296–1312. https://doi.org/10.1037/0022-3514.77.6.1296

Pennebaker, J. W., Mehl, M. R., & Niederhoffer, K. G. (2003). Psychological aspects of natural language use: Our words, our selves. *Annual Review of Psychology, 54*, 547–577. https://doi.org/10.1146/annurev.psych.54.101601.145041

Philippot, P., Feldman, R. S., & Coats, E. J. (Eds.) (2003). *Nonverbal behavior in clinical settings.* Oxford University Press.

Piper, W. E., Ogrodniczuk, J. S., Joyce, A. S., McCallum, M., Rosie, J. S., O'Kelly, J. G., & Steinberg, P. I. (1999). Prediction of dropping out in time-limited, interpretive individual psychotherapy. Psychotherapy: Theory, Research, Practice, Training, 36(2), 114–122. https://doi.org/10.1037/h0087787

Polkinghorne, D. E. (2015). The self and humanistic psychology. In K. J. Schneider, J. F. Pierson, & J. F. T. Bugental (Eds.), *The handbook of humanistic psychology: Theory, research, and practice* (pp. 87–104). Sage Publications, Inc.

Ramseyer, F. T. (2020). Exploring the evolution of nonverbal synchrony in psychotherapy: The idiographic perspective provides a different picture. *Psychotherapy Research, 30*(5), 622–634. https://doi.org/10.1080/10503307.2019.1676932

Ramseyer, F. T., & Tschacher, W. (2011). Nonverbal synchrony in psychotherapy: Coordinated body movement reflects relationship quality and outcome. *Journal of Consulting and Clinical Psychology, 79*(3), 284–295. https://doi.org/10.1037/a0023419

Rasmussen, H. F., Borelli, J. L., Smiley, P. A., Cohen, C., Cheung, R. C. M., Fox, S., Marvin, M., & Blackard, B. (2017). Mother-child language style matching predicts children's and mothers' emotion reactivity. *Behavioural Brain Research, 325*(Pt B), 203–213. https://doi.org/10.1016/j.bbr.2016.12.036

Reich, C. M., Berman, J. S., Dale, R., & Levitt, H. M. (2014). Vocal synchrony in psychotherapy. *Journal of Social and Clinical Psychology, 33*(5), 481–494. https://doi.org/10.1521/jscp.2014.33.5.481

Reik, T. (1948). *Listening with the third ear; the inner experience of a psychoanalyst.* Farrar, Strauss & Co.

Reyes, L., Aristegui, R., Krause, M., Strasser, K., Tomicic, A., Valdés, N., Altimir, C., Ramirez, I., De La Parra, G., Dagnino, P., Echávarri, O., Vilches, O., & Ben-Dov, P. (2008). Language and therapeutic change: A speech acts analysis. *Psychotherapy Research, 18*(3), 355–362. https://doi.org/10.1080/10503300701576360

Rochman, D., & Amir, O. (2013). Examining in-session expressions of emotions with speech/vocal acoustic measures: An introductory guide. *Psychotherapy Research, 23*(4), 381–393. https://doi.org/10.1080/10503307.2013.784421

Rogers, C. R. (1939). *Counseling and psychotherapy.* Houghton Mifflin.

Rogers, C. R. (1951). *Client-centered therapy: Its current practice, implications, and theory.* Constable.

Rogers, C. R. (1957). The necessary and sufficient conditions of therapeutic personality change. *Journal of Consulting Psychology, 21*(2), 95–103. https://doi.org/10.1037/h0045357

Rogers, C. R. (1961). *On becoming a person.* Houghton Mifflin.

Safran, J. D., & Kraus, J. (2014). Alliance ruptures, impasses, and enactments: A relational perspective. *Psychotherapy, 51*(3), 381–387. https://doi.org/10.1037/a0036815

Safran, J. D., & Muran, J. C. (2000). *Negotiating the therapeutic alliance: A relational treatment guide.* Guilford Press.

Safran, J. D., & Muran, J. C. (2006). Has the concept of the therapeutic alliance outlived its usefulness? *Psychotherapy: Theory, Research, Practice, Training, 43*(3), 286–291. https://doi.org/10.1037/0033-3204.43.3.286

Safran, J. D., Muran, J. C., & Eubanks-Carter, C. (2011a). Repairing alliance ruptures. *Psychotherapy: Theory, Research, and Practice, 48*(1), 80–87. https://doi.org/10.1037/a0022140

Safran, J., Muran, C., & Eubanks-Carter, C. (2011b). Repairing alliance ruptures. In J. Norcross (Ed.), *Psychotherapy relationships that work: Evidence-based responsiveness* (2nd ed., pp. 224–238). Oxford University Press. https://doi.org/10.1093/acprof:oso/9780199737208.003.0011

Safran, J. D., Muran, J. C., Samstag, L. W., & Stevens, C. (2001). Repairing alliance ruptures. *Psychotherapy: Theory, Research, Practice, Training, 38*(4), 406–412. https://doi.org/10.1037/0033-3204.38.4.406

Safran, J. D., & Reading, R. (2008). Mindfulness, metacommunication, and affect regulation in psychoanalytic treatment. In S. F. Hick & T. Bien (Eds.), *Mindfulness and the therapeutic relationship* (pp.122–140). Guilford Press.

Safran, J. D., & Segal, Z. V. (1996). *Interpersonal process in cognitive therapy.* Jason Aronson.

Schoenherr, D., Paulick, J., Strauss, B. M., Deisenhofer, A.-K., Schwartz, B., Rubel, J. A., Lutz, W., Stangier, U., & Altmann, U. (2019). Nonverbal synchrony predicts premature termination of psychotherapy for social anxiety disorder. *Psychotherapy, 56*(4), 503–513. https://doi.org/10.1037/pst0000216

Schwartz, H. A., Eichstaedt, J., Kern, M. L., Park, G., Sap, M., Stillwell, D., Kosinski, M., & Ungar, L. (2014, June). Towards assessing changes in degree of depression through Facebook. *Proceedings of the workshop on computational linguistics and clinical psychology: From linguistic signal to clinical reality* (pp. 118–125). Association for Computational Linguistics. https://doi.org/10.3115/v1/W14-3214

Seraj, S., Blackburn, K. G., & Pennebaker, J. W. (2021, February). Language left behind on social media exposes the emotional and cognitive costs of a romantic breakup. Proceedings of the National Academy of Sciences of the United States of America, *118*(7), e2017154118. https://doi.org/10.1073/pnas.2017154118

Shapira, N., Atzil-Slonim, D., Tuval-Mashiach, R., & Shapira, O. (2022, July). Measuring linguistic synchrony in psychotherapy. *Proceedings of the Eighth Workshop on Computational Linguistics and Clinical Psychology* (Association for Computational Linguistics, pp. 158–176). https://doi.org/10.18653/v1/2022.clpsych-1.14

Sharf, J., Primavera, L. H., & Diener, M. J. (2010). Dropout and therapeutic alliance: A meta-analysis of adult individual psychotherapy. *Psychotherapy: Theory, Research, Practice, Training, 47*(4), 637–645. https://doi.org/10.1037/a0021175

Sikorski, W. (2012). Paralinguistic communication in the therapeutic relationship. *Archives of Psychiatry and Psychotherapy, 14*(1), 49–54.

Stalnaker, R. (2002). Common ground. *Linguistics and Philosophy, 25*(5/6), 701–721. https://doi.org/10.1023/A:1020867916902

Stern, D. B. (1997). *Unformulated experience: From dissociation to imagination in psychoanalysis.* Analytic Press.

Sutton, A. (2020). Living the good life: A meta-analysis of authenticity, well-being and engagement. *Personality and Individual Differences, 153*, 109645. https://doi.org/10.1016/j.paid.2019.109645

Tannen, D. (1986). *That's not what I meant!: How conversational style makes or breaks relationships.* Ballantine.

Tay, D., & Qiu, H. (2022). Modeling linguistic (a)synchrony: A case study of therapist–client interaction. *Frontiers in Psychology, 13*, Article 903227. https://www.doi.org/10.3389/fpsyg.2022.903227

Trager, G. L. (1958). Paralanguage: A first approximation. *Studies in Linguistics, 13*, 1–12.

Voutilainen, L., Peräkylä, A., & Ruusuvuori, J. E. (2011). Therapeutic change in interaction: Conversation analysis of a transforming sequence, *Psychotherapy Research, 21*(3), 348–365. https://doi.org/10.1080/10503307.2011.573509

Wampold, B. E., & Flückiger, C. (2023). The alliance in mental health care: Conceptualization, evidence and clinical applications. *World Psychiatry, 22*(1), 25–41. https://doi.org/10.1002/wps.21035

Watson, J. C., & Greenberg, L. S. (2000). Alliance ruptures and repairs in experiential therapy. *Journal of Clinical Psychology, 56*(2), 175–186. https://doi.org/10.1002/(sici)1097-4679(200002)56:2<175::aid-jclp4>3.0.co;2-5

Weiste, E., & Peräkylä, A. (2014). Prosody and empathic communication in psychotherapy interaction, *Psychotherapy Research, 24*(6), 687–701. https://doi.org/10.1080/10503307.2013.879619

Winther, F., & Dindler, C. (2018). Two models of ethical alignment through metacommunication in clinical situations. *Communication & Medicine – An Interdisciplinary Journal of HealthCare, Ethics and Society, 14*(2), 188–198. https://doi.org/10.1558/cam.32314

Wolf, A. W., Goldfried, M. R., & Muran, J. C. (Eds.). (2013). *Transforming negative reactions to clients: From frustration to compassion.* American Psychological Association. https://doi.org/10.1037/13940-000

Yildirim, I. Orazbekova, Z., & Unal, Y. (2014). About a role and value of nonverbal communication in psycholinguistics. *Asian Social Science, 10*(4), 27–30. https://www.doi.org/10.5539/ass.v10n4p27

Zlotnick, E., Strauss, A. Y., Ellis, P., Abargil, M., Tishby, O., & Huppert, J. D. (2020). Reevaluating ruptures and repairs in alliance: Between- and within-session processes in cognitive–behavioral therapy and short-term psychodynamic psychotherapy. *Journal of Consulting and Clinical Psychology, 88*(9), 859–869. https://doi.org/10.1037ccp0000598

The I$_{rt}$ – CARE Transtheoretical, Psycholinguistic Model of Termination: The Termination or the Ending Process of Therapy

6

Introduction

Many therapists feel grateful to have the opportunity to observe their patients grow gradually and make important changes. At some point, whether the members of the therapeutic dyad discuss termination during a rupture or in the absence of a disagreement, therapy draws to an end. It is during the termination phase in therapy, whether mutually agreed or unilateral, that the psychotherapy relationship moves toward its close for the client and the therapist. For example, a forced termination that is initiated by the therapist may generate a patient's feelings of loss, intrusion, protection, liberation, rejection, or guilt, and a patient's symptom resurgence is not infrequent at this time (Power, 2016). Mourning the loss of the therapist and/or the relationship where the patient internalizes the object that is lost contrasts with denial where the patient looks for substitutes, and when the patient is not ready to mourn and cannot express disappointment over the real situation of the therapist's departure, a forced termination may be felt

DOI: 10.4324/9781003128489-9

as an intrusion (Power, 2016). Power (2016, p. 85) notes that denial may take different forms such as leaving rapidly or extending the process of leaving for a long time in order to hold onto the therapist and/or the relationship (e.g., Loewald, 1962). Whereas in their attempt to deny the therapist who has been valuable for them, patients with a dismissive attachment style may deny the past by leaving rapidly, patients with a preoccupied attachment style tend to deny the future by denying that the parting with the therapist needs to occur (Loewald, 1962; Power, 2016). Power (2016) explains that it is possible for a patient with an avoidant style and a therapist with avoidant characteristics to conspire to underestimate the effects of a coerced ending initiated by the therapist, for example, the therapist's retirement. She asserts that although forced endings elicit a variety of issues related to attachment, it is a coerced ending such as a therapist's pregnancy that prompts the most complex issues.

It is in the client's best interest for therapists to aim for gentle endings. How can therapists navigate a smooth ending phase of therapy? Swift and Greenberg (2015) suggest that assisting patients to think about the end of therapy from the beginning may decrease premature or unilateral termination by clients. They reason that when patients know the approximate length of therapy, it may be easier to cope with the high and low points of therapy, patients may not be as likely to think progress in the beginning is a full recovery, patients understand that their wishes to end treatment are common, and they may feel more comfortable to talk to their therapist about their wishes to end therapy.

Given that the therapeutic alliance predicts the outcome of therapy (e.g., Horvath et al., 2011), it is no wonder that it can contribute to premature or unilateral termination (Swift & Greenberg, 2015). Client dropout in therapy happens a lot. Phillips and colleagues (2018) point out that client dropout tends to occur in early sessions (e.g., Barrett et al., 2008; McMurran et al., 2010; Swift & Greenberg, 2012; Wierzbicki & Pekarik, 1993). In fact, it has been shown that approximately 50% of clients unilaterally terminate by the third therapy session, and almost a third drop out after the first session (Barrett et al., 2008).

Mylona and Avdi (2021, p. 229) note that the frequency of confrontation ruptures is more predictive of unilateral termination than withdrawal strains (e.g., Coutinho et al., 2014; Eubanks, Lubitz, et al., 2019), and the failure to resolve ruptures can predict dropout (e.g., Eubanks, Lubitz, et al., 2019). Swift and Greenberg (2015) found that 20% of clients discontinue therapy prematurely, that patient and therapist variables have been shown to contribute to client dropout from therapy, and in order to decrease premature termination, it is critical that practitioners understand the frequency with which dropout occurs and to delineate the types of situations, for example, patients higher in personality and eating disorders, associated with the risk of dropout. They explain that therapists need to attend to patient premature termination particularly with patients who are younger because this type of patient is more at risk for dropping out of therapy and that the therapists' age, gender, and ethnicity do not predict rates of client dropout; however, practitioners with less experience have been shown to have more difficulty in keeping their clients in therapy, and dropout is more likely to occur in clinics at universities. Therapists need not stand by during the process of premature termination, and cultivating the therapeutic relationship throughout therapy and tracking the progress of patients are high priorities as they can decrease dropout from therapy (Swift & Greenberg, 2015).

Are you a therapist, whether novice or seasoned, whose client has dropped out of therapy? You are not alone. Are you a patient who has decided to drop out of therapy? Your situation is not uncommon. Client dropout is a challenging experience for patients and therapists. The rates of patient premature discontinuation have not been found to significantly differ depending upon the theoretical perspective used in therapy, and therapists can anticipate that whatever type of intervention they employ, they will experience client dropout from therapy despite their conscientious efforts (Swift & Greenberg, 2015). Sometimes, it is the ruptures in therapy that can result in failure in the treatment or lead to premature termination (Safran & Muran, 1996). Previous chapters have focused on how therapists can learn to avoid deleterious downturns during therapy, such as client dropouts. These chapters emphasized the need for therapists to seek to avoid client dropout from therapy by learning to repair ruptures. It has been shown that working through tensions or ruptures may contribute to retention in treatment (Cirasola et al., 2022; Eubanks et al., 2018). It is critical that therapists learn to decrease dropout from therapy by promoting the patient's level of hope (Swift & Greenberg, 2015). How can therapists help patients during the termination process regardless of whether the ending is an agreed ending by the therapist and the patient or a unilateral ending by the therapist or the patient?

Key therapist termination behaviors that have been identified across theoretical orientations include facilitating the patient's growth subsequent to termination, consolidating improvements that the patient has made, encouraging the progress of the patient, adherence to the code of ethics, and underscoring the client's awareness of competence (Norcross et al., 2017). Knox and colleagues (2011) discuss the need for therapists to consider the following plan in order to help patients navigate the termination process, that is to help patients prepare for a positive therapy ending:

1. Set out time to plan for ending therapy.
2. Help patients to review what they have garnered from therapy.
3. Encourage patients to identify what work is left.
4. Explore future possibilities after therapy.
5. Elicit patients' feelings about termination.

Many individuals may feel that they need therapy. Some may feel conflicted about beginning therapy, such as the patient, Jennifer (in Chapter 3), who did not show up for her first therapy session. Some individuals feel satisfied and complete therapy. Yet, others may feel dissatisfied and drop out before experiencing a full course of therapy. Premature terminations in therapy are different from a mutually agreed ending where goals and tasks have been accomplished with a successful ending, are not the same as an ambiguous beginning, an ambiguity about beginning therapy, for example, where clients, for whatever reason, want therapy but decide not to call, and are different from a forced termination by the therapist, for example, a therapist's retirement or internship endings at a clinic (Swift & Greenberg, 2015). During a forced ending initiated by therapists, to service their own needs, therapists intrude upon the therapeutic space in the service of their own needs, and this manner of intruding on the therapy process is fraught with challenges, for example, the matter of how to protect clients from a scenario where therapists are no longer able to offer treatment (Power, 2016). Power (2016) explains that patients, generally, do not welcome a forced ending in therapy, and she recognizes that this rupture will affect therapists as well as patients. She asserts that the matter of a coerced ending where therapists retire may occur for clinicians at any age. Whereas some patients at the beginning of therapy may not feel as challenged when the therapist retires because they have not invested a lot emotionally at the beginning, other patients at the beginning may feel that the therapist has deceived them when the therapist announces a forced ending soon after beginning with them (Power, 2016). Patients at the end stages of therapy may not feel as challenged because they have garnered further insight; however, patients in the middle stage of therapy, will be most challenged (Power, 2016).

Previous chapters on termination in therapy have emphasized that therapy dropouts are not positive events, that they are problematic for patients and for therapists, and when patients discontinue therapy prematurely, patients and therapists may be left with a host of negative feelings such as, rejection, surprise, guilt, frustration, disappointment, anger, loss, failure, sadness, regret, and others (e.g., Ogrodniczuk et al., 2005). Nevertheless, in situations where dropout does occur, therapists can lessen the negative effect and seek to terminate on a positive note (Swift & Greenberg, 2015).

Do therapists attribute patients' premature endings in therapy to their own characteristics or to the characteristics of patients? The literature is mixed with respect to the reasons assigned for premature patient discontinuation in therapy. Dandachi-FitzGerald and colleagues (2022 p. 972) point out that some research shows that rather than attributing patients' unilateral endings in therapy to themselves, therapists attribute patients' premature endings in therapy to the characteristics of patients (e.g., Murdock et al., 2010), a self-serving bias; however, their own findings did not support a self-serving bias in the attributions of practitioners.

Why do patients drop out of therapy if they feel that they need therapy? Each patient has a different reason for dropout (Renk & Dinger, 2002). For example, Renk and Dinger (2002, p. 1174) point out that patients may prematurely terminate because, although they have not reached the goals of therapy, they feel that they have made adequate improvement, they may be facing an external constraint, or they are not satisfied with the services that the therapist provides (e.g., Carter et al., 1995; Kasoff et al., 2000). Muran and colleagues (2009, p. 234) note that for clients who completed their therapy sessions, only 54% of individuals with depression, 63% of individuals with panic disorder, and 52% of individuals with GAD improved at the end of therapy (e.g., Westen & Morrison, 2001).

It was found that dropout rates differed for the interaction of different diagnoses, for example, PTSD, depression, eating disorders, and therapist theoretical orientation, for example, cognitive-behavioral, humanistic, and psychodynamic (Swift & Greenberg, 2015). For example, for depression the highest rates of premature termination occurred with CBASP (23%), and the lowest average rate of premature termination took place with the integrative psychotherapy approaches (10.9%) (Swift & Greenberg, 2015). Swift and Greenberg (2015) found that for the eating disorders, the lowest average rate of premature termination (5.9%) occurred with dialectical behavior therapy (DBT), and for PTSD, the highest average rate of premature termination took place with CBT (28.5%), and the lowest average rate of premature termination occurred with the integrative therapy perspectives (8.8%).

Previous chapters have emphasized the relationship between ruptures or impasses (discussed in Chapters 1 and 2) and client dropout from therapy (discussed in Chapters 3 and 4). Ruptures or impasses that have not been resolved can lead to a poor therapeutic relationship, to poor outcome, and to a patient's premature termination (Henry et al., 1986; Safran & Kraus, 2014; Safran et al., 2005). On the other hand, repaired ruptures can result in less client dropout and positive outcomes for clients (Eubanks, Muran, et al., 2019).

The importance of the therapeutic relationship has been emphasized throughout the book. During different phases of therapy, the relationship between the client and the therapist may change, with the relationship being more prominent during the termination or ending phase of therapy (Abargil & Tishby, 2021). Chapters 3 and 4 remind therapists that the ending phase of therapy is a sensitive time for patients, and that it is critical that therapists facilitate gentle landings for the termination process of their patients. A poor therapy relationship between a patient and a therapist can result in difficult endings for the patient (Knox et al., 2011).

An important focus of the book has been on repairing ruptures in the therapeutic alliance. What is the connection between ruptures, the resolution of ruptures, and termination? Luo et al. (2022, p. 643) point out that ruptures that are not repaired may result in clients terminating therapy prematurely (e.g., Eubanks et al., 2018; Sharf et al., 2010). There has been renewed support for training therapists in AFT in order to supplement CBT (Castonguay et al., 2019; Muran et al., 2018). To decrease the possibility of client dropout, Swift and Greenberg (2015) propose the following eight evidence-based strategies:

1. Offer role induction (education about therapy to clients).
2. Integrate clients' preferences for interventions.
3. Incorporate a plan for the process of ending therapy.
4. Discuss the change process in therapy.
5. Validate hope or that the process of therapy will bring about change.
6. Facilitate motivation.
7. Cultivate the alliance.
8. Review patients' progress.

To limit the potential for problems in therapy such as premature terminations, Knox and colleagues (2011) suggest that therapists discuss with their patients their perceptions of therapy, a process that offers patients the opportunity to discuss positive and negative affects about how therapy is proceeding for them. To decrease premature terminations, Ogrodniczuk and colleagues (2005) propose several strategies, for example, develop a contract with the client that pertains to the length of treatment, focus on the therapeutic alliance during therapy, and others.

Chapter 5 discussed the part of the transtheoretical model, the I_{rt} – CARE Transtheoretical, Psycholinguistic Model of Ruptures and Repairs, that focused on ruptures and repairs within the therapeutic process. This chapter delves into the part of the model, the I_{rt} – CARE Transtheoretical, Psycholinguistic Model of Termination: The Termination or the Ending Process of Therapy, that focuses on the termination or ending phase of therapy, discusses the process used to navigate termination in the context of differing theoretical orientations, and explains how the transtheoretical, psycholinguistic part of the model can be useful across theories. Each of the letters of the model in its entirety, the I_{rt} – CARE Transtheoretical, Psycholinguistic Model of Ruptures, Repairs, and Termination, included in Chapters 5 and 6 represent different aspects or concepts of ruptures, repairs, and termination, and the concepts may interconnect. The part of the model included in this chapter, the I_{rt} – CARE Transtheoretical, Psycholinguistic Model of Termination: The Termination or the Ending Process of Therapy, underscores the need for therapists to recognize that what may not be said during therapy and at the end of therapy may be as important, if not more important, than what is said. Therapists, novice and seasoned, can avail themselves of the transtheoretical model of termination, the I_{rt} – CARE Transtheoretical, Psycholinguistic Model of Termination: The Termination or the Ending Process of Therapy, included in this chapter, a model that is informed by psycholinguistic elements, to learn about the importance of the termination process, the potentially deleterious effects of premature or unilateral termination, and strategies for facing the challenge of early client dropout. The model, in its reliance on psycholinguistic elements, emphasizes the verbal and nonverbal nuances of language as well as paralinguistic features necessary to understand what is happening in the therapeutic alliance and describes the relationship between the aforementioned language components and the termination process. Similar to, but somewhat different from, the representations of the letters of the model that were described in Chapter 5, in the psycholinguistic model described in this chapter, the I_{rt} – CARE Transtheoretical, Psycholinguistic Model of Termination: The Termination or the Ending Process of Therapy, the letter "I" stands for inner (covert), the letter "r" (subscript) of I_{rt} for rupture, the letter "t" (subscript) of I_{rt} for termination, the letter "C" for covert or consolidation, the letter "A" for awareness or alliance, the letter "R" for repair or resolution, and the letter "E" for ending or empathy. See Figure 6.1.

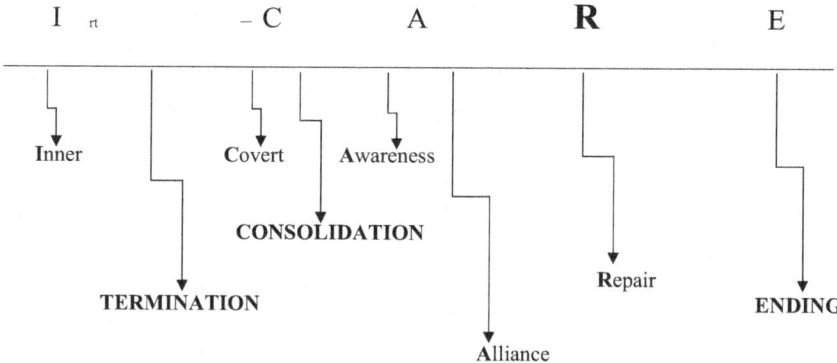

Figure 6.1 I$_{rt}$ – CARE Model of Termination

Note. This figure illustrates the components of the transtheoretical model, the I$_{rt}$ – CARE Transtheoretical, Psycholinguistic Model of Termination: The Termination or the Ending Process of Therapy.

The Subscript "T" of the I$_{rt}$ – CARE Term: T for Termination (or E for Ending)

The Termination or Ending of Therapy Sessions and Conversation Analysis

Chapter 5 explained how conversation analysis informs the I$_{rt}$ – CARE Transtheoretical, Psycholinguistic Model of Ruptures and Repairs. The I$_{rt}$ – CARE Transtheoretical, Psycholinguistic Model described in Chapter 5 suggests that therapists become familiar with psychotherapy discourse in order to help them to understand the reason for ruptures or conversations that deteriorate. Conversation analysis can be used as well to help therapists to become more aware of what transpires at the end of single therapy sessions, which may suggest important information about the "E" for ending or the "t" for termination phase of therapy itself. For example, Dittmann (2017) uses conversation analysis to examine the ending or closing of single therapy sessions or encounters and how these closings impact the therapy process. He explains that endings of single therapy sessions unfold within the dyad as discernible steps via three kinds of closing. In addressing the dilemma of how a session with open topics can be ended in a way that is helpful for the patient, he describes the following three types of closing during a session: Compact, stretched, and commented. The different types of closings speak to the issue of how therapists can end or close a session when the patient's material or topic is open (Dittmann, 2017). Topics may be open at the end of a therapy session, and Dittmann (2017) views these open topics as a dilemma. The I_{rt} – CARE Transtheoretical, Psycholinguistic Model of Termination: The Termination or the Ending Process of Therapy uses the subscript letter "t" of the I_{rt} – CARE term to represent termination (or E for ending). How can therapists help patients to end therapy in different circumstances when patients are ready to end, when there is a forced termination by the therapist, for example, retirement or an intern leaves at the end of the year and patients are not ready to end, or when patients wish to end, initiating premature termination, but are not ready to end because, in reality, they have not completed their work? Although Dittmann's (2017) work focuses on the ending process of single therapy sessions rather than on the termination phase of therapy, there may be some similarities to be gleaned for the ending or termination of therapy itself. In either case, conversation analysis is an approach that can inform the I_{rt} – CARE Model of Termination: The Termination or the Ending Process of Therapy, which relies on psycholinguistic elements to navigate the ending.

The Termination or Ending of Therapy Sessions and Grammatical Markers (Peterson, 2011)

Grammatical markers such as pronouns can help therapists discover the emergence of the patient's identity during the different phases of therapy (e.g., Peterson, 2011). The I_{rt} – CARE Transtheoretical, Psycholinguistic Model of Termination: The Termination or the Ending Process of Therapy incorporates the work of Peterson (2011) who underscores the need for therapists to be aware of grammatical markers used by patients during the different phases of therapy, for example, the beginning phase of therapy, or the termination or ending phase of therapy. This section addresses the importance of patients' usage of pronouns during therapy and specifically during termination. Peterson (2011) suggests that therapists who hover evenly over a patients' conversational utterances or silences during therapy sessions pay attention to the use of grammatical markers such as the patient's usage of pronouns throughout the course of therapy. He suggests that patients display predictable sequences in their usage of pronouns throughout treatment. He indicates that at the beginning of therapy, the pronoun, "they," is used; however, over the course of time, in the middle phase of treatment, the patients join the analyst in using, "we," and as the course of an analysis moves toward the termination, the first-person agency, the "I" is developed. Termination or ending in therapy implies a successful internalization of the analyst and the commencement of a separation from the therapist (Peterson, 2011). It is the establishment of a robust therapeutic alliance that facilitates the emergence of the patient's agency in the first person during the termination phase of treatment, and it is the grammatical markers that signal the beginning, middle, and termination phases so that a renewed patient identity can emerge (Peterson, 2011).

The Termination or Ending of Therapy Sessions and Linguistic Processing Methods: The Therapeutic Cycle Model (Mergenthaler, 1996)

In order for therapists to study the language of therapists and patients during the termination of therapy so that they can detect significant moments of change between themselves and their clients, and in order to learn to adjust their language and behavior to meet the needs of their patients, the I$_{rt}$ – CARE Transtheoretical, Psycholinguistic Model of Termination: The Termination or the Ending Process of Therapy suggests the usage of linguistic processing methods. Certain kinds of patient-therapist dialogue may facilitate deep changes in therapy (McCarthy et al., 2011). Linguistic processing methods can help therapists to assess clinical progress by examining the language in therapy sessions in order to delineate gains, important change moments during sessions and incidents related to clinical progress (Comninos & Grenyer, 2007; McCarthy et al., 2011). For example, McCarthy and colleagues (2011) point out the research of Hölzer and colleagues (1996) and Mergenthaler (1996), research that illustrates how therapists can use language to study what takes place in therapy sessions. In 1996, Hölzer and colleagues showed that therapists accommodated to the language of clients more in successful therapy cases than in unsuccessful ones. In the same year, Mergenthaler's (1996) Therapeutic Cycle Model (TCM), a computer-assisted analysis of text, was shown to be able to delineate different affect-abstraction patterns that match various therapeutic phases depending upon the main kind of language used in a therapy session. The TCM applies to different psychotherapy approaches and can identify primary moments within therapies, and the theory of the TCM is not based on one specific kind of therapy, but on how progress unfolds during the course of therapy reflected by the verbalizations of patients and therapists (McCarthy et al., 2011; Mergenthaler, 1996, 2008). The subscript letter "t" of the I_{rt} – CARE term of the I_{rt} – CARE Transtheoretical, Psycholinguistic Model of Termination: The Termination or the Ending Process of Therapy focuses on the termination (or the E for ending in therapy). Consider the following example with a focus on the "t" or the termination phase of therapy. In a sequence of moments between a patient and therapist where the therapist is focusing on the "t" or termination, the patient resists termination, the therapist interprets the patient's resistance, and two sessions after the therapists' interpretations, the patient accepts the therapist's interpretations, and begins to grieve (McCarthy et al., 2011). At this point in the sequence, it is possible to identify an increase in the emotional tone of the output of the TCM, a connecting transition commences, and it suggested that this sequence contains important work in therapy (McCarthy et al., 2011; Mergenthaler, 2008; Milbrath et al., 1999).

I for Inner (or C for Covert): The Inner Thoughts of Therapists and Patients and Termination

Previous chapters provided examples of how impasses or tensions (ruptures) that occur in the therapeutic alliance can result in the premature termination of therapy by the patient or to a failed therapy outcome. Successful repairs of disagreements are related to a higher retention (lower premature termination) in therapy, as measured over the first six meetings of patient and therapist (Muran et al., 2009; Nof et al., 2021). The I_{rt} – CARE Transtheoretical, Psycholinguistic Model of Termination: The Termination or the Ending Process of Therapy uses the letter "I" of the I_{rt} – CARE term to represent inner, to underscore how the inner or covert thoughts of the therapist resonate with the patient. Becoming a therapist requires an exploration of one's own inner thoughts (Cozolino, 2004). This exploration is particularly important during the termination phase of therapy. Given the importance of the inner ("I") experiences to the progress of the patient throughout therapy, and particularly during ruptures and during termination, perhaps during the last rupture, novice therapists from psychoanalytic and psychodynamic theoretical backgrounds immerse themselves in an intense psychoanalysis prior to and/or while seeing patients (Bennett-Levy et al., 2003; Macran & Shapiro, 1998; Williams et al., 1999). Although novice therapists in cognitive and behavior therapies, generally, are not required to undergo personal therapy as part of their training, self-reflection is emphasized (Bennett-Levy et al., 2003; Laireiter, 1998). It is Yalom (2002) who considers one's personal therapy to be a critical component of training to become a therapist, and he emphasizes the importance of therapists seeking a diversity of theoretical perspectives (Norcross & Finnerty, 2019). Norcross and Finnerty (2019) point out that therapists, in many countries, consider their clinical experience to be the first most important aspect of their professional development and that therapists consider their analysis or personal therapy to be their second most critical part of their training (e.g., Orlinsky et al., 2001).

The next section discusses the "C" for consolidation of the I$_{rt}$ – CARE Transtheoretical Model. The I$_{rt}$ – CARE Transtheoretical, Psycholinguistic Model of Termination: The Termination or the Ending Process of Therapy provides a blueprint for the termination process, takes into consideration the internal experiences of patients and therapists, and entails a compass that can guide therapists and patients as they navigate difficult transitions during and at the end of therapy.

C for the Language of Consolidation (or E for Ending)

The I$_{rt}$ – CARE Transtheoretical, Psycholinguistic Model of Termination: The Termination or the Ending Process of Therapy is a framework that relies on core concepts from different theoretical orientations. The model suggests how therapists can meet patients where they are in the moment and can provide an intervention that has the potential to offer opportunity for change. That moment may be at the beginning, middle, or end of therapy, and the language that is suited for the termination or end phase of therapy, language that needs careful attention, may be viewed from the vantage point of the letter "C" for consolidation.

What role has termination played in the psychological literature? There is not much research on the termination phase of therapy, and some consider the term "termination" to be too harsh a term (Davis, 2008; Maples & Walker, 2014). Bartholomew and colleagues (2017, p. 82) point out that ending therapy is a key part of psychotherapy and an obligation that is ethical no matter the language used to describe termination (e.g., Davis & Younggren, 2009; Vasquez et al., 2008). The model in this chapter uses the letter "C" of the I$_{rt}$ – CARE term of the model to represent consolidation, to describe the ending of therapy. Consolidation refers to the process of ending therapy, which may take place in only one session or in a phase of many sessions, and during consolidation therapists aim toward a linguistic presentation of the ending of therapy that is future-oriented (Maples & Walker, 2014). Maples and Walker (2014) explain that a consolidation approach suggests that when therapy draws to an end, the therapist needs to focus on solidifying the gains that have been made during previous sessions and directing patients to the future, to a life outside the context of therapy (Maples & Walker, 2014). They recommend that during the consolidation or end phase of therapy, the therapist proceeds with cautious language that is suitable to the ending phase of treatment and that works toward the collaboration with patients in order to increase the patient's progress that was made during the course of therapy. Whereas it has been suggested that adopting the term, "consolidation" in place of "termination" could promote an effective end phase of therapy and can be reserved for when the goals of this phase are addressed in their entirety, the term "end" can be applied to treatment that concludes with no prior warning or without suitably consolidating the gains of the therapy (Maples & Walker, 2014). Maples and Walker (2014) recommend strategies for establishing the consolidation phase. They note that therapists who engaged in more frequent discussion about termination talked about the treatment course more and discussed the patient's emotional response to termination more in cases where the therapist considered the outcome to be successful than in cases where the therapist considered the outcome to be unsuccessful (e.g., Quintana & Holahan, 1992). A therapist's thoughts and emotions that emerge as termination approaches has an effect on their behaviors and influences the effectiveness of therapy, and that substituting the term, "consolidation" for the term "termination" may help therapists in the critical process of discussing the end phase of therapy for patients without successful outcomes (Maples & Walker, 2014; Quintana & Holahan, 1992). According to Maples and Walker (2014), the term "consolidation" is congruent with different theoretical approaches to psychotherapy. For example, Maples and Walker (2014) note that the concept of consolidation seems to fit with a client-centered focus of therapy, which embraces the notion of positive regard in order to facilitate the client's progress (e.g., Thorne, 2007), with relational psychodynamic frameworks that encourage patients to become their own therapists rather than attempting to settle the transference neurosis (e.g., Curtis & Hirsch, 2003), and with cognitive-behavioral therapy models that aim to help the client resolve problems and reinforce and strengthen the client (e.g., Dobson & Dobson, 2009). Therapists who think of the ending of therapy as consolidation can convey positivity for clients as they plan to move on (Maples & Walker, 2014).

A for Awareness or Alliance

Awareness

The I$_{rt}$ – CARE Transtheoretical, Psycholinguistic Model of Termination: The Termination or the Ending Process of Therapy uses the letter "A" of the I$_{rt}$ – CARE term to represent awareness during the termination phase of therapy, that is when therapists hold the last opportunity to be in touch with their inner thoughts as they experience them vis-à-vis patients who end therapy. At the end phase of therapy, how do therapists seek experiences that lead them to further awareness and knowledge about themselves, which, in turn, will provide them with a last chance to promote awareness for patients who are ending therapy? How aware are therapists of their patients meeting the goals of therapy and their satisfaction with therapy? During the termination phase of therapy, therapists need to assist patients to consolidate the changes that they have made during therapy, to help patients be aware of future challenges and how to cope with them, to focus on the prevention of relapse, and to be aware of their own feelings about ending their relationships with patients (da Silva et al., 2022). Therapists may be only somewhat aware of whether their clients are meeting their goals and of their patients' satisfaction with therapy (da Silva et al., 2022; Westmacott et al., 2010). According to da Silva and colleagues (2022), it is important for therapists to be aware that patients have different levels of trust and that trust needs to build gradually, to be aware of the reasons that patients choose to end therapy, to explore these reasons, to identify risks, and to let patients know that they may return if needed. If client dropout does occur, it is important for therapists to be self-aware or self-reflect in a positive way, with a focus on plans for growth, rather than rumination which may result in demoralization (Swift & Greenberg, 2015). Sometimes, however, discussions between clients and therapists may not be possible during the termination or ending phase of therapy as illustrated in some of the examples of Chapters 3 and 4 that depicted abrupt unilateral terminations by clients. In these cases, premature terminations occur, no matter what the level of therapists' or clients' self-awareness.

Alliance

THE THERAPEUTIC ALLIANCE, THE PARALINGUISTIC, AND TERMINATION

The I_{rt} – CARE Transtheoretical, Psycholinguistic Model of Termination: The Termination or the Ending Process of Therapy, a transtheoretical model, considers the importance of a common theme, a core component of psychotherapy, the therapeutic alliance. De Pasquale and colleagues (2019, p. 3043) point out that the therapeutic alliance is predictive of compliance, outcome, and rates of premature termination from therapy (e.g., Samstag et al., 1998). Nof and colleagues (2021) assert that there is a relationship between the therapeutic alliance and auditory cues. They explain that therapists need to consider that paralinguistic cues such as acoustic markers provided by clients during the therapy process can help them to avoid clients' premature terminations from therapy. For example, paralinguistic characteristics such as the pretreatment acoustic markers of the client's voice (e.g., a higher degree of pause proportion or speech intervals that are silent during speech and a higher degree of jitter or instability that derives from voicing variations, sometimes identified as hoarseness) in the first three minutes of the intake session, even prior to the client's meeting with the therapist, have been found to predict lower alliance strength during therapy (Nof et al., 2021; Rochman & Amir, 2013). Nof and colleagues (2021) note that the aforementioned finding is consistent with clinical research that shows that high levels of jitter during therapy sessions may suggest anger that is not resolved, which can obstruct the development of the therapeutic alliance (e.g., Diamond et al., 2010) and with clinical research that finds that silences during therapy sessions may suggest a dynamic of disengagement, which can weaken the therapeutic alliance (e.g., Levitt, 2001). The consideration of paralinguistic cues such as acoustic markers can help therapists to predict a client's early tendency to form a relationship with the therapist, and some markers may be detected more easily than others, e.g., the detection of pauses being more automatic than the analysis of jitter that requires a more intense investment (Nof et al., 2021). Until further technological advances can provide simultaneous pointers that offer therapists knowledge about the tendency for patients to form therapeutic alliances, therapists are encouraged to rely on their innate abilities to sort out prosody communication about a patient's psychological being (Nof et al., 2021; Wiethoff et al., 2008). The I_{rt} – CARE Transtheoretical, Psycholinguistic Model of Termination: The Termination or the Ending Process of Therapy considers the importance of paralinguistic cues and their relationship to the therapeutic alliance and to a client's premature ending in therapy.

The I$_{rt}$ – CARE Transtheoretical, Psycholinguistic Model of Termination: The Termination or the Ending Process of Therapy uses the letter "A" of the I$_{rt}$ – CARE term to represent alliance during the termination phase of therapy. Whereas other sections of this chapter describe the relationship between linguistic signals and termination, this section focuses on the relationship between paralinguistic signals and premature termination from therapy. The I$_{rt}$ – CARE Transtheoretical, Psycholinguistic Model of Termination: The Termination or the Ending Process of Therapy suggests that researchers and practitioners attend to the study of paralinguistic cues such as acoustic markers which can help therapists to predict a client's early tendencies to form a relationship with the therapist (e.g., Nof et al., 2021). Nof and colleagues (2021) point out that acoustic markers of patients that are acquired prior to treatment have been shown to predict the therapeutic alliance, and these findings suggest that such markers may be able to facilitate practitioners' ability to select treatment in a manner that could prevent the weakening of the therapeutic alliance (e.g., Barlow et al., 2017). Reich et al. (2014) assert that they were the first to study the association between synchrony of pitch and therapy process and outcome. Relevant to the development of the therapeutic alliance, they showed that there was a lower therapeutic relationship quality for therapeutic dyads with elevated degrees of pitch synchrony, and they suggest further study into the context of elevated and low moments of synchrony during therapy.

THE THERAPEUTIC ALLIANCE, NONVERBAL SYNCHRONY, AND PREMATURE TERMINATION

Synchrony can be expressed verbally, for example, in the use of words, and nonverbally, for example, in facial expression (Reich et al., 2014). This section underscores the importance of the therapeutic alliance and its association with client ruptures and client dropout or premature termination, and focuses on nonverbal synchrony, on how the study of nonverbal mannerisms of therapists and clients impacts therapy. Mylona and Avdi (2021, p. 230) point out that evidence for synchrony that is nonverbal in therapy, for example, the movement of the body and the expression of the face, underscores its importance for the therapeutic alliance (e.g., Koole & Tschacher, 2016). Koole and Tschacher (2016) emphasize the use of synchrony in the therapeutic alliance, that is how the members of the therapeutic dyad coordinate temporally.

Components of their Interpersonal Synchrony (I-Sync) model can be utilized to understand and facilitate the therapeutic alliance, its contribution to therapy, and the emotion-regulation capacity of clients. Theirs is a multidisciplinary approach to the therapeutic alliance that relies on constructs from linguistics, neuroscience, developmental, and psychophysiological elements. The development of a common language and emotional co-regulation between members of the therapeutic dyad can be facilitated through synchrony, and the movement synchrony of clients and therapists has been shown to be positively related to the alliance and to outcomes in therapy (Koole & Tschacher, 2016). Features of the I-Sync model of Koole and Tschacher (2016) can be included in training programs in psychotherapy. It is difficult for therapists to learn to build alliances when ratings of the alliance are subjective, and the In-Sync model could develop objective measures (common language and synchrony in movement) in order to facilitate feedback for therapists who seek to develop the therapeutic alliance with their clients (Koole & Tschacher, 2016).

Not all individuals benefit from therapy. Nof and colleagues (2021) point out that although many clients benefit from therapy, approximately 33% of clients do not benefit significantly (e.g., Lambert, 2013), and it is the therapeutic alliance that has been found to predict outcome in therapy (Flückiger et al., 2018). Chapter 5 introduced the psycholinguistic model, the I_{rt} – CARE Transtheoretical, Psycholinguistic Model of Ruptures and Repairs, that recognizes the relationship between changes in the therapeutic alliance and paralinguistic characteristics such as acoustic markers. This transtheoretical model relies on the benefits of establishing a strong therapeutic alliance, regardless of theoretical orientation. The ability of a therapist to predict the development of the therapeutic alliance that a client will form with a therapist, even prior to the first session, can help therapists to decrease the negative impact of a weak therapeutic alliance on the outcome and to prevent premature termination (Nof et al., 2021). Nof and colleagues (2021) point out that given that it is not easy to delineate a weakening in the therapeutic alliance, it is not possible to rely solely on the accuracy of therapists' evaluations of the alliance, particularly with regard to withdrawal ruptures (e.g., Eubanks et al., 2018). They note that there are new methods that can help to assess the therapeutic alliance (e.g., Imel et al., 2017) and that synchrony (in therapy, the correspondence between therapists' and clients' nonverbal mannerisms) is a focus of these contemporary methods. For example, they assert that therapist and client body movement synchrony can signify the quality of a relationship (e.g., Ramseyer & Tschacher, 2014) and that arousal synchrony that is vocally encoded can signify the empathy of a therapist (e.g., Imel et al., 2014).

Nonverbal Synchrony: Ruptures, Repairs, and Termination

Whereas Chapter 5 described the relationship between nonverbal or movement synchrony and alliance ruptures and previous sections of this chapter described the relationship between linguistic or paralinguistic elements and termination in therapy, this section addresses the association between nonverbal synchrony and the termination in therapy. The I_{rt} – CARE Transtheoretical, Psycholinguistic Model of Termination: The Termination or the Ending Process of Therapy relies on the study of nonverbal synchrony to gather information about the termination or ending phase of therapy. It has been suggested that nonverbal synchrony may help to spot patients who are likely to drop out from therapy (Paulick et al., 2018; Rubel et al., 2015). Ramseyer (2020, p. 624) notes that higher nonverbal synchrony was observed in CBT than in psychodynamic therapy, and synchrony that took place early in therapy was associated with a stronger alliance later in therapy and decreased interpersonal difficulties at termination (e.g., Altmann et al., 2020). Schoenherr and colleagues (2019, p. 504) point out that the level of nonverbal synchrony for individuals who prematurely terminate therapy was lower than for individuals who mutually agreed on terminating therapy and did not improve in therapy (e.g., Paulick et al., 2018).

What is the association between ruptures, repairs, and the termination or the ending phase of therapy? Deres-Cohen et al. (2021, p. 506) point out that ruptures that are not repaired may lead to premature termination (e.g., Eubanks et al., 2018; Gülüm et al., 2018). Dolev-Amit and colleagues (2022) assert that these ruptures, breaches, or impasses have the potential to lead to dropout or premature termination from therapy or to enrich the relationship and lead to success. They explain that if therapists are to repair ruptures, first they need to learn how to become aware of ruptures, particularly withdrawal ruptures as they are difficult to detect (e.g., Eubanks Lubitz, et al., 2019). Negri and colleagues (2019, p. 71) note that alliance ruptures can help therapists understand how clients function, can facilitate a therapeutic relationship, and can benefit outcome in therapy (e.g., Colli et al., 2019; Safran et al., 2011). The connection between ruptures, their resolution, and the termination or the ending phase of therapy, cannot be underestimated (Dolev-Amit et al., 2022; Eubanks et al., 2018).

Chapter Summary

Chapter 6 focuses on the I_{rt} – CARE Transtheoretical, Psycholinguistic Model of Termination: The Termination or the Ending Process of Therapy and how it can guide therapists who wish to reduce premature termination of patients from therapy. The chapter further expands on the association between the therapeutic alliance and the ending in therapy and the connection between ruptures, their resolution, and the termination or the ending phase of therapy. It is the alliance that has been found to be the most solid forecaster of therapy outcome, and some practitioners view psychotherapy as a conversation where the alliance is built via intersubjective means, such as the process of repairing ruptures or deteriorations, taking turns, and recognizing the other person's point of view (Horvath & Symonds, 1991; Knox, 2019). Disruptions or tensions (ruptures) in the therapeutic alliance, if not resolved, may result in clients' unilateral terminations from therapy (Abbass & Town, 2021; Eubanks et al., 2018). The I_{rt} – CARE Transtheoretical, Psycholinguistic Model of Termination: The Termination or the Ending Process of Therapy embraced in this chapter emphasizes the importance of the development of psycholinguistic investigations, for example, linguistic, paralinguistic, and nonverbal synchrony, regarding ruptures and premature terminations so that therapists can receive feedback about their sessions with their patients to better enable them to avoid these negative events, thereby decreasing the likelihood of clients' premature terminations from therapy. The takeaway is that if therapists are open to receiving cues from a psycholinguistic model that is transtheoretical, they can learn how to establish a durable therapeutic alliance in a few sessions so that clients can benefit as much as possible early on in the therapy, and therapists can be alerted during the termination phase of therapy about potentially negative turns.

See Figure 6.2.

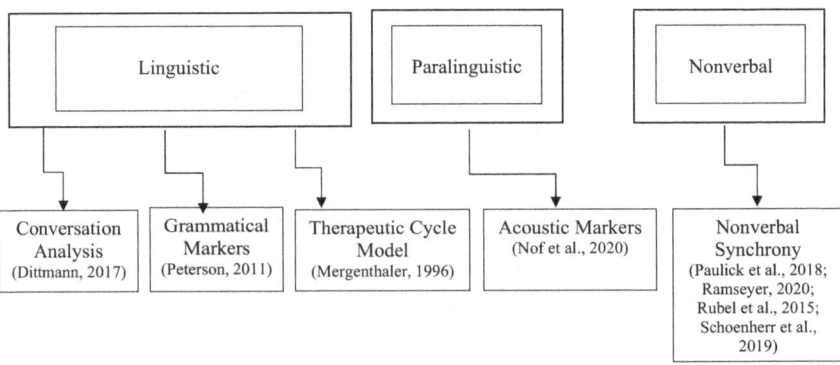

Figure 6.2 I_{rt} – CARE Transtheoretical, Psycholinguistic Model of Termination: The Termination or the Ending Process of Therapy

Note. This figure illustrates the different components of the psycholinguistic model.

References

Abargil, M., & Tishby, O. (2021). Countertransference as a reflection of the patient's inner relationship conflict. *Psychoanalytic Psychology, 38*(1), 68–78. https://doi.org/10.1037/pap0000312

Abbass, A. A., & Town, J. M. (2021). Alliance rupture-repair processes in intensive short-term dynamic psychotherapy: Working with resistance. *Journal of Clinical Psychology, 77*(2), 398–413. https://doi.org/10.1002/jclp.23115

Altmann, U., Schoenherr, D., Paulick, J., Deisenhofer, A.-K., Schwartz, B., Rubel, J. A., Stangier, U., Lutz, W., & Strauss, B. (2020). Associations between movement synchrony and outcome in patients with social anxiety disorder: Evidence for treatment specific effects. *Psychotherapy Research, 30*(5), 574–590. https://doi.org/10.1080/10503307.2019.1630779

Barlow, D. H., Farchione, T. J., Sauer-Zavala, S., Latin, H. M., Ellard, K. K., Bullis, J. R., Bentley, K. H., Boettcher, H. T., & Cassiello-Robbins, C. (2017). *Unified protocol for transdiagnostic treatment of emotional disorders: Therapist guide*. Oxford University Press.

Barrett, M. S., Chua, W.-J., Crits-Christoph, P., Gibbons, M. B., & Thompson, D. (2008). Early withdrawal from mental health treatment: Implications for psychotherapy practice. *Psychotherapy: Theory, Research, Practice, Training, 45*(2), 247–267. https://doi.org/10.1037/0033-3204.45.2.247

Bartholomew, T. T., Lockard, A. J., Folger, S. F., Low, B. E., Poet, A. D., Scofield, B. E., & Locke, B. D. (2019). Symptom reduction and termination: Client change and therapist identified reasons for saying goodbye. *Counselling Psychology Quarterly, 32*(1), 81–99. https://doi.org/10.1080/09515070.2017.1367272

Bennett-Levy, J., Lee, N., Travers, K., Pohlman, S., & Hamernik, E. (2003). Cognitive therapy from the inside: Enhancing therapist skills through practising what we preach. *Behavioural and Cognitive Psychotherapy, 31*(2), 143–158. https://doi.org/10.1017/S1352465803002029

Carter, M. M., Turovsky, J., Sbrocco, T., Meadows, E. A., & Barlow, D. H. (1995). Patient dropout from a couples' group treatment for panic disorder with agoraphobia. *Professional Psychology: Research and Practice, 26*(6), 626–628. https://doi.org/10.1037/0735-7028.26.6.626

Castonguay, L. G., Newman, M. G., & Holtforth, M. G. (2019). Cognitive-behavioral assimilative integration. In J. C. Norcross & M. R. Goldfried (Eds.), *Handbook of psychotherapy integration* (pp. 228–251). Oxford University Press. https://doi.org/10.1093/med-psych/9780190690465.003.0011

Cirasola, A., Martin, P., Fonagy, P., Eubanks, C., Muran, J. C., & Midgley, N. (2022). Alliance ruptures and resolutions in short-term psychoanalytic psychotherapy for adolescent depression: An empirical case study. *Psychotherapy Research, 32*(7), 951–968. https://doi.org/10.1080/10503307.2022.2061314

Colli, A., Gentile, D., Condino, V., & Lingiardi, V. (2019). Assessing alliance ruptures and resolutions: Reliability and validity of the Collaborative Interactions Scale-revised version. *Psychotherapy Research, 29*(3), 279–292. https://doi.org/10.1080/10503307.2017.1414331

Comninos, A., & Grenyer, B. F. S. (2007). The influence of interpersonal factors on the speed of recovery from major depression. *Psychotherapy Research, 17*(2), 230–239. https://doi.org/10.1080/10503300600849140

Coutinho, J., Ribeiro, E., Fernandes, C., Sousa, I., & Safran, J. D. (2014). The development of the therapeutic alliance and the emergence of alliance ruptures. *Anales de Psicología*, *30*(3), 985–994. https://doi.org/10.6018/analesps.30.3.168911

Cozolino, L. (2004). *The making of a therapist: A practical guide for the inner journey*. WW Norton & Company.

Curtis, R. C., & Hirsch, I. (2003). Relational psychoanalytic psychotherapy. In A. S. Gurman & S. B. Messer (Eds.), *Essential psychotherapies: Theory and practice* (pp. 69–106). Guilford Press.

Dandachi-FitzGerald, B., Meijs, L., Moonen, I. M. A. J., & Merckelbach, H. (2022). No self-serving bias in therapists' evaluations of clients' premature treatment termination: An approximate replication of Murdock et al. (2010). *Clinical Psychology & Psychotherapy*, *29*(3), 972–981. https://doi.org/10.1002/cpp.2677

da Silva, A. N., Ferreira, J. F., Conceição, N., Vaz Velho, C., & Vasco, A. B. (2022). Termination in psychotherapy: Contributions of an integrative metamodel. *Journal of Psychotherapy Integration*, *32*(2), 175–189. https://doi.org/10.1037/int0000235

Davis, D. D. (2008). *Terminating therapy: A professional guide to ending on a positive note*. Wiley.

Davis, D. D., & Younggren, J. N. (2009). Ethical competence in psychotherapy termination. *Professional Psychology: Research and Practice*, *40*(6), 572–578. https://doi.org/10.1037/a0017699

De Pasquale, C., Cullen, C., & Vaughan, B. (2019, September 15–19). An investigation of therapeutic rapport through prosody in brief psychodynamic psychotherapy. *Proceedings of INTERSPEECH*, Graz, Austria, 3043–3047. https://doi.org/10.21437/Interspeech.2019-2551

Deres-Cohen, K., Dolev-Amit, T., Peysachov, G., Ramseyer, F. T., & Zilcha-Mano, S. (2021). Nonverbal synchrony as a marker of alliance ruptures. *Psychotherapy*, *58*(4), 499–509. https://doi.org/10.1037/pst0000384

Diamond, G. M., Rochman, D., & Amir, O. (2010). Arousing primary vulnerable emotions in the context of unresolved anger: "Speaking about" versus "speaking to." *Journal of Counseling Psychology*, *57*(4), 402–410. https://doi.org/10.1037/a0021115

Dittmann, M. M. (2017). Moving closer. A conversation analytic perspective on how a psychotherapeutic dyad works on closing their encounters. *Language and Psychoanalysis*, *5*(2), 46–61. https://doi.org/10.7565/landp.v5i2.1560

Dobson, D. J. G., & Dobson, K. S. (2009). *Evidence-based practice of cognitive-behavioral therapy*. Guilford Press.

Dolev-Amit, T., Nof, A., Asaad, A., Tchizick, A., & Zilcha-Mano, S. (2022). The melody of ruptures: Identifying ruptures through acoustic markers. *Counselling Psychology Quarterly*, *35*(4), 724–743. https://doi.org/10.1080/09515070.2020.1860906

Eubanks, C. F., Lubitz, J., Muran, J. C., & Safran, J. D. (2019). Rupture resolution rating system (3RS): Development and validation. *Psychotherapy Research*, *29*(3), 306–319. https://doi.org/10.1080/10503307.2018.1552034

Eubanks, C. F., Muran, C. J., & Safran, J. D. (2018). Alliance rupture repair: A meta-analysis. *Psychotherapy*, *55*(4), 508–519. https://doi.org/10.1037/pst0000185

Eubanks, C. F., Muran, J. C., & Safran, J. D. (2019). Repairing alliance ruptures. In J. C. Norcross & M. J. Lambert (Eds.), *Psychotherapy relationships that work: Evidence-based therapist contributions* (pp. 549–579). Oxford University Press. https://doi.org/10.1093/med-psych/9780190843953.003.0016

Flückiger, C., Del Re, A. C., Wampold, B. E., & Horvath, A. O. (2018). The alliance in adult psychotherapy: A meta-analytic synthesis. *Psychotherapy, 55*(4), 316–340. https://doi.org/10.1037/pst0000172

Gülüm, I. V., Soygüt, G., & Safran, J. D. (2018). A comparison of pre-dropout and temporary rupture sessions in psychotherapy. *Psychotherapy Research, 28*(5), 685–707. https://doi.org/10.1080/10503307.2016.1246765

Henry, W. P., Schacht, T. E., & Strupp, H. H. (1986). Structural analysis of social behavior: Application to a study of interpersonal process in differential psychotherapeutic outcome. *Journal of Consulting and Clinical Psychology, 54*(1), 27–31. https://doi.org/10.1037/0022-006X.54.1.27

Hölzer, M., Mergenthaler, E., Pokorny, D., Kächele, H., & Luborsky, L. (1996). Vocabulary measures for the evaluation of therapy outcome: Re-studying transcripts from the Penn Psychotherapy Project. *Psychotherapy Research, 6*(2), 95–108. https://doi.org/10.1080/10503309612331331618

Horvath, A. O., Re, A. C. D., Flückiger, C., & Symonds, D. (2011). Alliance in individual psychotherapy. In J. C. Norcross (Ed.), *Psychotherapy relationships that work: Evidence-based responsiveness* (pp. 25–69). Oxford University Press. https://doi.org/10.1093/acprof:oso/9780199737208.003.0002

Horvath, A. O., & Symonds, B. D. (1991). Relation between working alliance and outcome in psychotherapy: A meta-analysis. *Journal of Counseling Psychology, 38*(2), 139–149. https://doi.org/10.1037/0022-0167.38.2.139

Imel, Z. E., Barco, J. S., Brown, H. J., Baucom, B. R., Baer, J. S., Kircher, J. C., & Atkins, D. C. (2014). The association of therapist empathy and synchrony in vocally encoded arousal. *Journal of Counseling Psychology, 61*(1), 146–153. https://doi.org/10.1037/a0034943

Imel, Z. E., Caperton, D. D., Tanana, M., & Atkins, D. C. (2017). Technology-enhanced human interaction in psychotherapy. *Journal of Counseling Psychology, 64*(4), 385–393. https://doi.org/10.1037/cou0000213

Kasoff, M. B., Castonguay, L. G., Horowitz, L. M., Luboski, J. A., & Boutselis, M. A. (2000, August). *Investigating client's reasons for terminating psychotherapy*. Poster presented at the Annual meeting of American Psychological Association, Washington, D.C..

Knox, J. (2019). The harmful effects of psychotherapy: When the therapeutic alliance fails. *British Journal of Psychotherapy, 35*(2), 245–262. https://doi.org10.1111/bjp.12445

Knox, S., Adrians, N., Everson, E., Hess, S., Hill, C., & Crook-Lyon, R. (2011). Clients' perspectives on therapy termination. *Psychotherapy Research, 21*(2), 154–167. https://doi.org/10.1080/10503307.2010.534509

Koole, S. L., & Tschacher, W. (2016) Synchrony in psychotherapy: A review and integrative framework for the therapeutic alliance. *Frontiers in Psychology, 7*, 862. https://doi.org/10.3389/fpsyg.2016.00862

Laireiter, A.-P. (1998). Self-directed experience and personal therapy: The situation in the German-speaking countries and "the state of the art" of empirical research. In E. Sanavio (Ed.), *Behaviour and cognitive therapy today: Essay in honor of Hans J. Eysenck* (pp. 163–179). Pergamon.

Lambert, M. J. (2013). Outcome in psychotherapy: The past and important advances. *Psychotherapy, 50*(1), 42–51. https://doi.org/10.1037/a0030682

Levitt, H. M. (2001). Sounds of silence in psychotherapy: The categorization of clients' pauses. *Psychotherapy Research, 11*(3), 295–309. https://doi.org/10.1080/713663985

Loewald, H. W. (1962). Internalization, separation, mourning, and the super-ego. *The Psychoanalytic Quarterly, 31*(4), 483–504.

Luo, X., Liu, S., Levendosky, A. A., Good, E. W., Turchan, J. E., & Hopwood, C. J. (2022). Idiographic and nomothetic relationships between momentary interpersonal behaviors, interpersonal complementarity, and alliance ruptures in psychotherapy. *Journal of Counseling Psychology, 69*(5), 642–655. https://doi.org/10.1037/cou0000619

Macran, S., & Shapiro, D. A. (1998). The role of personal therapy for therapists: A review. *British Journal of Medical Psychology, 71*(Pt 1), 13–25. https://doi.org/10.1111/j.2044-8341.1998.tb01364.x

Maples, J. L., & Walker, R. L. (2014). Consolidation rather than termination: Rethinking how psychologists label and conceptualize the final phase of psychological treatment. *Professional Psychology: Research and Practice, 45*(2), 104–110. https://doi.org/10.1037/a0036250

McCarthy, K. L., Mergenthaler, E., Schneider, S., & Grenyer, B. F. S. (2011). Psychodynamic change in psychotherapy: Cycles of patient–therapist linguistic interactions and interventions. *Psychotherapy Research, 21*(6), 722–731. https://doi.org/10.1080/10503307.2011.615070

McMurran, M., Huband, N., & Overton, E. (2010). Non-completion of personality disorder treatments: A systematic review of correlates, consequences, and interventions. *Clinical Psychology Review, 30*(3), 277–287. https://doi.org/10.1016/j.cpr.2009.12.002

Mergenthaler, E. (1996). Emotion-abstraction patterns in verbatim protocols: A new way of describing psychotherapeutic processes. *Journal of Consulting and Clinical Psychology, 64*(6), 1306–1315. https://doi.org/10.1037//0022-006x.64.6.1306

Mergenthaler, E. (2008). Resonating minds: A school-independent theoretical conception and its empirical application to psychotherapeutic processes. *Psychotherapy Research, 18*(2), 109–126. https://doi.org/10.1080/10503300701883741

Milbrath, C., Bond, M., Cooper, S., Znoj, H. J., Horowitz, M. J., & Perry, J. C. (1999). Sequential consequences of therapists' interventions. *The Journal of Psychotherapy Practice and Research, 8*(1), 40–54.

Muran, J. C., Safran, J. D., Eubanks, C. F., & Gorman, B. S. (2018). The effect of alliance-focused training on a cognitive-behavioral therapy for personality disorders. *Journal of Consulting and Clinical Psychology, 86*(4), 384–397. https://doi.org/10.1037/ccp0000284

Muran, J. C., Safran, J. D., Gorman, B. S., Samstag, L. W., Eubanks-Carter, C., & Winston, A. (2009). The relationship of early alliance ruptures and their resolution to process and outcome in three time-limited psychotherapies for personality disorders. *Psychotherapy: Theory, Research, Practice, Training, 46*(2), 233–248. https://doi.org/10.1037/a0016085

Murdock, N. L., Edwards, C., & Murdock, T. B. (2010). Therapists' attributions for client premature termination: Are they self-serving? *Psychotherapy: Theory, Research, Practice, Training, 47*(2), 221–234. https://doi.org/10.1037/a0019786

Mylona, A., & Avdi, E. (2021). Alliance ruptures and embodied arousal in psychodynamic psychotherapy: An exploratory study. *Hellenic Journal of Psychology, 18*(2), 226–248. https://doi.org/10.26262/hjp.v18i2.8193

Negri, A., Christian, C., Mariani, R., Belotti, L., Andreoli, G., & Danskin, K. (2019). Linguistic features of the therapeutic alliance in the first session: A psychotherapy process study. *Research in Psychotherapy: Psychopathology, Process and Outcome, 22*(1), 71–82. https://doi.org/10.4081/ripppo.2019.374

Nof, A., Amir, O., Goldstein, P., & Zilcha-Mano, S. (2021). What do these sounds tell us about the therapeutic alliance: Acoustic markers as predictors of alliance. *Clinical Psychology & Psychotherapy, 28*(4), 807–817. https://doi.org/10.1002/cpp.2534

Norcross, J. C., & Finnerty, M. (2019). Training and supervision in psychotherapy integration. In J. C. Norcross & M. R. Goldfried (Eds.), *Handbook of psychotherapy integration* (pp. 377–404). Oxford University Press. https://doi.org/10.1093/med-psych/9780190690465.003.0018

Norcross, J. C., Zimmerman, B. E., Greenberg, R. P., & Swift, J. K. (2017). Do all therapists do that when saying goodbye? A study of commonalities in termination behaviors. *Psychotherapy, 54*(1), 66–75. https://doi.org/10.1037/pst0000097

Ogrodniczuk, J. S., Joyce, A. S., & Piper, W. E. (2005). Strategies for reducing patient-initiated premature termination of psychotherapy. *Harvard Review of Psychiatry, 13*(2), 57–70. https://doi.org/10.1080/10673220590956429

Orlinsky, D. E., Botermans, J.-F., & Rønnestad, M. H. (2001). Towards an empirically grounded model of psychotherapy training: Four thousand therapists rate influences on their development. *Australian Psychologist, 36*(2), 139–148. https://doi.org/10.1080/00050060108259646

Paulick, J., Deisenhofer, A.-K., Ramseyer, F., Tschacher, W., Boyle, K., Rubel, J., & Lutz, W. (2018). Nonverbal synchrony: A new approach to better understand psychotherapeutic processes and drop-out. *Journal of Psychotherapy Integration, 28*(3), 367–384 https://doi.org/10.1037/int0000099

Peterson, C. A. (2011). Pronouns and progress: A psychoanalytic primer. *The Psychoanalytic Review, 98*(4), 515–530. https://doi.org/10.1521/prev.2011.98.4.515

Philips, B., Karlsson, R., Nygren, R., Rother-Schirren, A., & Werbart, A. (2018). Early therapeutic process related to dropout in mentalization-based treatment with dual diagnosis patients. *Psychoanalytic Psychology, 35*(2), 205–216. https://doi.org/10.1037/pap0000170

Power, A. (2016). *Forced endings in psychotherapy and psychoanalysis: Attachment and loss in retirement.* Routledge/Taylor & Francis Group.

Quintana, S. M., & Holahan, W. (1992). Termination in short-term counseling: Comparison of successful and unsuccessful cases. *Journal of Counseling Psychology, 39*(3), 299–305. https://doi.org/10.1037/0022-0167.39.3.299

Ramseyer, F. T. (2020). Exploring the evolution of nonverbal synchrony in psychotherapy: The idiographic perspective provides a different picture. *Psychotherapy Research, 30*(5), 622–634. https://doi.org/10.1080/10503307.2019.1676932

Ramseyer, F., & Tschacher, W. (2014). Nonverbal synchrony of head- and body-movement in psychotherapy: Different signals have different associations with outcome. *Frontiers in Psychology, 5*, Article 979, 1–9. https://doi.org/10.3389/fpsyg.2014.00979

Reich, C. M., Berman, J. S., Dale, R., & Levitt, H. M. (2014). Vocal synchrony in psychotherapy. *Journal of Social and Clinical Psychology, 33*(5), 481–494. https://doi.org/10.1521/jscp.2014.33.5.481

Renk, K., & Dinger, T. M. (2002). Reasons for therapy termination in a university psychology clinic. *Journal of Clinical Psychology, 58*(9), 1173–1181. https://doi.org/10.1002/jclp.10075

Rochman, D., & Amir, O. (2013). Examining in-session expressions of emotions with speech/vocal acoustic measures: An introductory guide. *Psychotherapy Research, 23*(4), 381–393. https://doi.org/10.1080/10503307.2013.784421

Rubel, J., Lutz, W., Kopta, S. M., Köck, K., Minami, T., Zimmermann, D., & Saunders, S. M. (2015). Defining early positive response to psychotherapy: An empirical comparison between clinically significant change criteria and growth mixture modeling. *Psychological Assessment, 27*(2), 478–488. https://doi.org/10.1037/pas0000060

Safran, J. D., & Kraus, J. (2014). Alliance ruptures, impasses, and enactments: A relational perspective. *Psychotherapy, 51*(3), 381–387. https://doi.org/10.1037/a0036815

Safran, J. D., & Muran, J. C. (1996). The resolution of ruptures in the therapeutic alliance. *Journal of Consulting and Clinical Psychology, 64*(3), 447–458. https://doi.org/10.1037/0022-006X.64.3.447

Safran, J. D., Muran, J. C., & Eubanks-Carter, C. (2011). Repairing alliance ruptures. *Psychotherapy, 48*(1), 80–87. https://doi.org/10.1037/a0022140

Safran, J. D., Muran, J. C., Samstag, L. W., & Winston, A. (2005). Evaluating alliance-focused treatment for potential treatment failures: A feasibility study and descriptive analysis. *Psychotherapy: Theory, Research, Practice, Training, 42*(4), 512–531. https://doi.org/10.1037/0033-3204.42.4.512

Samstag, L. W., Batchelder, S. T., Muran, J. C., Safran, J. D., & Winston, A. (1998). Early identification of treatment failures in short-term psychotherapy: An assessment of therapeutic alliance and interpersonal behavior. *Journal of Psychotherapy Practice & Research, 7*(2), 126–143.

Schoenherr, D., Paulick, J., Strauss, B. M., Deisenhofer, A.-K., Schwartz, B., Rubel, J. A., Lutz, W., Stangier, U., & Altmann, U. (2019). Nonverbal synchrony predicts premature termination of psychotherapy for social anxiety disorder. *Psychotherapy, 56*(4), 503–513. https://doi.org/10.1037/pst0000216

Sharf, J., Primavera, L. H., & Diener, M. J. (2010). Dropout and therapeutic alliance: A meta-analysis of adult individual psychotherapy. *Psychotherapy: Theory, Research, and Practice, 47*(4), 637–645. https://doi.org/10.1037/a0021175

Swift, J. K., & Greenberg, R. P. (2012). Premature discontinuation in adult psychotherapy: A meta-analysis. *Journal of Consulting and Clinical Psychology, 80*(4), 547–559. https://doi.org/10.1037/a0028226

Swift, J. K., & Greenberg, R. P. (2015). Premature termination in psychotherapy: Strategies for engaging clients and improving outcomes. American Psychological Association. https://doi.org/10.1037/14469-000

Thorne, B. (2007). Person-centered therapy. In W. Dryden (Ed.), *Dryden's handbook of individual therapy* (pp. 144–172). Sage Publications Ltd.

Vasquez, M. J. T., Bingham, R. P., & Barnett, J. E. (2008). Psychotherapy termination: Clinical and ethical responsibilities. *Journal of Clinical Psychology, 64*(5), 653–665. https://doi.org/10.1002/jclp.20478

Westen, D., & Morrison, K. (2001). A multidimensional meta-analysis of treatments for depression, panic, and generalized anxiety disorder: An empirical examination of the status of empirically supported therapies. *Journal of Consulting and Clinical Psychology, 69*(6), 875–899. https://doi.org/10.1037/0022-006X.69.6.875

Westmacott, R., Hunsley, J., Best, M., Rumstein-McKean, O., & Schindler, D. (2010). Client and therapist views of contextual factors related to termination from psychotherapy: A comparison between unilateral and mutual terminators. *Psychotherapy Research, 20*(4), 423–435. https://doi.org/10.1080/10503301003645796

Wierzbicki, M., & Pekarik, G. (1993). A meta-analysis of psychotherapy dropout. *Professional Psychology: Research and Practice, 24*(2), 190–195. https://doi.org/10.1037/0735-7028.24.2.190

Wiethoff, S., Wildgruber, D., Kreifelts, B., Becker, H., Herbert, C., Grodd, W., & Ethofer, T. (2008). Cerebral processing of emotional prosody – influence of acoustic parameters and arousal. *NeuroImage, 39*(2), 885–893. https://doi.org/10.1016/j.neuroimage.2007.09.028

Williams, F., Coyle, A., & Lyons, E. (1999). How counselling psychologists view their personal therapy. *British Journal of Medical Psychology, 72*(4), 545–555. https://doi.org/10.1348/000711299160112

Yalom, I. D. (2002). *The gift of therapy: An open letter to a new generation of therapists and their patients.* HarperCollins Publishers.

Conclusion

Sometimes individuals begin therapy, but then it is difficult for them to see their way through their course of therapy. They encounter bumps in the road, and the journey becomes anything but smooth sailing. *Why did she/he say this to me? Why now? What am I even doing here? What to do? Oh, gee, unreal.* These may be some of the inner thoughts of patients and therapists during and/or after a rupture or an impasse in the therapeutic relationship. A deterioration in the therapeutic or working alliance, whether a withdrawal, confrontation, or a mixed rupture, can disrupt the therapy work of patients and therapists (Mylona & Avdi, 2021). Lipner and colleagues (2020, 2023) explain that the frequency of ruptures can vary widely (3%–84%) subject to the methodology utilized to discern these disagreements, suggesting that rupture definitions vary. The book, *Navigating Ruptures, Repairs, and Termination Within the Therapeutic Process*, suggests that the therapeutic or working alliance ruptures, tensions, or breaches that occur during therapy, although frequently negative, may be more manageable than anticipated. Sometimes they unfold in ways that are difficult to comprehend and at times that are inopportune. When ruptures or tensions happen, therapists can view them as a chance for a change or as a setback, depending on the capacity of the therapist to discern the ruptures and unpack them (Lipner et al., 2023).

The failure of therapists to develop, establish, and/or maintain a strong therapeutic alliance can be a cause for the premature termination of patients from therapy (Vail et al., 2021), and dropouts from therapy are not uncommon (Kullgard et al., 2022). The book, *Navigating Ruptures, Repairs, and Termination Within the Therapeutic Process*, describes some feelings that patients have when

DOI: 10.4324/9781003128489-10

they drop out of therapy, for example, feelings of anger, hopelessness, confusion, and/or relief, and these patients may have difficulty trusting another therapist if they try therapy again. Therapists, too, may feel defenseless, sad, puzzled, and/or relieved, and may select to seek consultation or may be reluctant to do so. The following may be the inner thoughts of both members of the therapeutic dyad after the negative event of a patient dropout: *What has happened? How did we get here?*

In a survey of approximately 84,000 therapy clients, it was found that almost a fifth dropped out of therapy, and there was no difference in rates of premature termination among theoretical perspectives, for example, humanistic, cognitive-behavioral, or psychodynamic (Leichsenring et al., 2019). Attention to the inner life of therapists and patients throughout the book, *Navigating Ruptures, Repairs, and Termination Within the Therapeutic Process*, affords therapists an opportunity to examine the association between the therapeutic or working alliance and its connection to premature termination and to realize that the process of termination or ending in therapy is not as simple as it looks, and, at times, is fraught with complexity.

The book, *Navigating Ruptures, Repairs, and Termination Within the Therapeutic Process*, describes different types of endings in therapy, for example, mutually agreed, planned terminations, unplanned, premature terminations initiated by patients or patient dropouts, forced or coerced terminations initiated by therapists, and it provides the inner thoughts of patients and therapists that accompany the examples of the different kinds of endings in therapy. Although a mutually agreed, planned termination is voluntary, it is difficult for patients to leave therapists who are an important part of their lives, and, at the same time, a termination that is mutually agreed can offer patients the opportunity to end a meaningful connection to another individual while being in a constructive relationship (Schlesinger, 2014). Therapists, from the beginning of and throughout therapy, are faced with issues related to the ending of therapy, for example, an ending that is apparent to patients when therapists take a vacation or a pause in the conversation during a therapy session, and the aforementioned delicate moments suggest a future ending for therapy to patients and provide a chance during therapy to rehearse the termination phase (Knafo, 2018).

There are therapists, and there are therapists. The book, *Navigating Ruptures, Repairs, and Termination Within the Therapeutic Process*, emphasizes that therapists who are attuned have the capacity to recognize their own inner thoughts and to explore the evolving inner feelings of their patients. The vignettes show how therapists who are curious are able to inquire about patients' thoughts and experiences and can ask how their patients have evolved to become the human beings they are today. Patients who are non-responders to therapy can inform by offering therapists the opportunity to explore why and how therapy works and with whom it works (Leichsenring et al., 2019). Tschuschke and colleagues (2022) find support for the notion that the person of the therapist is more important than has been previously thought (e.g., Baldwin & Imel, 2013; Barkham et al., 2017; Wampold et al., 2017). Therapists who are effective are able to develop a therapeutic alliance across a broad scope of individuals, and these therapists have advanced interpersonal skills that they can use in the face of challenging circumstances (Wampold et al., 2017).

The two-part model included in this book, the I_{rt} – CARE Transtheoretical, Psycholinguistic Model of Ruptures, Repairs, and Termination, encourages therapists across different theoretical approaches to rely on rupture-repair strategies in order to adjust negative feelings toward patients. The transtheoretical model, in its illustration of how practitioners navigate during therapy sessions and in its exploration of the verbal, paralinguistic, and nonverbal dynamics of the therapeutic process (the verbal and nonverbal synchrony between members of the therapeutic dyad) has implications for training therapists and their supervisors or consultants to expand their understanding of alliance ruptures, their repair, and the connection of ruptures or disagreements and their resolutions to the termination phase of therapy.

References

Baldwin, S. A., & Imel, Z. E. (2013). Therapist effects: Findings and methods. In M. J. Lambert (Ed.), *Bergin and Garfield's handbook of psychotherapy and behavior change* (6th ed., pp. 258–297). Wiley.

Barkham, M., Lutz, W., Lambert, M. J., & Saxon, D. (2017). Therapist effects, effective therapists, and the law of variability. In L. G. Castonguay & C. E. Hill (Eds.), *How and why are some therapists better than others?: Understanding therapist effects* (pp. 13–36). American Psychological Association. https://doi.org/10.1037/0000034-002

De Pasquale, C., Cullen, C., & Vaughan, B. (2019, September 15–19). An investigation of therapeutic rapport through prosody in brief psychodynamic psychotherapy. *Proceedings of INTERSPEECH*, Graz, Austria, 3043–3047. https://doi.org/10.21437/Interspeech.2019-2551

Knafo, D. (2018). Beginnings and endings: Time and termination in psychoanalysis. *Psychoanalytic Psychology, 35*(1), 8–14. https://doi.org/10.1037/pap0000125

Kullgard, N., Holmqvist, R., & Andersson, G. (2022). Premature dropout from psychotherapy: Prevalence, perceived reasons and consequences as rated by clinicians. *Clinical Psychology in Europe, 4*(2), 1–16. https://doi.org/10.32872/CPE.6695

Laireiter, A.-P. (1998). Self-directed experience and personal therapy: The situation in the German-speaking countries and "the state of the art" of empirical research. In E. Sanavio (Ed.), Behaviour and cognitive therapy today: Essay in honor of Hans J. Eysenck (pp. 163–179). Pergamon.

Leichsenring, F., Sarrar, L., & Steinert, C. (2019). Drop-outs in psychotherapy: A change of perspective. World Psychiatry, 18(1), 32–33. https://doi.org/10.1002/wps.20588

Lipner, L. M. (2020). Needle in the haystack: The identification of ruptures in the therapeutic alliance with implications for psychotherapy outcome (Publication No. 27541568) [Doctoral Dissertation, Adelphi University]. ProQuest Dissertations Publishing.

Lipner, L. M., Liu, D., Cassell, S., Hunter, E., Eubanks, C. F., & Muran, J. C. (2023). V-episodes in the alliance: A single-case application of multiple methods to identify rupture repair. Psychotherapy, 60(1), 119–129. https://doi.org/10.1037/pst0000469

Mylona, A., & Avdi, E. (2021). Alliance ruptures and embodied arousal in psychodynamic psychotherapy: An exploratory study. Hellenic Journal of Psychology, 18(2), 226–248. https://doi.org/10.26262/hjp.v18i2.8193

Schlesinger, H. J. (2014). Endings and beginnings: On terminating psychotherapy and psychoanalysis (2nd ed.). Routledge/Taylor & Francis Group.

Tschuschke, V., Koemeda-Lutz, M., von Wyl, A., Crameri, A., & Schulthess, P. (2022). The impact of clients' and therapists' characteristics on therapeutic alliance and outcome. Journal of Contemporary Psychotherapy, 52(2), 145–154. https://doi.org/10.1007/s10879-021-09527-2

Vail, A. K., Girard, J., Bylsma, L., Cohn, J., Fournier, J., Swartz, H., & Morency, L.-P. (2021, December). Goals, tasks, and bonds: Toward the computational assessment of therapist versus client perception of working alliance. In 2021 16th IEEE Proceedings of the International Conference on Automatic Face and Gesture Recognition (FG 2021) (pp. 1–8). IEEE Computer Society. https://doi.org/10.1109/fg52635.2021.9667021

Wampold, B. E., Baldwin, S. A., Holtforth, M. g., & Imel, Z. E. (2017). What characterizes effective therapists? In L. G. Castonguay & C. E. Hill (Eds.), How and why are some therapists better than others?: Understanding therapist effects (pp. 37–53). American Psychological Association. https://doi.org/10.1037/0000034-003

Index

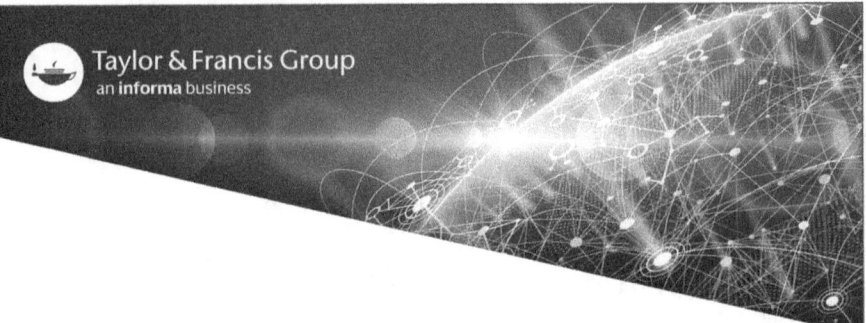
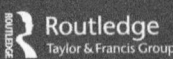
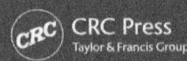